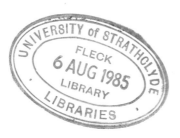

Laser Diagnostics
and Photochemical Processing
for Semiconductor Devices

MATERIALS RESEARCH SOCIETY SYMPOSIA PROCEEDINGS   VOLUME 17

ISSN 0272-9172

Volume 1—Laser and Electron-Beam Solid Interactions and Materials Processing, J.F. Gibbons, L.D. Hess, T.W. Sigmon, 1981

Volume 2—Defects in Semiconductors, J. Narayan, T.Y. Tan, 1981

Volume 3—Nuclear and Electron Resonance Spectroscopies Applied to Materials Science, E.N. Kaufmann, G.K. Shenoy, 1981

Volume 4—Laser and Electron-Beam Interactions with Solids, B.R. Appleton, G.K. Cellar, 1982

Volume 5—Grain Boundaries in Semiconductors, H.J. Leamy, G.E. Pike, C.H. Seager, 1982

Volume 6—Scientific Basis for Nuclear Waste Management, S.V. Topp, 1982

Volume 7—Metastable Materials Formation by Ion Implantation, S.T. Picraux, W.J. Choyke, 1982

Volume 8—Rapidly Solidified Amorphous and Crystalline Alloys, B.H. Kear, B.C. Giessen, M. Cohen, 1982

Volume 9—Materials Processing in the Reduced Gravity Environment of Space, G.E. Rindone, 1982

Volume 10—Thin Films and Interfaces, P.S. Ho, K.N. Tu, 1982

Volume 11—Scientific Basis for Nuclear Waste Management V, W. Lutze, 1982

Volume 12—In Situ Composites IV, F.D. Lemkey, H.E. Cline, M. McLean, 1982

Volume 13—Laser-Solid Interactions and Transient Thermal Processing of Materials, J. Narayan, W.L. Brown, R.A. Lemons, 1983

Volume 14—Defects in Semiconductors, S. Mahajan, J.W. Corbett, 1983

Volume 15—Scientific Basis for Nuclear Waste Management VI, D.G. Brookins, 1983

Volume 16—Nuclear Radiation Detector Materials, E.E. Haller, H.W. Kraner, W.A. Higinbotham, 1983

Volume 17—Laser Diagnostics and Photochemical Processing for Semiconductor Devices, R.M. Osgood, S.R.J. Brueck, H.R. Schlossberg, 1983

Volume 18—Interfaces and Contacts, R. Ludeke, K. Rose, 1983

Volume 19—Alloy Phase Diagrams, L.H. Bennett, T.B. Massalski, B.C. Giessen, 1983

Volume 20—Intercalated Graphite, M.S. Dresselhaus, G. Dresselhaus, J.E. Fischer, M.J. Moran, 1983

Volume 21—Phase Transformation in Solids, T. Tsakalakos, 1983

MATERIALS RESEARCH SOCIETY SYMPOSIA PROCEEDINGS   VOLUME 17

Laser Diagnostics and Photochemical Processing for Semiconductor Devices

Symposium held November 1982 in Boston, Massachusetts, U.S.A.

EDITORS:

R.M. Osgood
Department of Electrical Engineering, Columbia University
New York, New York, U.S.A.

S.R.J. Brueck
Massachusetts Institute of Technology—Lincoln Laboratory
Lexington, Massachusetts, U.S.A.

and

H.R. Schlossberg
Air Force Office of Scientific Research
Bowling Air Force Base, Washington, D.C., U.S.A.

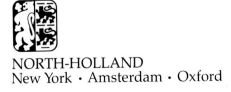

NORTH-HOLLAND
New York · Amsterdam · Oxford

Symposium sponsored by the Air Force Office of Scientific Research, Air Force Systems Command, USAF, under Grant Number AFOSR 82-0353. The United States Government is authorized to reproduce and distribute reprints for Governmental purposes notwithstanding any copyright notation thereon.

©1983 by Elsevier Science Publishing Co., Inc.
All rights reserved.

Published by:
Elsevier Science Publishing Company, Inc.
52 Vanderbilt Avenue, New York, New York 10017

Sole distributors outside the USA and Canada:
Elsevier Science Publishers B.V.
P.O. Box 211, 1000 AE Amsterdam, The Netherlands

Library of Congress Cataloging in Publications Data

Main entry under title:

    Laser diagnostics and photochemical processing for semiconductor devices.

    (Materials Research Society symposia proceedings; v. 17)
    "Sponsored by the Air Force Office of Scientific Research"—P. iv.
    Includes index.
    1. Lasers—Industrial applications—Congresses. 2. Semiconductors—Congresses.
    I. Osgood, R.M. II. Brueck, S.R.J. III. Schlossberg, H.R. IV. United States. Air Force. Office of Scientific Research. V. Series.
TA1673.L355   1983   621.3815'2   83-8028
ISBN 0-444-00782-2
ISSN 0272-9172

Manufactured in the United States of America

Contents

Introduction ix

Acknowledgements xiii

SECTION I. PHOTODEPOSITION OF METAL STRUCTURES

*LASER FABRICATION OF MICROSTRUCTURES: EFFECT OF GEOMETRICAL
SCALING ON CHEMICAL REACTION RATES
D.J. Ehrlich and J.Y. Tsao   3

WAFER-SCALE LASER LITHOGRAPHY: I. PYROLYTIC DEPOSITION OF METAL
MICROSTRUCTURES
I.P. Herman, R.A. Hyde, B.M. McWilliams,
A.H. Weisberg and L.L. Wood   9

PRODUCTION OF MICROSTRUCTURES BY LASER PYROLYSIS
D. Bauerle   19

LASER-INITIATED Ga-DEPOSITION ON QUARTZ SUBSTRATES
Y. Rytz-Froidevaux, R.P. Salathe and H.H. Gilgen   29

UV PHOTODECOMPOSITION FOR METAL DEPOSITION: GAS VS. SURFACE PHASE
PROCESSES
T.H. WOOD, J.C. WHITE AND B.A. THACKER   35

SECTION II. PHOTOETCHING OF ELECTRONIC MATERIALS

*LASER CHEMICAL ETCHING OF CONDUCTING AND SEMICONDUCTING MATERIALS
T.J. Chuang   45

HIGH RESOLUTION ETCHING OF GaAs AND CdS Crystals
D.V. Podlesnik, H.H. Gilgen, R.M. Osgood, A. Sanchez and V. Daneu   57

LIGHT INDUCED ETCHING OF GaAs IN A ZINC ATMOSPHERE
R.P. Salathe and G.B. Rao   65

LASER-CONTROLLED ETCHING OF CHROMIUM-DOPED AND n-DOPED <100> GaAs
G.C. Tisone and A.W. Johnson   73

SECTION III. DIAGNOSTICS OF SEMICONDUCTOR STRUCTURES

*OPTICAL MICROANALYSIS OF SMALL SEMICONDUCTOR STRUCTURES
D.V. Murphy and S.R.J. Brueck   81

RAMAN SCATTERING AS A TEMPERATURE PROBE FOR LASER HEATING OF Si
D. Kirillov and J.L. Merz   95

*Invited Papers

MEASUREMENT OF GRAIN BOUNDARY PARAMETERS BY LASER-SPOT
PHOTOCONDUCTIVITY
E. Poon, H.L. Evans, W. Hwang, R.M. Osgood and E.S. Yang 103

HIGH RESOLUTION LASER DIAGNOSTICS FOR DIRECT GAP SEMICONDUCTOR
MATERIALS
R.P. Salathe and H.H. Gilgen 109

Section IV. PHOTOFORMATION OF INSULATORS

*LASER PHOTOLYTIC DEPOSITION OF THIN FILMS
P.K. Boyer, C.A. Moore, R. Solanki, W.K. Ritchie, G.A. Roche
and G.J. Collins 119

UV LASER-INITIATED FORMATION OF Si_3N_4/
T.F. Deutsch, D.J. Silversmith and R.W. Mountain 129

EVIDENCE FOR LASER INDUCED SURFACE SILANOL FORMATION
D.F. Muller, M. Rothschild and C.K. Rhodes 135

SELECTIVE Mn DOPING OF THIN FILM ZnS:Mn ELECTROLUMINESCENT
DEVICES BY LASER PHOTOCHEMICAL VAPOR DEPOSITION
A. Kitai and G.J. Wolga 141

SECTION V. DIAGNOSTICS OF CONVENTIONAL AND LASER PROCESSING

*LASER SPECTROSCOPIC INVESTIGATION OF GAS-PHASE PROCESSES RELEVANT
TO SEMICONDUCTOR DEVICE FABRICATION
R.F. Karlicek, Jr., V.M. Donnelly and W.D. Johnston, Jr. 151

LASER-INDUCED FLUORESCENCE DIAGNOSTICS OF $CF_4/O_2/H_2$ PLASMA ETCHING
S. Pang and S.R.J. Brueck 161

SPECTROSCOPY AND PHOTOREACTIONS OF ORGANOMETALLIC MOLECULES ON
SURFACES
C.J. Chen and R.M. Osgood 169

THE SPECTROSCOPY AND PHOTOLYSIS OF METALLO-ORGANIC PRECURSORS TO
III-V COMPOUNDS
M.R. Aylett and J. Haigh 177

SECTION VI. PHOTODEPOSITION OF SEMICONDUCTORS

*SEMICONDUCTOR THIN FILMS GROWN BY LASER PHOTOLYSIS
J.G. Eden, J.E. Greene, J.F. Osmundsen, D. Lubben, C.C. Abele,
S. Gorbatkin and H.D. Desai 185

*Invited Papers

LASER STIMULATED GROWTH OF EPITAXIAL GaAs
W. Roth, H. Krautle, A. Krings and H. Beneking   193

LASER INDUCED CHEMICAL VAPOR DEPOSITION OF HYDROGENATED AMORPHOUS SILICON
R. Bilenchi, I. Gianinoni, M. Musci and R. Murri   199

DIRECT WRITING USING LASER CHEMICAL VAPOR DEPOSITION
S.D. Allen, A.B. Trigubo and R.Y. Jan   207

IR LASER-INDUCED DEPOSITION OF SILICON THIN FILMS
T.R. Gattuso, M. Meunier, D. Adler and J.S. Haggerty   215

SECTION VII. PHOTOCHEMICAL DOPING

*PULSED UV EXCIMER LASER DOPING OF SEMICONDUCTORS
T.F. Deutsch   225

SUBMICROMETER-LINEWIDTH LASER DOPING
J.Y. Tsao and D.J. Ehrlich   235

CHARACTERISTICS OF LASER IMPLANTATION DOPING
K.G. Ibbs and M.L. Lloyd   243

USING OPTICAL FIBERS IN LASER PROCESSING
L.D. Laude, L. Baufay and A. Pigeolet   249

SECTION VIII. NOVEL PROCESSES

LASER-PULSED PLASMA CHEMISTRY: SURFACE OXIDATION OF NIOBIUM
R.F. Marks, R.A. Pollak and Ph. Avouris   257

PHOTOELECTROCHEMICAL DEPOSITION OF METAL PATTERNS ON SEMICONDUCTORS
T.L. Rose, R.H. Micheels, D.H. Longendorfer and R.D. Rauh   265

ANALYSIS OF LASER-ENHANCED ADSORPTION/DESORPTION PROCESSES ON SEMICONDUCTOR SURFACES VIA ELECTRONIC SURFACE STATE EXCITATION
W.C. Murphy, A.C. Beri, T.F. George and Jui-Teng Lin   273

FORMATION OF CdO AND Cu_2O FILMS BY LASER IRRADIATION OF THE CORRESPONDING METALLIC FILMS IN AIR
R. Andrew, L. Baufay, A. Pigeolet and M. Wautelet   283

*Invited Papers

AUTHOR INDEX   291

SUBJECT INDEX   295

Introduction

Microelectronics technology is in the midst of a materials revolution. The requirements for ultrafine resolution, high reliability, and sophisticated circuit layout and device designs which are inherent in VLSI circuits are forcing electronic-materials specialists to turn to new materials systems and new processing techniques.

Laser sources and techniques have been receiving increasing attention, both directly as a means for materials processing, as well as a means for diagnosing and controlling other materials processing procedures. The applications of lasers which have been examined are both novel and diverse. For example, in processing, an ultraviolet laser has been used to write directly sub-micrometer-wide metal lines on various semiconductor and insulator quartz substrates. As diagnostics, lasers have been used for example, to monitor, in situ, the reactive species and chemical dynamics of a silicon CVD reactor. The eventual consequence of these and other related developments will be the ability to prepare precisely, both in terms of chemistry and spatial dimensions, materials for microelectronics devices.

The common element in this new area of materials research is the compatibility of light, whether at UV, visible, or infrared frequencies, with the requirements of a chemical processing system. Because of this match lasers have become a pervasive and powerful research tool in physical chemistry. The specific advantages of lasers include : 1) their ability to penetrate a relatively dense material media, 2) their extremely narrow spectral output, and hence, chemical specificity, and 3) their high spatial coherence and brightness.

Unlike electron and ion beams, laser beams propagate through a wide variety of solids and dense gases. For semiconductor processing in particular, practical processing rates can only be achieved for gas densities $\#10^{15}$ cm^{-3} or higher. Typically, the dominant species involved in such processing are molecules or free radicals. The optical path length at these molecular densities is sufficiently long to allow both laser processing and probing.

The narrow spectral output available from lasers makes them ideal sources for exciting a specific electronic transition in the processing medium. The combination of excitation and emission spectra provides a powerful technique for identifying chemical species and their excited state distributions with high sensitivity. In the case of laser photochemistry, the spectral specificity of the laser output allows one to sever selectively a specific molecular bond, and, thus, drive a predetermined chemical reaction. In many instances one may wish to drive a thermally initiated surface reaction. The depth of the thermal excitation can be controlled by making use of the orders of magnitude variation of semiconductor absorption coefficients over the infrared to visible spectral region.

The spatial coherence of the laser permits focusing of the laser beam to micrometer scale lengths. For processing applications this allows laser beams to be used to "write" on a solid surface with the material products of a microscopic chemical reaction. For laser diagnostics, local probing of device substructure or small regions of the processing volume can be accomplished.

The utility of lasers in microelectronics is shown by the substantial rise in activity and the number of technical advancements in laser processing and diagnostics over the last few years. Using laser diagnostics, it has become possible, for the first time, to identify and measure, in situ, many of the active species in a plasma etcher and CVD deposition chamber. Further progress in these experiments will make it possible to link unambiguously the properties of material grown or modified in the processing chamber to the particular species and excitation levels present in the processing atmosphere. Similarly, by using tightly focussed laser beams it has become possible to study the spatial variation in the material properties of micrometer-sized electron devices. A particular instance is the measurement of the variation in the silicon-on-sapphire stress field with Raman spectroscopy.

Laser processing has advanced in two main areas: the development of new chemical processing techniques and the demonstration of high resolution processing. Laser-driven chemistry has now been used as the basis for many of the fundamental processing steps required in microelectronics fabrication including: deposition of metals, semiconductors, and insulators; etching of semiconductors and insulators; and doping of semiconductors. In these processing steps, the chemical reactions are driven either by selective-bond breakage via UV or infrared photodissociation, transient surface heating, or even by laser-produced plasma formation. Each of these forms of processing offers one or more unique characteristics which make it potentially valuable for microelectronic fabrication. In general, the main advantages of the laser chemical processing can be tied to lower processing temperature, more controlled environment, or simply to the absence of any other processing options. One particularly important development has been the demonstration of submicron spatial resolution in a number of these processes. This allows changes in VLSI electronic circuits or the fabrication of high quality electrooptic components. Localized laser processing can be carried out even after metalization steps have been performed. This allows an interactive development of new device designs; a facility which is not readily available with more conventional planar processing technologies.

Research on laser processing and diagnostics is clearly an interdisciplinary enterprise involving areas normally considered physical chemistry, solid-state physics, optical physics, and device engineering. It is also an endeavor in which basic research and immediate applications are, more than usually, intertwined. As a specific case in point consider current research on photochemical deposition of metals, in which the output from an ultraviolet laser is used to photodissociate metallorganic molecules near a passive solid surface. A metal film results from local condensation of the photodissociated metal atoms. Metal photodeposition can be used to direct-write metal lines for many applications including repair of photolithographic masks and fabrication of interconnects for customized programmable logic arrays (PLA's). At the same time, experimental results on UV photodeposition have raised many basic questions about the influence of ultraviolet radiation on molecule-and-atom surface chemistry and kinetics. The research spurred by these questions has led to important discoveries such as stimulated growth of metal microstructures due to scattering by surface electromagnetic waves, plasma enhanced photochemical reactions, and the properties of physisorbed metalalkyl molecules. Similarly, concurrent work in both the basic and applied aspects of laser chemical processing is occurring in other areas such as laser etching and doping.

To conclude this introduction, we would like briefly to look into the near future, and make several predictions as to the advances in laser processing and diagnostics which can be expected to occur. Our estimates are conservative and are based purely on what we think are advantages of lasers as probes and processing beams. We anticipate the following:

1) Greater research on the use of lasers as ancillary processing tools on other complex but "conventional" processing equipment such as MOCVD chambers.

2) Near-routine use of lasers as diagnostic aids in conventional growth or etching chambers.

3) Commercialization of at least one laser chemical processing technology. From the current results this would be most probably either laser etching or doping.

4) Development of new laser devices and techniques for specific use in laser processing and diagnostics.

Acknowledgments

Organization of a new symposium in an area which has only recently developed is a perilous undertaking. Not only are the organizational traditions totally lacking, but even as the conference is being planned, the very subject of the conference may change and a wholly unexpected area of emphasis may move to the forefront. We were extremely fortunate in this first symposium on Laser Diagnostics and Photochemical Processing for Semiconductor Devices to have a program committee which provided us with broad guidance on recent developments in the technical area of the symposium. The same program committee performed "double" duty at the symposium by chairing the sessions in a timely and professional manner, and also acting as <u>in situ</u> reviewers of many of the symposia manuscripts. The Program Committee included:

> Vince Donnelly
> Greg Stillman
> Jim Merz
> George Wright
> Dan Ehrlich
> Rene Salathé

In addition, Dave Nelson from ONR substituted at the meeting for George Wright, who was unexpectedly unable to attend.

A key part of any symposium is the selection of invited speakers. Typically they set the tone and provide perspective for each session. Again we were fortunate. Each of the invited speakers provided an excellent review of his areas and, in many cases, presented new and exciting results from his research group. The invited speakers were:

> Dan Ehrlich
> Tung Chuang
> Dan Murphy
> Rene Salathé
> Kirk Boyer
> Bob Karlicek
> Gary Eden
> Tom Deutsch

As is usual, most of the difficult, detailed work of organizing the conference fell to the unheralded administrative personnel. Ms. Vicki Zell of the Columbia Radiation Lab along with her staff, Ms. Insook Moon and Ms. Sharon Larchuk, admirably handled the mailing, typing, and financial matters. In a very real sense, their efforts allowed us to focus on the technical organization alone.

Finally we are indebted to the Air Force Office of Scientific Research for providing the main financial support for this symposium and to Helionetics and TRW for each providing important additional financial aid.

Laser Diagnostics and Photochemical Processing for Semiconductor Devices

SECTION I
PHOTODEPOSITION OF METAL STRUCTURES

LASER FABRICATION OF MICROSTRUCTURES: EFFECT OF GEOMETRICAL SCALING ON CHEMICAL REACTION RATES*

D. J. EHRLICH AND J. Y. TSAO
Lincoln Laboratory, Massachusetts Institute of Technology
Lexington, Massachusetts 02173

ABSTRACT

Laser-chemical processing for microfabrication makes use of chemical reactions and phase changes confined to micrometer-scale dimensions at vapor/solid and liquid/solid interfaces. When conditions are established for rapid interfacial reactions, processing speeds can become limited by diffusive transport. These diffusion-limited rates, however, increase by many orders of magnitude as the microreaction geometry is reduced to micrometer lengths using well-focused visible and UV beams. A calculation of the geometric scaling of such rates is summarized here. For realistic conditions, rate increases of up to four decades are predicted relative to corresponding reactions on semi-infinite plane surfaces.

INTRODUCTION

With the use of tightly focused laser beams it is possible to excite highly localized "microchemical" reactions on surfaces [1]. For example, in typical etching, deposition and doping processes a TEM_{00} visible or UV laser beam is focused to a ~ 1-μm-diameter spot using high-numerical-aperture optics. This corresponds to the minimum focal-spot size which can be obtained practically under constraints on field of view, working distance and cost for the optics, although particularly in the UV such a diameter is substantially larger than the diffraction limit. Therefore, 1 μm is a common scale length for a laser-excited gas volume or surface area. This is largely independent of the mode of excitation, which may be photolysis of a vapor or surface-adsorbed molecular layer, or may be direct substrate heating to activate pyrolysis or solid-state diffusion. Process nonlinearities permit even shorter scale lengths; linewidths as small as ~ 0.3-0.4 μm have been achieved in cw laser doping of Si [2], and in laser-controlled deposition [7] or etching [3]. A listing of the current minimum feature sizes possible for well controlled laser-writing processes is given in Table I.

In the last several years a wide range of photochemically and thermally activated microchemical processes have been studied, from the points of view of understanding molecule-surface interactions and of exploring the possibilities in microfabrication which derive from this highly localized form of chemistry. In many cases surface reactions of importance in established planar microelectronics processing technology have been studied in the regime of small laser-excited geometries. From observations on a variety of reactions, it has been found that new considerations must enter into the chemical kinetics. Examples where such considerations are important are laser-enhanced electrochemical reactions between solids and liquids [4], and visible-laser-induced pyrolytic reactions on surfaces [5-7]. The purpose of this short paper is to outline one of the implications stemming from limiting gas/surface or liquid/surface reaction dimensions to micrometer and submicrometer lengths.

---

*This work was supported by the Army Research Office, the Department of the Air Force, in part under a specific program sponsored by the Air Force Office of Scientific Research, and by the Defense Advanced Research Projects Agency.

TABLE I
Spatial resolution of several laser-writing processes

Process	Minimum Linewidth (Well Controlled)	Previous References
Photodeposition (photolytic)	0.8 μm	Ref. 1
Pyrolytic Deposition (Si)	0.4 μm	Ref. 7
Si Etching in Cl_2	0.4 μm	Ref. 3
Si Doping (B,P)	0.25 μm	Ref. 2
Polymerization (PMMA)	0.8 μm	Ref. 8

SCALING OF DIFFUSION LIMITED RATES

As a fairly general observation, the rates of microchemical processes often greatly exceed conventional diffusion limits. To illustrate this point, Table 2 collects some process rates for various focused-beam induced reactions. These are several orders of magnitude larger than typical fast diffusion-limited reactions on extended surfaces. To explain these results we have modeled the effects of dimensional scaling on the diffusion-limited reaction flux for conditions of rapid surface etching or deposition. The resulting rates for small laser-beam spot sizes are sufficient to explain the unusually rapid rates (e.g., > 10^3-μm/s vertical etch rates) observed in fast laser-microchemical reactions. A summary of this model is presented here; a more detailed treatment is to be the subject of a future publication [8]. The results are relevant to both gas- and liquid-phase reactions, although additional effects due to enhanced convection and boiling (in liquids) can also be important at high temperatures [4].

Table II
Steady-State Process Rates

Process	Maximum Observed Rate*	Previous References
Si Etching in Cl_2	4×10^3 μm/s	Ref. 3
Pyrolytic Deposition (Si)	~ 50 μm/s	Ref. 6,7
Electrochemical Plating (Etching)	10-50 μm/s	Ref. 4,10

*Geometry dependent, quasi-planar geometries listed here

In the absence of convective flow, all heterogeneous-reaction rates are determined by a balance between the mass transport by diffusion of reactants and products to and from the surface, and the surface reaction itself. For large-area planar reactions this balance is generally modeled by solving the one-dimensional diffusion equation subject to a boundary condition at the surface which specifies the reaction rate vs the surface concentration, and a boundary condition at a plane within the gas which specifies the concentration of reactants or products as fixed by convective flow outside the plane.

If the reaction is limited to a small area on a surface, however, mass transport by gas-phase diffusion must be modeled by the full three-dimensional diffusion equation, subject to the more complicated boundary conditions (1) the reaction rate is proportional to the surface concentration of reactants only within a small zone on the surface, and (2) the concentration far away from the surface is fixed. In condition (1) the small zone can be taken, without loss in applicability, to be circular and of radius ω_0. Condition (2) reflects actual experimental arrangements, in which static, and not flowing, gas cells are generally used. In this treatment we neglect surface diffusion, although in many cases it can be significant. We also treat only the simple case where reactant diffusion is slower than product diffusion, e.g., the case of SiH_4 decomposition into Si and H_2. The geometry is shown in Fig. 1.

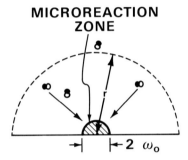

Fig. 1. Geometry for diffusive transport of molecules near a laser-microchemical reaction zone.

Under these conditions it can be shown [8] that the general solution for the time-dependent surface-reaction flux is

$$j_{surf}(t) = \frac{Dn_0}{r_0+\omega_0} \left\{ 1 + \frac{\omega_0}{r_0} e^{(1/r_0+1/\omega_0)^2 Dt} \operatorname{erfc}\left[\left(\frac{1}{r_0}+\frac{1}{\omega_0}\right)\sqrt{Dt}\right] \right\}. \quad (1)$$

In this expression D is the (spatially invariant) molecular diffusivity, n_0 is the molecular density initially, or well away from the microreaction site, and $r_0 \equiv 2D/\eta\, v$ is a length scale proportional to the mean-free path in the gas. The quantity η is the reaction efficiency per surface collision, and v is the r.m.s. velocity of reactant molecules near the surface. This expression contains no unknown scale factors or free parameters. In general the surface-reaction efficiency, η, can be measured directly under low-pressure, single-collision conditions; values for SiH_4 pyrolysis, for example, can be found in Ref. 9. Effects of inert vapor or liquid (solvent) diluents are included via their implications on the value of the diffusivity, D.

To illustrate the predictions of this model Figs. 2 and 3 show the time evolution of the reaction flux for various values of the reaction-zone radius. The conditions chosen are representative of vapor-phase laser etching and CVD reactions. As can be seen there is a rapid dependence of the time required to approach steady-state conditions on radius. This time can be specified by a parameter

$$\tau \sim \frac{1}{D}\left(\frac{1}{1/r_o + 1/\omega_o}\right)^2 \qquad (2)$$

that is linearly related to pressure for small spots ($\omega_o \ll r_o$), but becomes inversely related to pressure (in undiluted gases) for large spots ($\omega_0 \gg r_o$). The equilibration time can be < 10 ns for small spot sizes and moderate (< 1000 Torr) pressures; for small spots even pulsed-laser experiments will generally be in a regime of steady-state conditions. In most cases, the film deposited or etched during the equilibration time is far too thin (~ 3 nm) to be of practical importance. Therefore the overall kinetics of film deposition is generally dominated by the steady-state solution to the diffusion equation.

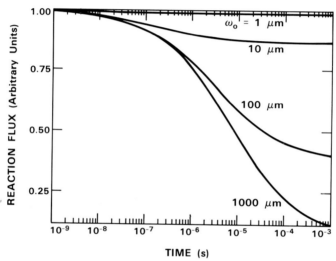

Fig. 2. Temporal dependence given by Eq. (1) for the surface-reaction molecular flux into a microreaction zone of radius ω_o. The plots are for a pressure of 100 Torr, a temperature of 1000°C, a diffusion coefficient, D, of 2.8 cm^2 s^{-1}, and a reaction efficiency, η, of 0.1.

The pressure dependence of the steady-state reaction rate for various reaction-zone radii is plotted in Fig. 4. The plots are for an undiluted vapor at 1000°C with η = 0.1. For all radii the reaction flux follows an initial linear dependence on pressure typical of interface-limited kinetics, and then saturates as the reaction becomes diffusion limited at high pressures. However, the pressure at which saturation occurs is dependent strongly on the zone radius. Since the reaction rate can be scaled with pressure to much larger values before reaching the diffusion limit, very substantial rates are possible for small reaction-zone radii. In this example, the fluxes predicted under conditions of a 1-µm radius and a pressure ~ 500 Torr are ~ 10^{22} molecules cm^{-2} s^{-1}; which corresponds to a deposition or etch rate of several mm/s. This magnitude is sufficient, for example, to explain the most rapid etching results of Table 2.

In the extreme limit, the ratio of the reaction rate on a small sphere to that on a planar surface approaches infinity. In practice, as mentioned above, reactions on planar surfaces are always carried out in flowing reactors, in which diffusive transport need only occur across a thin boundary layer of width

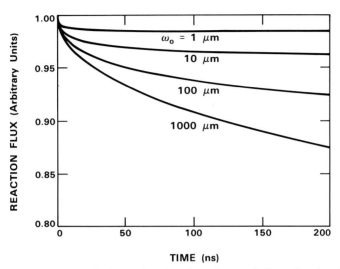

Fig. 3. Expanded plots of the early-time dependence of the molecular flux shown in Fig. 2.

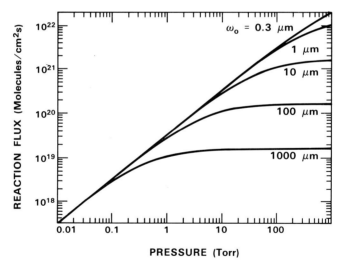

Fig. 4. Steady-state values for the molecular reaction flux as a function of pressure given by Eq. (1) at times $t \gg \tau$. Curves are plotted for a diffusivity $D = \alpha/P$, $\alpha = 2 \times 10^2$ Torr cm^2 s^{-1}, and length scale factor $r_o = \beta/P$, $\beta = 5 \times 10^{-2}$ Torr cm, under the conditions $T = 1000°C$ and $\eta = 0.1$. These values are typical of thermally activated laser etching.

$\delta \simeq 5\sqrt{\nu x/u}$, where ν is the kinematic viscosity, x is a characteristic size of the surface, and u is the velocity of the flow far from the surface. The small-hemisphere enhancement then becomes δ/ω_0. For typical values of $\delta \sim 3$ mm and $\omega_0 \sim 1$ μm, the enhancement is approximately four orders of magnitude.

Finally, we note that although the effects of enhanced diffusive transport have been calculated in a sufficiently general way to model microreactions in high-pressure gases and in liquids, in dense media additional transport mechanisms become important under the strong thermal gradients of many thermally activated microreactions. Some of these are described in Ref. [10].

CONCLUSION

In conclusion, we have summarized an analysis of the kinetics of highly localized, laser-induced microchemical reactions at a gas/surface interface. The analysis is based upon three-dimensional diffusion of reactants towards a small reaction zone on a plane surface, followed by surface reaction. The overall reaction kinetics depend markedly on the size of the reaction zone. For diffusion-limited reactions, the steady-state rates are inversely proportional to reaction-zone size, and are adequately fast to explain the up to four orders-of-magnitude enhancement observed experimentally for laser microreactions relative to corresponding reactions on a semi-infinite plane.

REFERENCES

1. D. J. Ehrlich, R. M. Osgood, Jr., and T. F. Deutsch, IEEE J. Quantum Electron. QE-16, 1233 (1980).

2. D. J. Ehrlich and J. Y. Tsao, Appl. Phys. Lett. 41, 297 (1982); see also J. Y. Tsao and D. J. Ehrlich (this volume).

3. D. J. Ehrlich, R. M. Osgood, Jr. and T. F. Deutsch, Appl. Phys. Lett. 38, 946 (1981).

4. R. J. von Gutfeld and R. T. Hodgson, Appl. Phys. Lett. 40, 352 (1982).

5. S. D. Allen and M. Bass, J. Vac. Sci. Technol. 16, 431 (1979).

6. D. Baurle, P. Irsigler, G. Leyendecker, H. Noll and D. Wagner, Appl. Phys. Lett. 40, 819 (1982).

7. D. J. Ehrlich, R. M. Osgood, Jr. and T. F. Deutsch, Appl. Phys. Lett. 39, 957 (1981).

8. J. Y. Tsao and D. J. Ehrlich (to be published).

9. R. F. C. Farrow, J. Electrochem. Soc. 110, 1235 (1963).

10. R. J. von Gutfeld, R. E. Acosta and L. T. Romankiw, IBM J. Res. Dev. 26, 136 (1982).

WAFER-SCALE LASER LITHOGRAPHY: I. PYROLYTIC DEPOSITION OF METAL MICROSTRUCTURES[*]

IRVING P. HERMAN, RODERICK A. HYDE, BRUCE M. MCWILLIAMS, ANDREW H. WEISBERG and LOWELL L. WOOD.
Physics Department, Lawrence Livermore National Laboratory, P.O. Box 808-L-278, Livermore, CA 94550

ABSTRACT

Mechanisms for laser-driven pyrolytic deposition of micron-scale metal structures on crystalline silicon have been studied. Models have been developed to predict temporal and spatial properties of laser-induced pyrolytic deposition processes. An argon ion laser-based apparatus has been used to deposit metal by pyrolytic decomposition of metal alkyl and carbonyl compounds, in order to evaluate the models. These results of these studies are discussed, along with their implications for the high-speed creation of micron-scale metal structures in ULSI systems.

INTRODUCTION

In order that state-of-the-art computers can reproduce with less human interference and thus with lower error rates and latencies, it is necessary for them to be able to micropattern semiconductor substrates directly and at high speed. Contemporary supercomputer systems composed of 10^8 transistors, each constituted of as many as 10^2 'tiles' of various materials stacked in particular arrangements, contain as many as 10^{10} 'tiles' in their ultra-large scale integrated (ULSI) patterns. In order that latencies involved in computer-directed generation of new computer-scale micropatterns be not much greater than a day, creation of a single 'tile' must be accomplished in an interval of the order of 10^{-5} seconds.

In the series of papers of which this is the first, we will report on means for accomplishing such processing in this context. This paper reports on that aspect of laser micropatterning which is possibly the least advanced through the present: the discretionary, high-speed generation of lines of metal—paths of metallic 'tiles' laid edge-to-edge—suitable for interconnecting active devices in ULSI circuits.

Monolithically implemented computers of the present era consist of sheets of metal traces of micron-scale width and thickness, separated almost (but not quite) everywhere from each other by nearly hole-free dielectric sheets, and occasionally touching the terminals of transistor devices which are embedded for convenience in a semiconductor substrate common to all such devices. The large majority of the structure (indexed by the fraction of total 'tiles' in the pattern) of computers implemented in the ever more popular metal-oxide semiconductor (MOS) family of technologies is expressed in metal (or in surrogate metal, highly doped polysilicon). It is thus quite crucial to greatly extend the hitherto highly limited ability to create suitable metal microstructures directly with laser processing techniques, as this approach is qualitatively superior to all other current

---
[*] Work performed under the auspices of the U.S. Department of Energy by the Lawrence Livermore National Laboratory under contract number W-7405-ENG-48.

prospects for high-speed, computer-controlled micropattern generation directly on semiconductor substrates.

We report here an order of magnitude enhancement in the rate of metal micropatterning in the ULSI context, relative to the highest rates previously reported. Taken together with results from other workers on rapid semiconductor substrate doping and dielectric layer creation, this advance makes feasible in principle the generation of monolithic, ULSI supercomputers on day time scales.

The laser-driven metal deposition processes of interest consist of a semiconductor substrate surfaced with the reactant gas, with a laser beam focused to the region on the substrate where metal is to be deposited. Two different types of laser-induced metal deposition processes are candidates for this role: pyrolysis and photolysis. The pyrolytic processes are based on thermal decomposition reactions which occur due to laser-induced heating of the substrate, while the photolytic processes entail gas phase photolytic decomposition reactions occurring in the laser-irradiated gas-filled region above the substrate.

The ultimate limit on the rate of metal deposition by either pyrolytic or photolytic processes is determined by the maximum possible rate of mass transport of the reactant gas to the substrate. Pyrolytic processes may usefully be thought of as unimolecular decompositions, while photolytic ones are two-body (binary) ones in the same sense—both gas molecules and photons must occupy the same space-time volume for photolysis to occur.

In order for photolysis to occur in unit time, the photon fluence must equal the reciprocal of the cross-section for the metal-bearing molecule to photolytically absorb the photon. Since the unit of time is that for the molecule to transit the reaction zone—about 10 nanoseconds for molecular weights of the order of 100 amu and reaction zone scales of the order of 1 micron—and since the largest photolytic cross-sections of interest less than 10^{-17} cm^2, the photon fluxes required for mass transport-limited photolysis are of the order of 10^{25} photons cm^{-2} sec^{-1}, or about 10 megawatt cm^{-2}, which implies a minimum input of 0.1 watts of hard-won 4-6 eV laser photons.

By way of comparison, the laser intensity required for pyrolysis of metal-bearing gases of interest at a comparable mass-processing rate is just that needed to maintain a square micron of substrate at a temperature of the order of 1000°K, which is again about 10^7 watts cm^{-2}, but now involves an input of 0.1 watts of readily available, wavelength-insensitive optical laser spectral power. Thus, even when using metal-bearing gases with the highest UV photolytic cross-sections, the laser intensity regime for efficient photolysis already completely overlaps the one for pyrolysis, but is accessed with substantially greater technical difficulty. When using gases with more typical photolytic cross-sections, the laser intensities required for efficient photolysis will boil the substrate on nanosecond time scales. Intensity reduction to more acceptable levels will slow the photolysis rate, relative to the photolytic one, by the ratio of the photolytic cross-section to the peak value of 10^{-17} cm^2, e.g., for aluminum trimethyl with its photolytic cross-section of 10^{-20} cm^{-2}($\lambda \simeq 0.26$ μm), photolytic deposition of aluminum metal will be approximately three orders of magnitude slower than will pyrolytic.

We therefore restrict our attention to pyrolytic mechanisms of metal micropatterning of semiconductor substrates. Earlier work has demonstrated photolytic deposition of Al, Cd, Zn and Sn from gas-phase and surface decomposition of the respective alkyls[R1], and of Fe, W, Cr, and Mo from the respective carbonyls[R2,R3], using ultraviolet ($\lambda \leq 0.26$ μm) laser light. Previous workers have pyrolytically deposited large, dendrite-rich strips of Al, Zn and Cd at low speeds on GaAs surfaces with focussed radiation from a krypton-ion laser[R4], and deposited large scale Ni[R5] and W[R6] films with CO$_2$ laser radiation focused on silica surfaces.

Mass transport-limited, laser-driven pyrolysis of dimethyl zinc, trimethyl aluminum and nickel carbonyl to form metal traces with micron-scale widths and thicknesses on silicon wafers by focused argon-ion laser light ($\lambda = 0.5145~\mu m$) is reported in the present paper. Because of its superior properties—high Ni(CO)$_4$ vapor pressure, high melting point, high electrical conductivity and excellent corrosion resistance of metallic nickel, and good model qualities for other systems of interest—this nickel system has been singled out for extensive study. We interpret these results with theories of quantitative predictive quality, and thereby extrapolate them to ULSI applications of ultimate interest.

THEORY OF LASER-INDUCED PYROLYTIC DEPOSITION PROCESSES

The laser-induced pyrolytic metal deposition processes under consideration are based on thermal decomposition reactions of the form:

$$[MX_n] \rightarrow [M] + n[X] \qquad (1)$$

where MX$_n$ is the reactant gas molecule (e.g., a metal alkyl or carbonyl), M is the metal atom being deposited, and X is a product gas of the reaction. The process can be thought of as involving five consecutive steps:

a. Diffusion of the reactant gas to the heated portion of the substrate;
b. Adsorption of reactant;
c. Decomposition of the reactant;
d. Desorption of the volatile product; and
e. Diffusion of the product gas away from the substrate.

At lower temperatures, the rate-determining step of the process is usually (c); at higher temperatures, where the decomposition reaction rate becomes substantial, (a) and (e) become the rate-limiting steps.

We present a generally applicable model for high-speed deposition of metal microstructures by pyrolysis of a metal-bearing gas, emphasizing generation of micron-scale nickel traces by pyrolysis of Ni(CO)$_4$.

The kinetics of processes (b) through (d) have been analyzed by Carlton and Oxley[R7]. Their expression for the overall reaction rate is:

$$R(p_1, p_2, T) = R_0(T) f(p_1, p_2, T) \qquad (2)$$

where

$$R_0(T) = 5.1 \times 10^{29} exp\{-T_0/T\} \quad cm^{-2}sec^{-1}; \quad T_0 = 11,022°K \qquad (3)$$

$$f(p_1, p_2, T) = k_1^2 [p_1^2 - (p_2^4/K_{eq})^2]/[1 + k_1 p_1 + k_2 p_2]^2 \qquad (4)$$

$$\begin{aligned} k_1 &= 0.089 exp\{T_1/T\} \quad Torr^{-1}; \quad T_1 = 352°K \\ k_2 &= 0.00152 exp\{T_2/T\} \quad Torr^{-1}; \quad T_2 = 2,013°K \\ K_{eq} &= 1.4 \times 10^{31} exp\{-T_3/T\} \quad Torr^3; \quad T_3 = 18,800°K \quad [R8] \end{aligned} \qquad (5)$$

Here p_1 is the Ni(CO)$_4$ partial pressure, while p_2 is that of CO. The reaction is second order and is choked at high pressure by adsorbed Ni(CO)$_4$ and CO. Since f is always less than one, R_0 represents the peak rate possible, which is attained at high p_1 and low p_2. We can neglect the reverse reaction, since at the temperatures needed to make R_0 large, the equilibrium constant for the reaction, K_{eq}, is also large; the recombination reaction is thus negligible for present purposes.

Examination of (2) shows that, as we increase surface temperature, the rate will climb due to the activation energy factor R_0. Eventually, though, we will reach an asymptotic condition where gas diffusion is insufficient either to maintain p_1 near its far-field value, or to disperse CO and keep p_2 low near the deposition site. Both of these effects will cause f to fall. Our model must therefore relate T to laser power, and must consider gas diffusive mass transport. First we obtain $R_0(T)$.

The temperature field produced in a plane slab of solid silicon by a linearly swept laser beam of Gaussian profile has been treated previously[R9, R10]. Using a Kirchhoff transform we define a linearized temperature:

$$\theta(T) = \int_{T_r}^{T} \frac{K(T')}{K(T_r)} dT', \tag{6}$$

where T_r is the reference (initial) temperature. Writing the space- and time-dependent laser intensity I as

$$I(x - vt, y) = \frac{P}{\pi r_0^2} exp\left\{-\frac{(x-vt)^2 + y^2}{r_0^2}\right\} \tag{7}$$

where P is the incident laser power and v s the laser focal spot sweep rate, then

$$\theta(X, Y, Z; V) = \frac{2}{\pi}\theta_c \int_0^{\infty} exp\left\{-\frac{(X + Vu^2)^2 + Y^2}{1 + u^2} - \frac{Z^2}{u^2}\right\} \frac{du}{1 + u^2} \tag{8}$$

where

$$X = \frac{x}{r_0} \quad Y = \frac{y}{r_0} \quad Z = \frac{z}{r_0} \quad V = \frac{vr_0}{\sqrt{8D}} \tag{9}$$

$$\theta_c = \frac{P(1 - \Re_S)}{2\sqrt{\pi}K(T_r)r_0} \tag{10}$$

This temperature solution is found via a Green's function route. This approach is not exactly correct, since the silicon thermal diffusivity D is temperature-dependent, but for "relatively slow" scan velocities, D fades from significance.

The reflectivity $\Re_S$ has been assumed constant over the laser beam focal spot, which is reasonable for solid Si. The term θ_c is the peak value of θ for the static case; to relate it to the actual temperature, we must assume an expression for thermal conductivity. We use $K(T)$ and $\Re_S$ from[R9]:

$$K(T) = \frac{k}{T - T_k}; \quad k = 299 \, W/cm; \quad T_k = 99°K \tag{11}$$

$$\Re_S(T) = 0.367 + 4.29 \times 10^{-5} T$$

Solving (6) gives

$$\theta(T) = (T_r - T_k) ln\frac{T - T_k}{T_r - T_k}. \tag{12}$$

$$T(\theta) = T_k + (T_r - T_k) exp\left\{\frac{\theta}{T_r - T_k}\right\} \tag{13}$$

$$T_c = T_k + (T_r - T_k) exp\left\{\frac{P(1 - \Re_S)}{2\sqrt{\pi}kr_0}\right\} \tag{14}$$

For $P = 300$ mW and $r_0 = 2 \, \mu m$, we find $T_c = 575°K$.

The simplest expression for metal deposition rate is obtained by assuming a relatively slow laser focal spot scan rate and looking at the center of the spot; placing (14) in rate

(3) we obtain the rate of increase of the metal film thickness $\dot{W}_c$:

$$\dot{W}_c = 5.6 \times 10^{10} exp\{-T_0/T_c\} \quad \mu m/sec \tag{15}$$

This is plotted in Figure 1 as a function of specific laser power P/r_0, using $T_r = 300°K$. This model can also predict the spatial variation of growth rate by combining (3), (8) and (13). We can obtain a simple relation by Taylor expansion, which is useful since $T \ll T_0$

$$\theta(r) \approx \theta_c[1 - \frac{r^2}{2r_0^2}] \tag{16}$$

$$T(r) \approx T_c - \theta_c \frac{T_c - T_k}{T_r - T_k} \frac{r^2}{2r_0^2} \tag{17}$$

so

$$\dot{W} \approx \dot{W}_c exp\{-r^2/\rho^2\} \tag{18}$$

where ρ is the effective interaction radius

$$\frac{\rho}{r_0} = \frac{T_c}{\sqrt{T_0 \theta_c}} \sqrt{2 \frac{T_r - T_k}{T_c - T_k}} \tag{19}$$

For example, at $P/r_0 = 0.15$ $W/\mu m$, we find $\rho/r_0 = 0.38$, so the Ni spot size should be about 2.5 times smaller than that of the laser.

The growth rates of Figure 1, based on Equation 15, are invalid at high temperatures, because gas diffusion cannot supply $Ni(CO)_4$ or remove CO sufficiently rapidly. Therefore, we need to obtain $f(p_1, p_2, T)$ and do so by analyzing gas diffusion by a Green's function approach analogous to (8). Solving for the "relatively slow" scan case using a reaction rate spatial variation as in (18), the species population changes at spot center are

$$\Delta n_i = \frac{\sqrt{\pi}}{2} \rho \frac{R_i}{D_i} \quad cm^{-3}; \quad i = 1, 2 \tag{20}$$

Here the rate for $Ni(CO)_4$, R_1, is $-R$ from (2), while R_2 for CO is $+4R$. The gas diffusivities are D_1 and D_2, while Δn_1 and Δn_2 are the Ni and CO population changes from their far-field values. If we convert populations to pressures, we arrive at equations which must be solved self-consistently:

$$p_1 = p_{1\infty} - 5.35 \times 10^{10} exp\{-T_0/T_c\} \frac{\rho T_r}{D_1} f(p_1, p_2, T_c) \quad Torr \tag{21}$$

$$p_2 = 4\frac{D_1}{D_2}(p_{1\infty} - p_1) \quad Torr \tag{22}$$

where $p_{1\infty}$ is the pressure far from the laser beam focal spot in Torr, and other variables have units as noted above.

The effects of diffusion are illustrated in Figure 1 for a 2 μm radius laser spot. We assume that the gas was at $T_r = 300°K$, not at T_c. For D_1 and D_2, we assume a 1 atm He buffer gas background, a common choice in our early experiments. Using the method of[R11], we obtain

$$D_1 = 0.23 \ cm^2/sec; \quad D_2 = 0.93 \ cm^2/sec \tag{23}$$

The inaccuracy in using (15) at low laser beam power levels is due to neglecting $f(p_{1\infty}, 0, T_c)$. Of more fundamental interest are the high power asymptotic results. This diffusion-limited

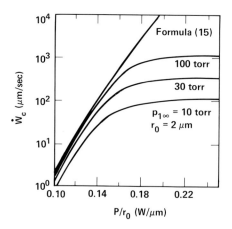

Figure 1 - Calculated Ni growth rate on Si substrate. The three right-most curves assume $r_0 = 2\ \mu m$.

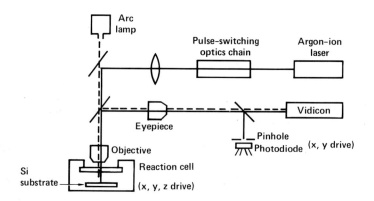

Figure 2 - Experimental arrangement for laser-pyrolytic deposition of metal microstructures.

rate is

$$R \lesssim \frac{2}{\sqrt{\pi}} \frac{D_1}{\rho} n_{1\infty} \qquad (24)$$

Expressed in terms of metal-bearing gas pressure and growth rate of metal thickness, it is

$$\dot{W}_c \lesssim 9.1 \times 10^{-4} p_{1\infty}/\rho \quad \mu m/sec, \qquad (25)$$

where $p_{1\infty}$ is in Torr and ρ is in cm. This limit is set by gas transport to the laser-heated spot on the surface; other factors enter only weakly through the radius of the metal spot, ρ. Small spot sizes and high partial pressures of Ni(CO)$_4$ are desirable in order to realize high metal trace growth rates. Fortunately, this is the regime of most interest to us.

This analysis assumes that the laser spot is being scanned "relatively slowly" over the substrate—$v \lesssim 500$ cm/sec—and that deposition is taking place onto Si. Obviously, most of the Ni metal deposition occurs on top of existing Ni. Since only a thin metallic layer ($\lesssim 0.01$ μm) is necessary to dominate reflectivity and absorption of laser light, we can assume that the entire laser spot sees the Ni reflectivity, $\Re_N$. Making the reasonable assumption that heat absorbed by the Ni transports primarily downward with little lateral conduction, then our analysis of the local Si temperature remains applicable for thin Ni layers, save for using $\Re_N$ in place of $\Re_S$. Using $\Re_N = 0.62$, the abscissa variable in Figure 1 now becomes $0.63 P/r_0$. But our T_c is at the Si surface; the Ni surface is at a higher temperature and thus conducts the incident power down into the Si substrate. We can obtain a thickness limitation on the deposited metal film at which point the Ni starts to melt on its upper, laser-irradiated surface:

$$W_M = \frac{\pi r_0^2 K_N}{P(1 - \Re_N)} (T_{mp} - T_c) \quad cm \qquad (26)$$

Here T_{mp} is the Ni melting point of $1728°K$, K_N is its thermal conductivity of 0.7 $W/cm/°K$, and T_c is found from (14), using a value of $\Re_N$ of 0.62. As an example, consider a r_0 laser spot radius of 2 μm with a 0.6 watt incident laser beam power. We find that W_M in this case is 4.0 μm. This deposit thickness is attained quickly: a side effect of the large thermal gradient in the Ni is to drive the deposition process to the diffusion growth limit, so using (25) and (26), we find that melting occurs in a time t_M

$$t_M = 6.4 \times 10^7 \left(\frac{\rho}{r_0}\right) r_0^3 \frac{T_{mp} - T_c}{P p_{1\infty}} \quad sec \qquad (27)$$

For 10 Torr Ni(CO)$_4$, $t_M = 34$ msec for the conditions just stated.

Dwelling at a location for longer than this time will cause melting of the top surface of the Ni. If the molten Ni spreads out, the line width of the metal trace being laid down will grow; if it doesn't have time to spread then, as more Ni is deposited, further temperature rise occurs, which can culminate in vaporization and spattering of superheated liquid Ni.

As a result, a single pass *minimum* scan rate V_{min} which just avoids melting under the stated conditions is

$$V_{min} \gtrsim 2\rho/t_M = 3.1 \times 10^{-8} \frac{P p_{1\infty}}{r_0^2 (T_{mp} - T_c)} \quad cm/sec \qquad (28)$$

EXPERIMENTAL STUDY

Description of Apparatus

Polished n-type silicon targets, typically oriented in [100] with 30 Ω-cm conductivity, were suitably cleaned and placed in a reaction cell having a sapphire entrance window. The cell was filled with the desired partial pressures of buffer gas and metal alkyl or carbonyl, and then irradiated by an argon-ion laser ($\lambda = 0.5145\ \mu m$) focused by one of two microscope objectives (10X, NA = 0.25; 36X, NA = 0.50).

Desired metal patterns (frequently lines) were created by moving the reaction cell with an x-y table stepper drive (1 μm steps; 1500 $\mu m/sec$ maximum speed), and by amplitude modulating the argon-ion laser beam by an optics chain which often included a half-wave plate followed by an electro-optics switch that was sandwiched between two Glan-Thompson prisms. During the course of each run, the laser patterns on the substrate and the deposited metal features were viewed through a microscope via a vidicon outputting to a color monitor. Laser beam profiles on the substrate were measured using a pinhole-photodiode arrangement mounted on a calibrated x-y drive located after the microscope. The samples were analyzed using optical and scanning electron microscopy (the latter with X-ray fluorescence capability) and stylus profilometry.

Results

Operating with present experimental conditions of ~ 10 Torr of metal alkyl or carbonyl and ~ 0.4 W of 0.5145 μm radiation focused to $r_0 = 2-3\ \mu m$ on the Si surface, we observed rapid and localized deposition of Zn, Al and Ni from $Zn(CH_3)_2$, $Al(CH_3)_3$ and $Ni(CO)_4$. For scanning rates of $\sim 400\ \mu m/sec$, $2-6\ \mu m$ wide and $0.2-10\ \mu m$ high metallic lines were obtained in ~ 4 sweeps. The aluminum lines possessed a $\sim 0.5-2\ \mu m$ diameter puffy, quasi-periodic substructure, in part due to the discrete stepping translation of the wafer, while the nickel substructure consisted of close-packed quasi-spherical beads of $\sim 0.5-4\ \mu m$ diameter. At high laser power levels, the line deposited of each metal contained a smooth-surfaced central axial depression due to melting and compaction of the beads within the depression, as discussed above. As was particularly evident in the Ni and Zn studies, there was significant vaporization of metal from this central valley and consequential prenucleation of the nearby substrate surface when high laser powers were employed.

Figure 3 demonstrates that the thickness of the deposited Ni strip is linear with the number of sweeps and with the dwell time per 1 μm stepper jump, as predicted by our theory. Figure 4 shows preliminary data concerning the height of the deposited Ni line versus laser power applied to the target area. These runs were performed with a gas mixture consisting of 11 Torr $Ni(CO)_4$ plus 700 Torr He. These data indicate that Ni was deposited at a rate of $\sim 100\ \mu m/sec$ at higher laser power, in agreement with the theoretical prediction of Eq. (25) and Figure 1.

Variations in height within a given metal line and between different lines drawn under similar conditions are attributed to the nature of nucleation on the surface. At lower power levels, the method of surface preparation (various methods of cleaning polished Si surfaces covered by its native oxide, including cleaning and stripping away the SiO_2) greatly affected the production of nucleation sites. Prenucleation due to boiling of metal from nearby nickel lines was observed to greatly lower the nucleation threshold for subsequent low laser power pyrolytic metal deposition runs. Nucleation effects are expected to be of much less importance in planned work involving substrate temperatures raised to far above threshold temperatures for sub-microsecond periods.

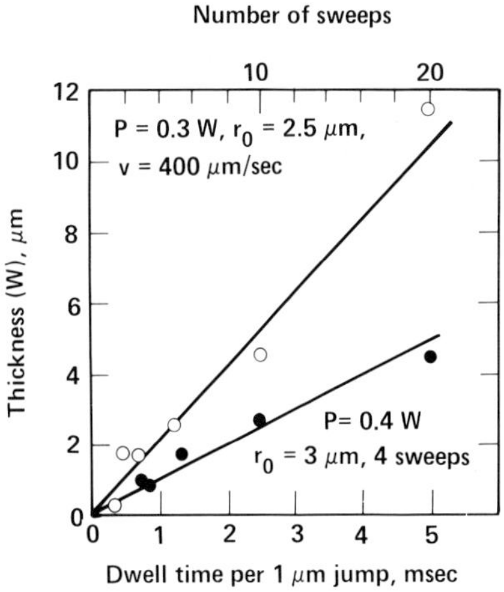

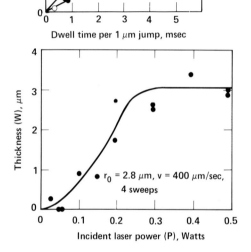

Figure 3 - Temporal dependence of nickel line deposition on silicon by laser pyrolysis (see text).

Figure 4 - Laser power dependence of pyrolytic deposition of nickel lines on silicon substrate (see text).

CONCLUSIONS

In this paper, we have reported a means for generating lines of metal suitable for use in ultra-large scale integrated (ULSI) circuits at rates which correspond to creating such circuits on times scales of a day. The best example of this approach involves the decomposition of metal, e.g., nickel or iron, carbonyl positioned above the (typically semiconductor) surface of interest at mass transport-limited rates, with the pyrolytic deposition of the metal being energized and localized by transiently heating the surface with a focussed visible laser beam of suitable power level.

The first-principles theory which we have presented is quantitatively predictive of the preliminary experimental results which we have obtained with respect to all measured aspects of metal deposition. It asserts that metal depth build-up rates of the order of centimeters per second can be attained with the use of nickel and iron carbonyls, with somewhat lower rates being attainable for the carbonyls of other metals of interest, such as molybdenum and tungsten.

Sweeping (or otherwise time-modulating) a micron-scale laser beam spot relative to a location being metallized on a time scale of the order of 10 nanoseconds is predicted to be sufficient to intrinsically confine the deposition to within a 1 micron spot diameter on a silicon substrate, moreover very crisply, due to the exponential dependence of the deposition rate with surface temperature over the range of interest. Substrates of lower thermal diffusivity (e.g., silica) are tolerant of more prolonged exposure before 'thermal transport blurring' of the laser beam spot will ensue.

Our present experimental results include creation of micron-scale metal lines at deposition rates of 0.1 millimeter thickness per second with argon-ion laser beam powers in the range 0.3-0.6 W incident on the silicon substrate with beam spot sweep rates of more than 500 microns per second.

At multi-watt incident laser beam power levels and saturated carbonyl pressure above the substrate, our experimentally validated theory predicts that nickel/iron lines with micron-scale widths and thicknesses of several tenths of a micron can be deposited on a substrate of choice at a sweep rate of 10 cm/sec. This is quite adequate for computer-driven creation of ULSI circuits at interestingly high rates.

ACKNOWLEDGMENTS

The authors would like to express their gratitude to Dr. Richard Osgood for useful discussions during the course of this work, to James Atkins, Donald Duerre, Mark Garrett, Fred Mitlitsky and Elon Ormsby for their expert technical assistance in the experimental aspects of this study, and to Christine Ghinazzi for assistance in preparing this paper for publication.

REFERENCES

[R1] D. J. Ehrlich, R. M. Osgood, Jr. and T. F. Deutsch, IEEE J. Quant. Electron. **QE-16**, 1233 (1980).

[R2] D. J. Ehrlich, R. M. Osgood, Jr. and T. F. Deutsch, J. Electrochem. Soc. **128**, 2039 (1981).

[R3] R. Solanki, P. K. Boyer, J. E. Mahan and G. J. Collins, Appl. Phys. Lett. **38**, 572 (1981).

[R4] Y. Rytz-Froidevaux, R. P. Salathe and H. H. Gilgen, Phys. Lett. **84A**, 216 (1981).

[R5] S. D. Allen, J. Appl. Phys. **52**, 6501 (1981).

[R6] R. S. Berg and D. M. Mattox, "Proceedings of the Fourth International Conference on Chemical Vapor Deposition", edited by F. A. Glaski (Am. Nucl. Soc., Hindsdale, Illinois, 1973), p. 196.

[R7] H. E. Carlton and J. H. Oxley, A.I.C.L.E. Journal **12**, 86 (1967).

[R8] W. M. Goldberger and D. F. Othmer, IECPDE **2**, 202 (1963).

[R9] J. E. Moody and R. H. Hendel, J. Appl. Phys., **53**, 4364 (1982).

[R10] Y. I. Nissim, A. Lietoila, R. B. Gold and J. F. Gibbons, J. Appl. Phys., **51**, 274 (1980).

[R11] J. O. Hirschfelder, C. F. Curtiss and R. B. Bird, *Molecular Theory of Gases and Liquids* (John Wiley and Sons, New York, 1954) p. 14.

PRODUCTION OF MICROSTRUCTURES BY LASER PYROLYSIS

DIETER BÄUERLE
Angewandte Physik, University of Linz, 4040 Linz, Austria

ABSTRACT

Laser pyrolysis at short wavelengths is a powerful tool for micron-sized one-step local deposition of insulating, semiconducting and metallic materials from the gas phase. Various structures, e.g. stripes on different substrates, and rods of various lengths and diameters, have been produced. The morphology of the deposited material, the deposition rate, and the dimensions (typically 1-300 µm) of the structures were investigated quantitatively as functions of laser irradiance, local temperature, laser focus diameter, scanning velocity, and gas pressure.

INTRODUCTION

Laser induced chemical vapor deposition (LCVD) can be achieved either by pyrolytic or by photolytic decomposition of molecules from the gas phase. Pyrolytic LCVD is based on local substrate heating by means of laser light which is not absorbed by the gaseous molecular species. Infrared (IR) [1-6] and visible (VIS) [7-13] laser light has been used for such experiments. The microscopic mechanism for the decomposition process is the same as in conventional CVD techniques, namely thermal activation of the chemical reaction near or on the hot surface of the substrate. The situation is quite different for photolytic LCVD [14]. In this case, dissociation of the molecular species is achieved either by electronic excitation or by multiphoton vibrational excitation by means of a UV or an IR laser, respectively. Thus, in principle, deposition can be performed without appreciable substrate heating.

In contrast to the standard CVD process, which is widely used for the production of e x t e n d e d thin films on uniformly heated substrates [15], LCVD allows one step l o c a l deposition or direct writing of structures with widths down to at least 1 µm. Besides this "two dimensional" deposition or direct writing, the production of three dimensional structures of micron-size is possible.

In this paper we review recent results on the application of laser pyrolysis, especially those obtained at visible wavelengths, for the production of microstructures. After a comparison of pyrolytic LCVD with IR and with VIS laser radiation, and a brief description of a typical experimental setup, we discuss the parameters and limitations which determine the deposition rates in the phase of direct writing and in the phase of steady growth. Finally, we comment on the morphology and the physical properties of the deposited material.

PYROLYTIC LCVD AT IR- AND VIS-WAVELENGTHS

Pyrolytic laser induced chemical vapor deposition was performed for the first time by means of IR lasers, nearly exclusively with the 10,6 µm radiation of pulsed or cw CO_2 lasers [1-6], and more recently, using VIS light, mainly from cw Ar^+ and Kr^+ lasers [7-13]. The use of VIS lasers instead of IR lasers is advantageous, whenever microstructures with the smallest possible lateral dimensions are to be produced. This is evident, because the diffraction limited diameter of the laser focus is proportional to the wavelength of the light, λ. For 488 nm Ar^+ and 10,6 μm CO_2 radiation, for example, this diameter differs by about a factor of 20 (!). Therefore, localization of heating is very much improved when using VIS light. Furthermore, because of the transparency of almost all gases in the VIS region, no problems arise with spontaneous reactions within the bulk. Such reactions may occur whenever the reacting species or possible admixtures or gaseous impurity molecules absorb the IR radiation and multiphoton vibrational excitation/dissociation of a species becomes possible. Finally, the optics and adjustments are much simpler for VIS radiation in comparison to IR radiation.

Because of the advantages mentioned, we concentrate henceforth on laser pyrolysis by means of VIS light. Detailed investigations have been performed on the deposition of C from C_2H_2, C_2H_4, and CH_4 [7-9], of Si from SiH_4 [8,10,11], of Cd from $Cd(CH_3)_2$ [12] and of Ni from $Ni(CO)_4$ [13]. The pyrolytic dissociation mechanism has been established from quantitative investigations of the dependence of the deposition rate on the local temperature, which is correlated to the laser irradiance. It was clearly shown that after an initial phase of nucleation one observes a phase of growth in which the deposition process is t h e r m a l l y activated and characterized by an apparent chemical activation energy [8,9]. On the other hand, in the very first step, the phase of nucleation, multiphoton dissociation of reactant molecules, which are adsorbed at the surface of the substrate, may play - at least in cases of weakly absorbing substrates - a dominant or even decisive role. Evidence for that was obtained during the deposition of Cd from $Cd(CH_3)_2$ on transparent glass substrates [12]. It is clear, however, that also quite different mechanisms, as e.g. absorption by defects or impurities in or on the surface of the substrate can be decisive as to whether nucleation, and hence deposition, occurs or not.

EXPERIMENTAL

A typical setup used in the LCVD experiments is schematically shown in Fig.1. The beam of a laser, here an Ar^+ or Kr^+ laser, is expanded to a diameter a, and then focused onto the substrate by a lens of focal length f. To avoid small changes in the beam diameter, the laser power is kept constant and the irradiance on the substrate is varied by means of a tunable neutral filter. For a Gaussian beam, the irradiance across the focus can be written in the form $I(w) = I(o) \exp\{-2w^2/w_o^2\}$, where $2w_o$ is the diameter of the laser beam in the focal plane, and is given by $w_o = 2f\lambda/\pi a$. The length of the focus, L, is the distance over which the power density varies by a factor of 2 and is given by $L = 2\pi w_o^2/\lambda$.

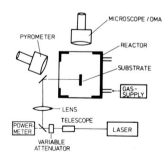

Fig. 1. Typical experimental setup for LCVD.

Local temperature measurements were made using a pyrometer (above 900 K). A detailed description is given in Ref. [9]. The reactor was operated up to $\sim 10^3$ mbar, either with a steady flow of gas, which is conveniently regulated by mass flow controllers, or in a sealed off condition. In the latter case the volume of gas consumed during the reaction must be negligible compared to the total volume of gas within the reaction chamber.

DIRECT WRITING

When in the experimental setup of Fig. 1 either the substrate moves or the laser beam is scanned, one can generate material patterns whose shapes depend on the relative motion of the laser beam and the substrate. In the simplest case one obtains stripes. A typical example is shown in Fig. 2 for the case of Ni, which was deposited from an atmosphere of $Ni(CO)_4$ in He. The partial pressures were $p(Ni(CO)_4) \simeq 395$ mbar, and $p(He) \simeq 526$ mbar. The deposition was performed

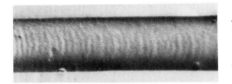

Fig. 2. Stripe of Ni deposited from $Ni(CO)_4$ (after Ref. [13]).

with $\lambda = 530.9$ nm Kr^+ laser radiation, $2w_o = 2.5$ μm, an irradiance of $I(0)=10.1$ kW/mm^2, and a scanning velocity of $v = 84$ μm/sec. The substrate was a 1000 Å thick film of a-Si on glass. When increasing the laser irradiance - at otherwise constant conditions - both the width, d, and the thickness, h, of the stripes increase. However, the growth rates are not determined only by the reactant species and the gas pressure, but will strongly depend also on the physical properties of the substrate, especially on its reflectivity and thermal conductivity. As a consequence, the thickness of the film during deposition also determines the growth rates. Fig. 3 not only shows the increase in width of stripes with increasing laser irradiance, but also reflects the differences in the physical properties of the substrates used. The figure shows a further interesting feature. In the low power regime, the width of the stripes may become smaller than the diameter of the laser focus, $2w_o$. This enhancement in spatial resolution is typical, and it could originate either from the nonlinear dependence of the deposition rate on temperature (see next section and Refs. [8,9,11], or from a threshold irradiance necessary for nucleation. The cross sections of the Ni stripes deposited on 1000 Å a-Si show a cylindrical surface, whose thickness, measured interferometrically by means of 589 nm Na radiation, increases about linearly with increasing width. For the example of Fig. 2 one finds d = 6 μm, and h = 0.27 μm. Thereby, the estimated rate of growth in film thickness is for this system and in this case of medium laser irradiance about 5 μm/sec. When increasing the scanning velocity - at constant laser irradiance - both the width and the thickness of the Ni stripes decrease [13].

It is clear that as a consequence of the many parameters which enter the deposition of stripes, quantitative results always refer only to the special system investigated. For instance, stripes of Si deposited on Si surfaces covered with 10-20 Å native oxide show a flat-topped mesa-like thickness profile - in contrast to the example mentioned above - and in addition the dependence of the deposited thickness on laser power seems in this case much more

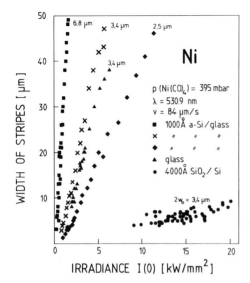

Fig. 3. Widths of Ni stripes as function of laser irradiance (after Ref. [13]).

complicated [10]. However, even for "identical" systems and parameters, tremendous differences in results may occur due to small differences in handling, as e.g. the procedure of substrate cleaning, or small differences in experimental conditions, such as incomplete blocking of the UV radiation from the gas discharge in the laser tube [12,13]. On the other hand, the qualitative features of the deposition are quite similar to those mentioned above for other systems investigated, as e.g. for C [7,8], Si [10,11], and SiO_2 [16] on various substrates. In particular, in all cases the deposition rates are by a factor of 10^2 to 10^3 larger than the maximal growth rates obtained in normal CVD large-area flow reactors [15]. This enormous enhancement in growth rates, which is characteristic for pyrolytic LCVD, is based on the strong localization of heating and thereby of the reaction zone. This essential difference between pyrolytic LCVD and conventional CVD will be presented in the next section where we discuss the deposition rates in the phase of steady growth.

The physical properties of the substrate together with the other parameters mentioned above, and, in addition, the chemical activation energy, which is typical for the particular chemical system used (see next section), determine also the lower limit for detectable film growth. In the actual process of direct writing, however, the laser irradiances used should be well above threshold. Otherwise, small changes in the surface quality of the substrate, or small inhomogeneities in its composition, may result in a break-off in film deposition. The upper limit for the deposition rates which can be achieved, depends on the thermal stability of the substrate and on the melting point and rate of evaporation of the deposited material. However, homogeneous cluster formation in the gas volume adjoining the surface may prevent controlled deposition even well below this limit. Of course, well defined deposition of micron-sized material patterns requires perfect mechanical stability of the experimental setup.

DEPOSITION RATES

When the positions of the laser beam and the substrate are both fixed, one observes the deposition of a circular spot. The beginning of nucleation is indicated by the occurence of a characteristic speckle pattern which reveals the appearance of scattering centers of submicrometer size. With the onset of speckle movement controlled growth of the deposit starts. Further irradiation results in the growth of a rod. A typical example is shown in Fig. 4 for the case of Si, which was grown in an atmosphere of SiH_4. Two phases of growth can clearly be observed: first, a phase during which the rod grows both parallel and perpendicular to the laser beam, and second a phase of steady growth. The first phase of growth, which is also relevant for the deposition of stripes, was discussed above. In the second phase the deposition rate depends only on the laser irradiance and on the reflectivity, and the thermal conductivity of the deposited material and n o t on the physical and chemical properties of the substrate. This was verified for the deposition of C, Si and Ni on various substrates [7,9,11,13]. As long as the axial growth in length, $\Delta\ell$, remains much less than the length of the focus, i.e. $\Delta\ell \ll L$, the phase of steady growth is characterized by a constant rod diameter. For the case of the rod shown in Fig. 4 this condition was satisfied within good approximation.

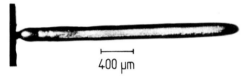

Fig. 4. Silicon rod grown from SiH_4. $I(o) = 4$ kW/mm^2, $\lambda = 488$ nm, $p(SiH_4) = 133$ mbar. Al_2O_3 ceramic substrate.

Quantitative investigations of the deposition rate in the phase of steady growth require correlation with the laser irradiance and the local temperature. While this correlation is trivial in the case of normal CVD, where the substrate is held at a uniform temperature, the situation is less obvious here, where deposition occurs at the tip of the growing rod, which naturally shows a strong temperature gradient. It is clear from the shape of the tip of the rod that the growth rate, $V(r)$, defined as the rate of translation of a surface element along its perpendicular, shows a maximum at the center of the tip, i.e. at r=0. This maximal growth rate, $V(r=0)$, is identical with the rate of increase of length of the rod, $W(T)$, and, when the surface temperature is always measured in the center of the rod, uniquely determined by $T \equiv T_s(r=0)$. One may therefore define the deposition rate by

$$W(T) = \frac{\Delta\ell}{\Delta t} \equiv V(r=0,T) \qquad (1)$$

With the experimental setup shown in Fig. 1, $\Delta\ell$, Δt and T could be measured simultaneously. Care must be taken that the time interval for measurements, Δt, is sufficiently short that $\Delta\ell \ll L$ is satisfied. Under these experimental conditions, the effective laser irradiance, and thereby the temperature T, remains constant within the interval Δt, and within accuracy of measurements. A very elegant method is to measure the changes in $\Delta\ell/\Delta t$ and T quasicontinuously during the growth of the rod along the axis of the laser focus. In this way a large number of data points can be generated as the irradiance varies along the focus, which was typically about 1 mm in these experiments [9].

For a thermally activated process, the deposition rate should follow an Arrhenius-type relation of the form

$$W = W_o \exp\{-\Delta E/kT\} \qquad (2)$$

where ΔE is the apparent activation energy, and W_o is a constant when the concentrations of the reacting species are constant. A typical example for an Arrhenius plot according to eq. (2) - assuming W_o to be independent of temperature - is shown in Fig. 5 for the case of C which was deposited from a C_2H_2 atmosphere at various pressures. Here, each data point marked was obtained by averaging about 30 single data points measured quasicontinuously according to the technique already mentioned above. The error bars represent the standard deviation, and directly indicate the excellent reproducibility of the data. Two

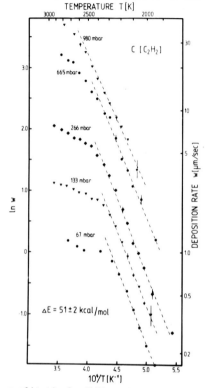

Fig. 5. Arrhenius plot for laser induced deposition of C from C_2H_2 (after Ref. [8]).

qualitatively different temperature regimes, which are typical also for other systems, are observed: The linear regime up to about 2300K reflects an exponential increase of the deposition rate with temperature. From the slope of the dashed line, which is a least squares fit through the data points in this regime, an activation energy of ΔE = 47±2 kcal/mol is derived. Within the accuracy indicated, this activation energy is independent of gas pressure. However, in the LCVD experiments the concentration of species within the reaction volume is not constant but temperature dependent. Correcting W_o by assuming the ansatz $W_o \propto 1/T$ - according to the ideal gas law - one still obtains in the low temperature regime of the Arrhenius plot a straight line - within accuracy of measurement - the slope of which is slightly increased and yields an actual apparent activation energy of ΔE = 51±2 kcal/mol. Similar experiments for the deposition of Si from SiH_4 yielded for the corrected value ΔE = 46.6±4 kcal/mol. These values are within the range of activation energies which were derived from the thermal decomposition of C_2H_2 [17] and SiH_4 [15,18,19].

The characteristic decrease in slope observed above a certain temperature may indicate that the decomposition process is no longer controlled by the chemical kinetics, but instead becomes limited by transport. However, alternative explanations cannot be ruled out, e.g. the onset of particle formation, different chemical reaction pathways, or enrichment of reaction products near the growing surface due to thermodiffusion.

When comparing the deposition rates achieved in the LCVD experiments with those obtained in conventional CVD systems, it is essential to consider the significant differences in the conditions of deposition in both systems. The area where laser induced deposition occurs is typically only 10^{-8} to 10^{-4} cm^2 in comparison to several cm^2 in the normal CVD large-area flow reactors [15]. The LCVD reactor can be held at a well defined (low) temperature even at very high local temperatures. Therefore, no problems arise with deposition elsewhere than the localized hot spot - even at pressures of several hundred mbar. As a consequence of the much higher pressures that can be used in the LCVD experiments, the deposition rates are higher by a factor of 10^2-10^3 compared to those reported for the corresponding CVD systems. Also because of the strong localization of heating, three dimensional diffusion of molecules to and from the reaction zone is possible, while in the normal CVD large-area slab-geometry only one dimensional diffusion is effective. Furthermore, convective transport of species will be much more important. This explains the much wider extension of the kinetically controlled regime, in which the slope of the curve is independent of pressure, gas velocity, reactor geometry etc. and is only determined by an apparent chemical activation energy which is typical for the system under investigation, and which characterizes the rate limiting step in the chain of chemical reactions involved in the deposition process. Because data points can be measured quasicontinuously - a consequence of the fast growth rates - we believe that pyrolytic LCVD will become a very powerful tool for rapid and accurate determination of such activation energies [9].

The lower and upper laser irradiance limits for deposition of rods are essentially of the same origin as those already discussed in the last section - except that not the physical properties of the substrate but only those of the deposited material enter. For the case of Si e.g., controlled deposition was limited by the large discontinuous increase in reflectivity at the melting point [20], which drastically reduces the absorbed power [11]. No increase in the deposition rate was observed even when doubling the laser irradiance.

Systematic investigations have also been performed on the dependence of the diameter of rods on laser irradiance. While in some cases, e.g. for C from C_2H_2 [7], a monotonic increase in rod diameter with increasing laser irradiance is observed, in other cases, e.g. for Ni from $Ni(CO)_4$ [13], a saturation type behaviour is found above a certain irradiance. This behaviour can be explained by the differences in thermal conductivity and reflectivity of deposited materials.

MORPHOLOGY AND PHYSICAL PROPERTIES OF DEPOSITS

The morphology and microstructure of the deposits was mainly investigated by optical microscopy, scanning electron microscopy (SEM), X-ray diffraction, and by Raman scattering techniques.

Stripes which are grown with irradiances well above threshold show a very fine weld seam like structure, which can clearly be observed in interference contrast micrographs, as in Fig. 2 for the case of Ni. SEM pictures taken from Ni stripes grown with various irradiances show a fine texture with a few nodules. For low irradiances the dimensions of this texture are typically <1000 Å ($I(0) \lesssim 2$ kW/mm^2, otherwise same parameters as in Fig. 2), and become more coarse, about 1000-3000 Å ($I(0) \approx 7$ kW/mm^2) at higher irradiances. The polycrystalline structure of the stripes was also established by X-ray diffraction, and, for the case of Si, by Raman scattering. In the Raman spectra one observes only a sharp line near 520 cm^{-1} which is typical for the T_{2g} transverse optical mode in crystalline or polycrystalline Si. In particular, no broad structure on the low energy side of this line, which would indicate the presence of an amorphous phase, was observed. Similar investigations on the morphology have also been performed on C, Si, and Ni rods. In all cases a crystalline structure of the material was found. Fig. 6 shows a SEM of a cross section of a Ni rod. Single, randomly oriented crystallites can clearly be observed. In summary one can say that all deposits investigated up to now, including those produced by non-resonant IR laser light, show a polycrystalline structure. The grain size depends strongly on the parameters used in the deposition process, especially on the laser irradiance and the gas pressure.

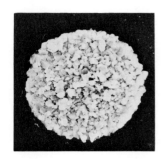

Fig. 6. SEM of a cross section of a Ni rod.

In most cases tested, the stripes adhered strongly on the various substrate materials. Sometimes difficulties did arise for high laser irradiances; e.g. Ni stripes grown on a-Si often peeled off when increasing the irradiance above about 16 kW/mm^2 ($2w_s \approx 2.5 \mu m$). The thermally induced lateral strain has been estimated for 1 µm Si stripes, which were deposited on 3500 Å thermally grown SiO_2 on Si, via the shift of the T_{2g} Raman line. The observed red shift of the line of about 1.5 cm^{-1} corresponds to a tensile stress of about 3 kbar [10].

The electrical resistivity of the Ni stripes was $(1.9\pm0.2) \cdot 10^{-5} \Omega$cm. This value is by about a factor of 2.8 larger than the bulk resistivity of pure Ni. There was no evidence for carbon inclusions [13]. Low resistivity stripes of Si have been produced by adding various doping gases to the silane [10]. It was found necessary to use doping gases with a pyrolysis rate close to that of the SiH_4. Appropriate dopants were BCl_3, and $B(CH_3)_3$. When doping with about 33 mbar of $B(CH_3)_3$ ($p(SiH_4) \approx 263$ mbar), the best films had resistivites of $1.5 \cdot 10^{-3} \Omega$cm. The doping gas did not change either the deposition rate or the morphology of the deposits.

CONCLUSION

   Laser pyrolysis at visible wavelengths allows one-step local deposition of micron-sized material patterns. The lateral dimensions of the deposits can easily be varied by at least a factor of 10^2 by simply varying the laser irradiance, scanning velocity etc.. The thickness profile can perhaps be tailored by proper choice of the incident irradiance distribution. The deposition rates exceed those achieved in normal CVD large-area flow reactors by a factor of 10^2 to 10^3. Therefore, pyrolytic LCVD may have a broad range of applications, e.g. in cases where at present microstructures are produced by standard CVD techniques combined with photolithographic methods, for the production of interconnects, ohmic contacts or coatings, or for mask and circuit repair etc..

ACKNOWLEDGMENTS

   We wish to thank the Fonds zur Förderung der wissenschaftlichen Forschung in Österreich for financial support.

REFERENCES

1. H. Lydtin in: Proc. 3rd Int. Conf. on Chemical Vapor Deposition, F. A. Glaski ed., Hinsdale 1972, pp. 121.

2. L. S. Nelson and N. L. Richardson, Mat. Res. Bull. 7, 971 (1972).

3. R. S. Berg and D. M. Mattox in: Proc. 4th Int. Conf. on Chemical Vapor Deposition, F. A. Glaski ed., Hinsdale 1973, pp. 196-204.

4. C. P. Christensen and K. M. Lakin, Appl. Phys. Lett. 32, 254 (1978).

5. S. D. Allen and M. Bass, J. Vac. Sci. Technol. 16, 431 (1979).

6. V. Baranauskas et al., Appl. Phys. Lett. 36, 930 (1980).

7. G. Leyendecker et al., Appl. Phys. Lett. 39, 921 (1981).

8. D. Bäuerle et al., Appl. Phys. B 28, 267 (1982).

9. G. Leyendecker et al., J. Electrochem. Soc. (1982).

10. D. J. Ehrlich et al., Appl. Phys. Lett. 39, 957 (1981).

11. D. Bäuerle et al., Appl. Phys. Lett. 40, 819 (1982).

12. Y. Rytz-Froidevaux et al., Appl. Phys. A 27, 133 (1982).

13. W. Kräuter and D. Bäuerle, Appl. Phys. (1982).

14. For a review see e. g.: D. J. Ehrlich et al., IEEE J. Quantum Electron., QE 16, 1233 (1980).

15. For a review see e. g.: J. Bloem and L. J. Giling in: Current Topics in Materials Science, E. Kaldis ed. (North-Holland, New York 1978) Vol. 1, pp. 147-342.

16. W. Kräuter et al., (to be published).

17. H. B. Palmer and C. F. Cullis, Chemistry and Physics of Carbon 1, 265 (1965).

18. F. C. Eversteijn, Philips Res. Repts. 26, 134 (1971).

19. J. H. Purnell and R. Walsh, Proc. R. Soc. A 293, 543 (1966).

20. M. O. Lampert et al., J. Appl. Phys. 52, 4975 (1981).

LASER-INITIATED Ga-DEPOSITION ON QUARTZ SUBSTRATES

Y. RYTZ-FROIDEVAUX, R.P. SALATHE, AND H.H. GILGEN
Institute of Applied Physics, University of Berne,
Sidlerstr. 5, 3012 Berne, Switzerland.

ABSTRACT

The deposition of Ga on quartz substrates by photodissociation of trimethylgallium has been investigated. Light from a frequency doubled Ar-ion laser beam (257.2 nm) was focused onto quartz substrates. The Ar-ion laser was operated under cw or mode-locking conditions. The deposition rate has been investigated as a function of averaged UV power densities in the range of 1.8 - 1750 W/cm^2 and is shown to depend critically on the laser operating mode. For cw operation, the maximum growth rate within the focal zone is limited to 17 Å/s whereas under mode-locking conditions, no saturation is observed and the growth rate increases linearly with the laser power up to 70 Å/s at 1.75 kW/cm^2.

1. INTRODUCTION

The laser-initiated etching or deposition of metals or semiconductors offers a new and interesting method for fabricating microstructures. This technique allows to structure the surface of a substrate in one step and thus presents a high economy of time and material. The process can be initiated by pyrolysis [1,2] or photolysis [1,3] of molecules near the surface. Semiconductors such as Si and Ge [1,4] and metals such as Al, Cd, Cr, Fe, Mo, W, and Zn [5-7] have been deposited. Here, we report on the deposition of Ga on quartz by photodissociation of trimethylgallium (Ga(CH$_3$)$_3$, TMGa) in the UV-range. Gallium is an interesting material because it has a much lower melting point than the metals investigated so far and because it is an important compound in different optoelectronic materials, e.g. GaAs, GaP, or GaN.

2. ABSORPTION MEASUREMENTS

The absorption of TMGa in the UV-range was measured with a Cary Mod. 219 spectrophotometer. Figure 1 shows a room temperature measurement of the absorption edge at small energies of TMGa diluted in H$_2$ under atmospheric pressure with a partial pressure of 29.4 Torr in a 1 cm long cell. The absorption cross section is on the order of 5.4 10^{-18} cm^2 at 193 nm and of 8.7 10^{-20} cm^2 at 257.2 nm. In the range of 210 - 230 nm, we observe a substructure similar to the one reported for Cd(CH$_3$)$_2$ [8].
Thin films of gallium on quartz substrates have been prepared by evaporation of elemental gallium. The films had a thickness of about 10 nm. They were used to evaluate the optical constants of solid gallium. With the spectrophotometer we measured a reflectivity of R = 0.54 and from transmission measurements an

absorption coefficient of $\alpha = 6.3 \; 10^5 \; cm^{-1}$ is evaluated at 257 nm.

Fig.1: Absorbance of trimethylgallium at 29,4 Torr in H_2 at 20 °C for an optical path length of 1 cm. (--->)

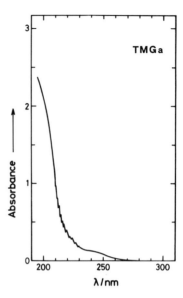

EXPERIMENTAL ARRANGEMENT

The experimental arrangement is shown in Fig. 2. An Ar-ion laser (Spectra Phys. Mod.171) operated at 514.5 nm under cw or mode-locking conditions (100 ps, 83.3 MHz) has been used in the experiment. The light is focused with lens L_1 (f = 500 mm) into the center of a 2 cm long potassium dihydrogen phosphate (KDP) crystal. Frequency doubling was achieved in the 90° configuration with the phases matched by tuning the temperature of the crystal to about -16 °C. The silica lens L_2 (f = 350 mm) is used to generate a parallel beam which is directed to the quartz prism P separating the frequency doubled beam (257.2 nm, solid line) from the argon laser beam (slim line). The frequency doubled beam is focused by means of the UV lens L_3 (Zeiss Ultrafluar, f=16.4 mm, N.A.=0.2) on the inner side of the entrance window of the gas cell Z. The focal spot diameter is diffraction limited and on the order of 8 μm in this case. The cell is flushed with a mixture of Pd-diffused H_2 (flow rate ~1 l/h) and TMGa (partial pressure of 58 Torr) at atmospheric pressure. The beam splitter BS and the

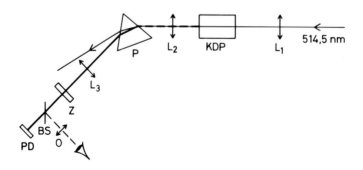

Fig. 2: Experimental arrangement. L_1, L_2, and L_3 are lenses, O a binocular. KDP is the frequency doubling crystal, P the quartz prism, Z the cell, BS the beam splitter, and PD the photodiode.

binocular O allow direct observation of the deposits. The growth of the metallic film is evaluated by measuring the transmitted UV-intensity with the photodiode PD (EG&G UV-444B).

RESULTS

Gallium has been deposited in cw operation at power densities of 120 - 400 W/cm^2 and in mode-locking operation at average densities of 0.15 - 1.75 kW/cm^2. The alkylmetallic molecules $M(CH_3)_n$ dissociate easily into the metal atom M and the methyl radicals which form CH_4 and some C_2H_6 [9]. Fig. 3 shows the transmission signal T as a function of the irradiation time t. The Ar-ion laser has been mode-locked in this case and the average UV power density was 1.75 kW/cm^2. The transmitted signal decreases immediately if the UV light is turned on. In contrast to the Cd deposition at visible wavelengths [8], no latent time could be observed. This indicates that the deposition is initiated directly from the gas phase. The growth rate R shown in Fig. 3 has been evaluated from the slope of the transmission curve with the measured absorption coefficient for gallium. R decreases with time because of absorption in the growing film in this particular configuration.

The maximum growth rate R_M (at t = 0) has been investigated as a function of the laser power density. Fig.4 shows the corresponding result for cw irradiation (dashed line) and for mode-locking pulses (solid line). R_M is proportional to the incident laser power for cw illumination at low densities. This dependency is expected for a deposition mode based on one photon excitation in the gas phase. With the measured cross-section for TMGa, we estimate from the

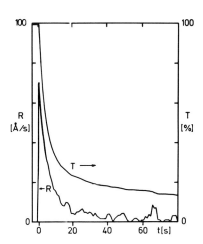
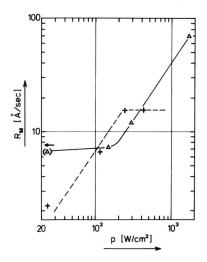

Fig.3: Transmission T and growth rate R vs. irradiation time t.

Fig.4: Maximum growth rate R_M vs. laser power density p for cw (dashed line) and pulsed (solid line) illumination. (Δ) refers to pulsed measurement at 1.8 W/cm^2.

measured growth rates that the gas volume of TMGa contributing to the deposition has a thickness of a few micrometers. For power densities greater than $P = 230$ W/cm^2, corresponding to a growth rate of 17 Å/s, a saturation for R_M is observed. This saturation can be explained by depletion of TMGa in the immediate vicinity of the surface or by a change in growth mode due to laser induced heating and liquefaction of the Ga deposit. Based on a laser spot radius of 4 μm, a measured reflectivity of 0.54 for solid gallium, and a thermal conductivity of 0.0132 W/cm·°C for the silica substrates [10], we calculate a temperature rise of 6.5 °C in the laser focus for the highest cw power level. For an ambient temperature of 24 deg.C the resulting maximum temperature would be above the melting point of gallium (29.8 °C).

Under mode-locking conditions, a linear increase in R_M is also observed in Fig.4. However, R_M is reduced by about 40 per cent with respect to the rates obtained with cw irradiation at comparable power densities. The FWHM of the mode-locked pulses (Δt = 100 psec) is below the average collision time in the gaz ($t_C \approx$ 150 psec). We thus attribute the lower rates to a reduction in the volume of TMGa contributing to deposition which is on the order of $\Delta t/t_C$. No saturation in R_M and a linear increase with average power density are observed up to 70 Å/s at 1.75 kW/cm^2, the maximum power density investigated in our case. The deposits generated at 200-300 W/cm^2 were thinner in the center and covered an area increased by 80 per cent with respect to deposits generated with cw illumination under identical conditions. These changes could be due to re-evaporation of TMGa in the center and to an increased peak power density in the outer regions. They lead to a considerably modified temperature profile during growth which could explain the absence of steady state melting in this case. At the low average power density of 1.8 W/cm^2 we measured a deposition rate of $\sim$ 7 Å/s. The peak power density ($\sim$ 200 W/cm^2) seems to be still above the threshold power density necessary for nucleation. The measurement demonstrates that it is easier to grow a nucleus of critical size under pulsed conditions.

A typical deposit obtained with a slightly defocused beam is shown in Fig.5a. The granular structure shown in this micrograph indicates that the deposition starts at individual Ga seeds. A similar "seed" structure has been observed in Cr deposition experiments [11]. The diameter of the seeds here is about 0.3 μm.

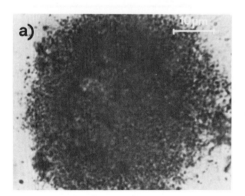
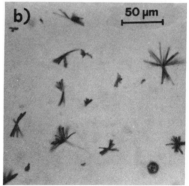

Fig. 5: Transmission micrographs : a) seeded feature of a Ga deposit obtained with a slightly defocused laser beam, b) spontaneously grown spins in the unilluminated regions.

The size and structure of the deposit depend on the power density and the illumination duration. For increasing powers and/or durations, the diameter and the thickness in the center of the deposit increase. Around thick deposits, interference structures were observed which exhibited a spatial resolution of 1.2 μm. Deutsch et al [5] obtained a similar resolution for the deposition of Cd. No particular difference in the morphology of the deposits was noted between the two modes of operation of the laser. The seeded structure originates from the preferred deposition of Ga on already seeded Ga. This preferential growth mechanism is further confirmed if unilluminated regions of the substrate are investigated. In these regions, spins of Ga form spontaneously (Fig. 5b); they appear above all at scratches on the surface. Their thickness and length are on the order of 1.5 - 2.2 μm and 20 - 28 μm, respectively. Ehrlich et al [7] have observed the same spontaneous growth in the case of the Fe deposition on quartz by photodissociation of $Fe(CO)_5$. It originates in the condensation of photoproducts which are produced "far" from the surface in the gas. This parasitic growth depends on the illumination power and on the mean free path length L. It can be reduced by decreasing the illumination power or by increasing the buffer gas pressure since the mean free path length L is inversely proportional to the density n of particules and their collision cross-sections σ ($L \propto 1/(n\sigma)$).

Based on this preferential growth, it is possible to limit the diameter of the deposition area to the inner part of the Gaussian beam profile. A low laser power and a long illumination duration have to be used in this case. Fig.6 shows the result of an experiment performed with pulsed illumination of TMGa in H_2 (58 Torr) with an average power density of 11 W/cm² and an illumination duration of 36 seconds. Here, the diameter of the deposit is 2.7 μm. This is a factor of 3 smaller than the halfwidth of the gaussian beam profile (8 μm). No attempt has been made so far to optimize the parameters of the preferential growth mechanism further.

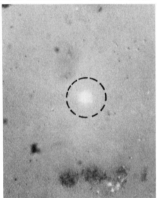

Fig.6: Ga deposit obtained at 11 W/cm² for 36 s. Ring indicates laser spot diameter.

In conclusion, we have obtained deposition of Ga by photodissociation of $Ga(CH_3)_3$ in frequency doubled Ar-ion laser light. In mode-locking operation, growth rates for the metallic film of 70 Å/s have been measured at average power densities of 1.75 kW/cm².

ACKNOWLEDGEMENTS:

The authors are grateful to Professor H.P. Weber for the opportunity to perform this work, to Dr. P. Anliker for the disposition of the mode-locking Ar-ion laser, B. Wicki for technical assistance, and the Swiss foundation for microtechnical research for financial support.

REFERENCES

[1] C.P. Christensen and K.M. Lakin, Appl. Phys. Lett. $\underline{32}$, 254 (1978)

[2] R.J. von Gutfeld, E.E. Tynan, and L.T. Romankiw, extended abstract n° 472, Electrochem. Soc. $\underline{79}$ (2) (1979)

[3] D.J. Ehrlich, R.M. Osgood, Jr., and T.F. Deutsch, Appl. Phys. Lett. $\underline{36}$, 698 (1980)

[4] R.W. Andreatta, C.C. Abele, J.F. Osmundsen, J.G. Eden, D. Lubben, and J.E. Greene, Appl. Phys. Lett. $\underline{40}$, 183 (1982)

[5] T.F. Deutsch, D.J. Ehrlich, and R.M. Osgood, Jr., Appl. Phys. Lett. $\underline{35}$, 175 (1979)

[6] R. Solanki, P.H. Boyer, J.E. Mahan, and G.J. Collins, Appl. Phys. Lett. $\underline{38}$, 572 (1981)

[7] D.J. Ehrlich, R.M. Osgood, Jr., and T.F. Deutsch, J. Electrochem. Soc. $\underline{128}$, 2039 (1981)

[8] Y. Rytz-Froidevaux, R.P. Salathe, H.H. Gilgen, and H.P. Weber, Appl. Phys. $\underline{A27}$, 133 (1982)

[9] E.W.R. Steacie, <u>Atomic and free radical reactions</u> (Reinhold Publishing Corporation, New York 1956)

[10] Landolt-Boernstein Vol.$\underline{IV}$,part $\underline{4b}$, <u>Waernetechnik</u> (Springer Verlag, Berlin 1972) p. 482

[11] J.R. Solanki, P.K.Boyer, J.E. Mahan, and G.J. Collins, Appl. Phys. Lett. $\underline{38}$, 572 (1981)

UV PHOTODECOMPOSITION FOR METAL DEPOSITION:
GAS VS. SURFACE PHASE PROCESSES

THOMAS H. WOOD, J. C. WHITE, AND B. A. THACKER
Bell Laboratories, Holmdel, New Jersey 07733

ABSTRACT

Photodecomposition of organometallic gases has been shown to be potentially useful for high resolution direct metal deposition. However, a number of problems, particularly the low writing rates, must first be solved. An understanding of the deposition mechanism is essential to this task. In particular, the decomposition must be shown to occur either in the gas phase or in the adsorbed layer. This question can be resolved by the dependence of the writing rate on spot size. Measurements of the process show that once the deposition begins the bulk of the deposit occurs from decomposition in the gas phase.

INTRODUCTION

Recently there has been a great deal of interest in ultraviolet photodecomposition for localized metal deposition and semiconductor etching. [1-5] Metal deposits with submicron features have been generated. [1] This "direct writing" method has applications to custom LSI fabrication, mask and wafer repair, etc. However, despite considerable work, little is known about the mechanism of the deposition. This is an important problem, since many potential applications are currently prohibited because of the slow writing rate (typically roughly 20 Å/sec in a 50 micron spot [1]).

In a typical experiment, a substrate is placed in a few torr of an organometallic gas such as dimethyl cadmium, and exposed to a focused UV, CW laser beam. Deposited metal is observed in the illuminated region. This metal may have been deposited by two different mechanisms. Organometallic molecules adsorbed on the surface may absorb a photon and decompose, leaving the metal behind on the substrate. Conversely, the decomposition may occur in the gas phase, followed by metal migration to and sticking on the substrate. As shown below, the number of molecules participating in these two reactions are comparable, so it is not possible to differentiate between them a priori without accurate measurements of the adsorbed and gas phase photodecomposition cross sections. Although gas phase decomposition has been suggested as the dominant factor, [4] no previous experiments directly address this question. Differentiation between these two processes is necessary to an understanding of the mechanisms of deposit localization, and to attempts to increase deposition rates.

Ehrlich et al. have proposed a two step model for writing in which the deposit is first localized by decomposition of adsorbed organometallic to form critical nuclei, followed by gas phase decomposition to form the bulk of the deposit. [4] Although this model successfully explains observation of localized deposits on prenucleated regions, the experimental observations do not indicate whether the bulk of the final deposited spot is due to decomposition in the gas or adsorbed phase. In this paper we show that these two hypotheses can be differentiated by the dependence of the deposition rate on laser spot size. Observations of this dependence indicate that the bulk of the writing process takes place due to gas phase decomposition.

THEORY

To differentiate between gas phase and surface phase decomposition, we derive formulas for the decomposition rate in each case. The surface phase decomposition rate can be found simply. We assume the substrate is illuminated by a laser beam of radius a. For simplicity, we consider the laser power profile to be uniform within the spot rather than gaussian. N_a is the number of surface adsorbed molecular per unit area, which is of the order of one monolayer density. [6] Then the deposition rate due to decomposition of adsorbed molecules, R_a, in atoms/cm^2-sec, is given by

$$R_a = \frac{N_a \sigma_a P_L}{h\nu \pi a^2}, \qquad (1)$$

where σ_a is the adsorbed dissociation cross section in cm^2, P_L is the laser power in Watts, and $h\nu$ is the laser photon energy in joules.

For gas phase decomposition, we neglect the divergence of the laser beam away from the substrate since, in our conditions, the confocal parameter is much greater than a, and the beam divergence angle is small. Then, within the illuminated cylinder, the rate of production of metal atoms/cm^3-sec, $\dot{\rho}_g$, is given by

$$\dot{\rho}_g = \frac{N_g \sigma_g P_L}{h\nu \pi a^2}, \qquad (2)$$

where σ_g is the gas phase dissociation cross section, and N_g is the number of reactant gas molecules per cm^3.

We now consider diffusion of metal atoms to the surface where they deposit. We assume each metal atom travels a distance $\emptyset$ in the gas phase before it is removed by a gas phase reaction. Measurements on the gas phase population decay indicate that $\emptyset \sim 10$ cm for typical reaction conditions. [2]

The deposition rate at the center of the laser spot due to gas phase decomposition, R_g, in atoms/cm^2-sec, can be found to be

$$R_g = \frac{\alpha}{4\pi} \int dV \frac{\dot{\rho}_g \cos\theta}{d^2}$$

$$= \frac{\alpha}{4\pi} \int_0^{2\pi} d\phi \int_0^{\emptyset} dz \int_0^a rdr \frac{z\dot{\rho}_g}{d^3}$$

$$= \frac{\alpha\dot{\rho}_g}{2} \left[\emptyset + a - \sqrt{\emptyset^2 + a^2} \right], \tag{3}$$

where α is the sticking probability of a metal atom incident on the substrate.

In the limit $\emptyset \gg a$, which is appropriate for all cases considered here,

$$R_g = \frac{1}{2} \alpha\dot{\rho}_g a. \tag{4}$$

This result can be understood qualitatively as indicating that those atoms created within a distance of order a/2 from the surface contribute to the deposition. Combining Eqn. (4) with Eqn. (2) gives

$$R_g = \frac{\alpha N_g \sigma_g P_L}{2\pi h \nu a}. \tag{5}$$

Thus, the deposition rate R should be observed to be of the form

$$R = ca^{-n}. \tag{6}$$

If n is observed to be 2, Eqn. (1) is valid and the decomposition is surface phase. If n is observed to be 1, Eqn. (5) is valid and the decomposition is gas phase.

EXPERIMENT AND RESULTS

We note that for the conditions used here, the gas and surface phase decomposition rates are of the same order of magnitude, assuming equal decomposition cross sections. [7]

The experimental layout is shown schematically in Fig. 1. Light at 5145Å from a Spectra-Physics 171 Argon ion laser is frequency doubled by a temperature regulated ADP crystal. The UV light is separated from the fundamental, filtered, and monitored before it is focused on the sample. Approximately 2 mW of UV light was obtained at the sample; the intensity was constant to within 5%. The light was focused on the quartz front window of a gas cell; deposition took place on this window's inner surface. The deposition thickness was monitored by the attenuation of the UV beam. Although some deposition did take place on the rear window, gas phase attenuation and the larger laser spot size meant this was not a significant contributor to the attenuation rate. Deposited spot sizes were adjusted by translating the focusing lens in the z direction. Gases were introduced into the cell through an all metal gas handling system. For this experiment, 1 of torr of electronic grade dimethyl cadmium was buffered with 750 torr of research grade helium. Pressures were read from a MKS model 220 capacitor manometer or a United Instruments diaphragm pressure gauge. After deposition, spot sizes were observed directly in a Zeiss light microscope.

The insert to Fig. 2 shows a typical transmission plot as a function of time. After a sharp rise at time $t = 0$, an exponential attenuation is observed. For each deposition, a time constant is calculated for the attenuation by measuring the initial slope of the transmission decay; these time constants are plotted as a function of spot size, a, in Fig. 2. The slope of the log-log plot gives the value of the exponent n in Eqn. 6. The observed value, $n = 0.73 \pm 0.15$, is most consistent with $n = 1$, which, as Eqn. (5) shows, implies gas phase decomposition. The fact that the observed value of n is slightly less than 1.0 implies that there is some error in the simplifying assumptions used in our analysis. These assumptions include neglect of nonuniformities of the beam intensity profile, both due to its gaussian nature and due to absorption as the deposit develops, and the calculation of the deposition rate only at the center of the deposit. Nevertheless, the analysis is sufficient to decide unambiguously between $n = 1$ and $n = 2$, and thus between gas and surface phase decomposition.

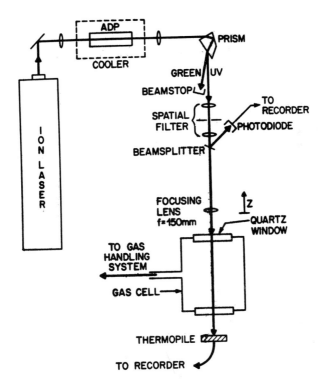

Figure 1   Optical schematic. The attenuation of the UV beam is used as a monitor of the deposition.

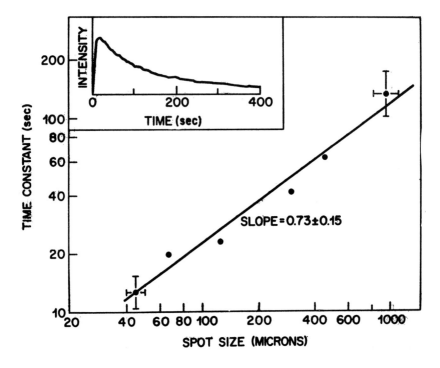

Figure 2   Insert shows UV transmitted intensity fall off as deposition proceeds, in the case of the largest dot. Main figure shows dependence of the fall off time constant on spot size, indicating the exponent relating the two is roughly n = 1.

Our data have been analyzed in terms of either pure gas phase or surface phase decomposition. In the context of the two stage writing model described by Ehrlich et al., [4] we show that the bulk of the decomposition does indeed take place in the gas phase, and that this decomposition is the rate limiting step. This fact indicates that molecules and laser wavelengths should be chosen for maximum gas phase decomposition cross sections. Finally, Eqn. (5) shows, at constant laser power density (such as would be achieved by illumination through a mask), the writing rates should be lower for small features than for large ones. This property, which is similar to the proximity effect observed in electron beam lithography, [7] will be particularly important to the understanding of growth of complex patterns, where all features are not the same size.

REFERENCES

[1] T. F. Deutsch, D. J. Ehrlich, and R. M. Osgood, Jr., Appl. Phys. Lett. 35, 175 (1979).

[2] D. J. Ehrlich, R. M. Osgood, and T. F. Deutsch, IEEE J. Quantum Electron. QE-16, 1233 (1980).

[3] D. J. Ehrlich, R. M. Osgood, Jr., and T. F. Deutsch, Appl. Phys. Lett. 36, 698 (1980).

[4] D. J. Ehrlich, R. M. Osgood, Jr., and T. F. Deutsch, Appl. Phys. Lett. 38, 946 (1981).

[5] R. Solanki, P. K. Boyer, J. E. Mahan, and G. J. Collins, Appl. Phys. Lett. 38, 572 (1981).

[6] D. J. Ehrlich and R. M. Osgood, Chem. Phys. Lett. 79, 381 (1981).

[7] T. H. P. Chang, J. Vac. Sci. Technol. 12, 1271 (1975).

SECTION II
PHOTOETCHING OF ELECTRONIC MATERIALS

LASER CHEMICAL ETCHING OF CONDUCTING
AND SEMICONDUCTING MATERIALS

T. J. CHUANG
IBM Research Laboratory, 5600 Cottle Road, San Jose, California, USA

ABSTRACT

The purpose of the paper is to examine the basic processes involved in the laser-enhanced chemical etching of solids. Specifically, the process of chemisorption, the reaction between the adsorbate and substrate atoms and the vaporization of product species affected by the laser radiation are discussed. It is shown that the laser method can provide important insight into the gas-surface reaction mechanisms. In addition, a number of examples are given to demonstrate the potential of the technique for applications to material processing. Some current studies on the laser-induced chemical etching of materials relevant to microelectronics are reviewed. Certain practical experimental approaches are also considered.

I. INTRODUCTION

There has been increasing interest in recent years in developing new techniques for processing electronic materials as possible supplements to existing methods of etching, doping and material deposition. The new techniques that have been explored are based primarily on the radiation-enhanced chemical interactions at gas-solid interfaces by energetic particles such as ions, electrons and photons [1-5]. Laser radiation due to its monochromatic and coherent characteristics can be readily focused or collimated onto solid surfaces and is well-suited to promoting surface reactions. Indeed, laser-induced chemical etching has been demonstrated in both gas-solid [6-8] and liquid-solid systems [9-11]. In many instances, it has been clearly shown that laser chemical etching technique not only can provide direct maskless etching at high etch rates but also can be applied to a wide variety of materials. In this paper, aspects related to laser-enhanced gas-surface chemical interactions pertinent to etching reactions will be discussed.

In general, the etching of a solid by the exposure to a gaseous chemical includes the processes of dissociative chemisorption, the reaction between the adsorbed species and solid atoms, and the removal of reaction products from the surfaces. The presence of laser radiation at a gas-solid interface can influence one or more than one of these processes. It thus seems conceptionally useful to divide the laser interaction with a gas-solid system into three basic processes, namely, the interaction of laser photons with (1) the gaseous species, (2) the species adsorbed on solid surfaces and (3) the solid substrate. The fundamental processes that are believed to play important roles in determining the laser-induced etching behavior will be discussed in Section II. In Section III, some experimental considerations in regards to optical arrangements and selection of laser systems will be given. Experimental results on some specific systems, in particular, on materials of practical interest to microfabrication such as Si, SiO_2, metals, magnetic materials and certain organic polymers will be presented in Section IV. In addition to the potential application of the laser chemical technique to material processing, we will also give examples to illustrate the usefulness of the laser technique for studying mechanisms involved in etching reactions, which are often obscured in complex plasma etching environments.

II. BASIC LASER-ENHANCED ETCHING PROCESSES

2.1 Laser excitation of gas phase species

In this mode of excitation, both the electronic and vibrational excitation of the gaseous etchant molecules can be involved. For halogen molecules, the electronic excitation in the ultraviolet and visible spectral region usually results in photodissociation to halogen atoms. The halogen atom being a radical is always more reactive than its parent molecule and can be readily chemisorbed on solid surfaces. Thus, a laser beam can induce photo-fragmentation of gaseous molecules and enhance dissociative chemisorption, a necessary first step in the etching processes. In many instances, the continuous photo-generation of halogen atoms can provide a sufficient high radical concentration to further promote the adsorbed atoms to react with substrate atoms to form reaction products. It is known that surface reaction rates often depend on the concentration of reactive species [12]. For example, F atoms and F_2 molecules at high pressure can spontaneously etch SiO_2 [13] and Si [14], respectively. At lower pressure, these reactions have not been detected. Similar effects have been observed in the laser-enhanced etching reactions. For instance, in SiO_2-Cl_2 system excited by an Ar laser at 457.9 nm focused on the solid substrate, the laser beam can photodissociate Cl_2 molecules into Cl atoms which subsequently react with SiO_2 [15]. In contrast, Cl_2 plasma which also produces Cl atoms does not show any significant etching of the solid [16]. Because a focused or collimated laser beam can generate a relatively high concentration of reactive atoms or radicals near the surface region, it can thus affect the surface chemistry more effectively.

The effect of vibrational activation of etchant molecules on surface reactivity has been demonstrated in Si-SF_6 reaction [17,18]. SF_6 molecules are inert to Si at 25°C but the molecules can be excited by multiple photon absorption with a pulsed CO_2 laser at 10.6 μm to react with the solid to form volatile products such as SiF_4 [17]. The bond strength between F and Si in SiF_4 (about 135 kcal/mole) is much greater than that of S-F bond in SF_6 (about 68 kcal/mole) [19]. Thus, thermodynamically, the reaction between SF_6 and Si to form SiF_4 and SiF_4 should be exothermic in nature. However, the activation barriers for reaction appears to be rather high. From Si-SF_6 thermal reaction studies, it was determined that the activation energy was about 17 kcal/mole in 950-1250°C temperature range [20,21]. In the CO_2 laser induced reaction at relatively low laser intensity, the level of SF_6 molecular excitation was found to involve perhaps 3 or 4 infrared photons, corresponding to about 9~12 kcal/mole. Furthermore, surface analyses with X-ray photoemission spectroscopy (XPS) showed that "SiF_2"-like species were formed on Si surfaces after reaction with laser-excited SF_6 molecules [5,22], indicating the possibility of the silicon-fluorine species being a surface reaction intermediate. The pulsed infrared laser can also be utilized in a different way to promote a different type of surface reaction. By focusing the CO_2 laser beam to a rather high intensity, it is possible to decompose the polyatomic molecule via multiple photon dissociation in its ground electron state [23,24]. The decomposition involving 30 or more CO_2 laser photons results in the production of F atoms [24] which subsequently react with Si surfaces [17]. A major difference between the Si-F reaction and the Si reaction with vibrationally excited SF_6 arises from the fact that F atoms once generated by photodissociation or by glow discharge can diffuse through the gas phase and remain active to Si. The excited SF_6 molecules, on the other hand, cannot remain activated after only a few collisions with other molecules or with a solid wall because of the rapid vibrational relaxation rates. Therefore, only the SF_6 molecules that are near the surface can be vibrationally excited to react with Si in the high pressure region. Similar studies involving CF_3 radical generation from multiple photon dissociation of CF_3Br molecules to react with SiO_2 have also been reported [8].

As illustrated with the examples given above, the level of molecular excitation and the generation of reactive species in the gas phase can be rather easily controlled by laser radiation. This enables us to identify the chemically active species and follow their reaction paths. The information would be much more difficult to obtain under plasma conditions. Again using

Si-SF_6 as an example, it is known that SF_6 plasma generated by electric discharge can rapidly etch the solid [25]. It was not clear, however, as to the active species involved in the etching reactions because many reactive neutral species and ions could be produced in the glow discharge. From the CO_2 laser excited Si-SF_6 experiments, it is found that both highly vibrationally excited SF_6 and F atoms can be readily chemisorbed on clean Si and react with the fluorinated Si surfaces to form SiF_4. There are experimental evidences to further suggest that the reaction products such as SiF_4 may be formed in excited states [5,26].

2.2 Laser excitation of adsorbed species

While SF_6 molecules do not chemisorb on Si at 25°C, the gas can be physisorbed on the solid at 90K. When the Si surface covered with 1-2 monolayers of SF_6 at low temperature is irradiated by CO_2 laser pulses in resonance with SF_6 ν_3 vibrational mode, we detect a substantial amount of SiF_4 produced from the laser-induced reaction. If the laser is tuned off resonance from SF_6 vibrational bands, no SiF_4 formation is observed. The results clearly show that vibrationally excited SF_6 is also reactive to Si even at 90K. The laser excitation and heating of Si substrate alone (without resonant SF_6 excitation) does not cause the surface reaction to occur. When the sample surface after reaction with SF_6 is examined by XPS, we detect a small shoulder about 2.5 eV higher in binding energy in the Si(2p) and Si(2s) spectra indicating the presence of "SiF_2"-like species, very similar to that observed in Si-XeF_2 reaction, also studied with XPS [22]. It thus appears that the formation of "SiF_2"-like surface species may be an important step in Si reaction with fluorine-containing species, whether the active species is in the form of F atoms [27], XeF_2 [22], or vibrationally excited SF_6 molecules [26].

2.3 Laser excitation of solid substrates

The initial interaction of the laser light with a solid is almost always with its electrons except in the medium and far infrared regions where direct lattice phonon excitation can occur. The photon energy absorbed by the electrons is ultimately shared with atoms of the solid as electronic excitation is transformed into lattice excitation. The exact sequence of photon-electron-phonon interactions depends on the detailed electronic structure of the solid and the intensity of the laser radiation field [28]. The complex coupling between the incident photon and the surface modes is not generally understood for most materials, particularly when the photon intensity is very high as in the focused laser beam. For chemical interactions on light absorbing substrates, direct laser-induced substrate heating effect definitely is an important factor in determining the surface reaction rates. The role played by the electronic excitation of the solid in directly influencing the etching reaction is less clear. In a laser-enhanced Si oxidation reaction studied by Schafer et al. [29], a small nonthermal component was detected. It was suggested that the nonthermal oxidation process might be due to the electrons injected by uv photons from Si into SiO_2 where charged oxygen species could be formed. The nonthermal oxidation effect induced by laser radiation has been found to be much more pronounced on GaAs surfaces [29,30]. In view of the fact that many aspects of surface etching reactions seem to be quite analogous to surface oxidation reactions [12], it is possible that nonthermal effect also exists in certain laser-induced etching reactions [31,32]. The nonthermal component could arise from direct interactions of the excited electronic states or the photon generated electron-hole pairs in the substrate with the adsorbate atoms or molecules.

It is by the direct laser excitation of the solid that most efficient chemical etching has been observed and often achieved with high spatial resolution. The resolution appears to be controlled primarily by the extent of the laser excitation and heating area on the surface. Thermal modeling predicts that the surface temperature at a distance about three times the beam radius would decrease to 1/e of the peak temperature at the center of the laser beam [33,34]. Since a laser beam in the uv and visible regions can be focused to a spot about or less than 1 μm in diameter, a spatial resolution in the order of 1 μm should not be very difficult to obtain. Indeed, a spatial resolution of about 1.5-1.7 μm has been demonstrated in both GaAs [7] and Si [35] etching reactions. Each rates greater than 10 μm/sec have been observed in Si [35,36], MnZn ferrites [37] and polyester systems [38].

2.4 Chemical etching and physical ablation

When an intense photon beam is incident on a solid surface, it can cause phase changes and surface melting in the irradiated region. In some instances, the induced surface tension can cause physical ablation to form holes and trenches as a result of laser heating [39]. The material removed from the hole usually accumulates around the rim of the hole. If the laser intensity is sufficiently high, it can even vaporize the material. Other physical effects of the high-power laser radiation have been quite thoroughly discussed by Ready [40]. It should be noted that physical ablation including melting and evaporation or vaporization usually does not produce sharp and smooth edges on the etched features. This may be caused by the inhomogeneous removal of materials and the redeposition of particles and clusters of various sizes in the ablation processes. Chemical etching, on the other hand, often produces smooth and well-defined edges and wall, particularly when the surface reaction products are readily vaporized. Sometimes, the combined effect of chemical etching and physical ablation can result in very high etch rate and still maintain reasonably good etching structures. This approach can be particularly powerful for materials such as Si [35]. It should also be realized that there are fundamental differences between laser-induced etching and plasma etching. When a laser beam is focused onto a solid surface, the material can be locally excited and heated to a rather high temperature. The chemical reactivity of the gas-solid system and the volatility of reaction products in laser stimulated reaction can be very different from the essentially low temperature reactions in plasma environments. With a few exceptions, plasma etching of metals are usually not very efficient. In many instances, laser-induced etching has been shown to be highly effective in etching metals (further discussed below).

III. EXPERIMENTAL CONSIDERATIONS

3.1 Optical arrangements

There are many possible ways to manipulate the laser beam into desirable experimental configurations. The laser can be readily focused with a lens or a combination of lenses into a spot or a line. It can be expanded and collimated for flood exposure of a sufficiently large area. The light can be spatially scanned with reflective optical elements. The irradiation geometry can be controlled with irises. In some applications, an optical mask with a desirable pattern may be employed. The pattern mask can be placed inside or outside the reaction cell. It should be emphatically pointed out that the laser-induced chemical method is a direct maskless etching technique. The idea of using a pattern mask which can be made of metals such as molybdenum or tungsten should not be confused with the photoresist masks commonly used in plasma and wet etching processes. The pattern mask which may or may not be in physical contact with the solid is utilized only for projecting a desirable light pattern on the sample surface and it can be reused from one process to another. Some of the simple optical arrangements are shown schematically in Figure 1. More sophisticated optical configurations can be adopted when needed. For practical purposes, the light beam incident normal to the surface is most efficient for inducing etching reactions.

3.2 Selection of laser systems

For molecular excitations involving electronic and vibrational transitions, specific lasers at frequencies in resonance with these transitions have to be used. For example, F_2, Cl_2 and Br_2 can be excited and dissociated by photons with wavelengths below 400, 500 and 700 nm, respectively [41]. Thus, uv and visible lasers such as excimer, N_2 and Ar lasers are suitable for studying the interactions of solids with the halogen atoms generated by single-photon photolysis of halogen molecules. CO_2 lasers have been widely used for multiple photon vibrational excitation and dissociation of polyatomic molecules such as SF_6, BCl_3, $CF_3X(X=Cl,Br,I)$, CF_2X_2, N_2F_4, etc. [24]. The active species produced by multiple photon absorption can be used for possible reactions with Si, SiO_2 and other solids. As discussed earlier, pure gas phase excitations are suitable for investigating surface reaction mechanisms. In most cases, however, this mode of excitation alone is ineffective in promoting efficient etching. If high reaction rates and high spatial resolution are the primary objectives, direct laser excitation of the solid should be employed. For this purpose, the laser wavelength requirement is not as restrictive as for molecular excitation because most solids have rather wide range of optical absorption bands with sufficiently large optical extinction coefficients. For instance, Si has a maximum absorption near 265 nm and can be excited by lasers with the wavelength shorter than 1 μm (band gap). SiO_2 does not absorb light from 0.2 to about 2.5 μm, but absorbs CO_2 laser photons strongly at 10 μm and vacuum uv photons below 180 nm. Practically all metals are opaque from uv to ir and can be readily excited by commonly available lasers. For industrial applications, CO_2 laser and Nd:YAG laser (1.06 μm) appear to be very useful. For very high resolution, uv light such as excimer lasers should be used because the spatial resolution is ultimately limited by the wavelength of the light beam.

Apart from the wavelength, the choice of a cw (continuous wave) or a pulsed laser should also be considered. A cw laser has the potential of achieving a high etch rate simply because it has continuous radiation effects. But it also has a potential problem of overheating the substrate. A pulsed laser has the advantage of high peak power but has the shortcoming of a shorter reaction period per pulse. The choice of a laser is likely to depend on the material properties. From our experience, a cw uv-visible laser works very well for chemical etching of Si wafers because the thermal conductivity of the solid is very high and laser heating does not cause serious damage to the material. For applications to thin film materials and materials of delicate thermal and mechanical properties, a pulsed laser is probably more suitable. Both high power CO_2 and Nd:YAG lasers are commercially available for cw and pulsed operations. In many applications, laser beam uniformity is also an important factor to consider. The output of a laser system can have a Gaussian intensity distribution or have a multiple mode pattern. There are transmission and reflection types of optical devices that can transform a Gaussian or an inhomogeneous light beam into a spatially more uniform beam. A uniform beam is particularly important for operations with flood exposure configurations. In short, for a given gas-solid system of interest, all these factors including the laser wavelength, cw and pulsed operations, laser power, pulse energy, pulse duration and pulse rate, mode structure and beam uniformity have to be taken into account in order to select a laser system that is capable of achieving effective results.

3.3 Reaction chamber and gas handling

Laser-induced chemical etching has been demonstrated with or without a reaction cell to confine the etchant gas in a finite volume. For certain etching reactions with oxygen, the experiments can be carried out in air. A gas jet with the etchant gas flowing through a nozzle directed at the sample surface has also been shown to be capable of etching the material by simultaneous laser irradiation of the gas-exposed area [42]. No reaction vessel is needed for such applications. For most of our experiments, the etching reactions are performed with a small stainless steel chamber equipped with a glass or a quartz window for uv-visible-near ir laser induced reactions, or an ir transparent window such as KCl for CO_2 laser excited reactions. Both flowing and stationary gas exposures have been tested depending on the chemical nature of the etchant gas. For stable molecules such as SF_6 and freon, the gas sealed in a closed chamber is adequate for small scale etching reactions. For molecules such as XeF_2, a flow system is usually used [31]. The small reaction cell can also be set on a motorized translation stage and thus allow us to generate desirable two or three dimensional etching patterns.

IV. RESULTS AND DISCUSSION ON SOME SOLID SYSTEMS

A fairly large range of materials have been studied with laser-enhanced dry chemical etching in recent years. This includes the etching of semiconductors such as Si, Ge, InP and GaAs, metals such as Ta, Te, Ni, Fe and W, magnetic and ceramic materials such as MnZn ferrites and TiC-Al_2O_3, and insulators such as SiO_2, all in various kinds of halogen-containing gases. Even some organic polymers can be efficiently etched in oxygen or air by uv or visible lasers. Table 1 summarizes recent studies on laser-induced gas-surface etching reactions. Primary etching characteristics including the laser systems, etch rates and spatial resolutions achieved with the laser technique are listed in the table. Some of the solids that we have studied are further discussed below.

4.1 Si and SiO_2

Silicon clearly can be etched by F, Cl and Br atoms generated by multiple photon dissociation of SF_6 [17], and single-photon dissociation of Cl_2 [36] and Br_2 [43]. It can also react with vibrationally excited SF_6 to form volatile products [6,17]. XeF_2 gas can spontaneously etch the solid [44], but the etch rate can be greatly enhanced by a pulsed CO_2 laser [31] or a cw Ar laser [32]. The most efficient etching has been achieved by focusing a laser beam on the solid in the ambiance of fluorine and chlorine containing species. The observed etch rates are greater than 10 μm/sec [36] or even higher [35]. It is interesting to note that the overall etch rates using fluorine-containing gases are usually faster than those using chlorine-containing chemicals. This is not surprising in view of the fact that F atoms can spontaneously react with Si at 25°C and low gas pressure, in contrast to Cl atoms which can hardly etch the solid under the same condition [2b]. A theoretical calculation performed by Seel and Bagus [45] on the F and Cl chemisorption on Si(111) assuming no surface reconstruction showed that while Cl atoms could readily chemisorb on Si surface, the potential barrier for surface penetration was very high (13 eV). The corresponding penetration barrier for F atoms was only about 1 eV. Diffusion of halogen atoms to positions beneath the surface layer may be an important part of the etching mechanism, since it would facilitate the surrounding of each Si atoms with enough halogen atoms to form the etch product. The different abilities of Cl and F atoms to penetrate the Si surface may be responsible for the differences in etch rates of the two halogen species either with or without the presence of laser radiation.

Etching of SiO_2 has been demonstrated by photodissociation of Cl_2 [15], and multiple photon dissociation of CF_3Br [8] and CDF_3 [46]. Figure 2 shows the result of SiO_2-Cl_2 reaction induced by a focused Ar laser beam [15]. A rather efficient SiO_2 etching was reported by direct CO_2 laser heating of the substrate exposed to a HF gas jet [42]. We have also observed the similar CO_2 laser-induced etching effect using a different type of fluorine-containing gas [47]. It is known that F atoms can readily adsorb on SiO_2 [44,47], but in the absence of external radiation, etching reaction occurs only at a rather high atom flux [13]. Laser excitation and heating clearly reduce the barrier for reaction. The laser technique can also provide high etching selectivity. For a thin SiO_2 layer on Si in Cl_2 gas, the differential laser-induced etch rate was found to be about 1:80 [36]. For a pure Si and a pure SiO_2 substrates in Cl_2 excited by a uv-visible laser, the etch rate ratio can be a factor of 10^3 or greater. In this case, the bulk SiO_2 is not significantly heated by the laser beam, in contrast to the SiO_2 layer on Si where the photon energy absorbed by the underlying Si is converted into substrate heating.

4.2 Metals and magnetic materials

Metals such as Ni-Fe alloy cannot be efficiently etched by plasma reactions presumably because the halide products are involatile at or near 25°C. It is observed that the transition metals can be effectively etched in Cl_2, CCl_4, CF_4 or SF_6 when the solid is irradiated by a

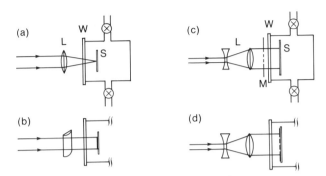

Figure 1. Some simple optical arrangements for laser-induced chemical etching of solids: (a) focused into a spot on the solid surface; (b) focused into a line on the surface; (c) laser beam expanded for flood exposure with a pattern mask outside the reaction cell and (d) with a pattern mask on the solid surface inside the reaction cell; L=lens, W=window and S=sample.

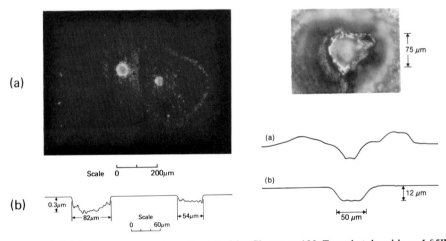

Figure 2 (left). Spots on a quartz wafer etched by Cl_2 gas at 100 Torr photolyzed by a 1.85W Ar laser at 457.9 nm focused with a 12 mm f.l. lens; (a) observed under a 100x microscope and (b) as determined with a diamond stylus. The larger spot is produced in 15 min. and the smaller spot in 5 min.

Figure 3 (right). A spot on Ni(80%)-Fe(20%) alloy etched by CF_4 at 100 Torr induced by a 6.3W Ar laser at 515 nm focused with a 12 mm f.l. lens; (a) determined with a diamond stylus for the sample before cleaning by organic solvents and (b) after cleaning by organic solvents showing that the reaction products initially deposited on the wall and outer edge of the etched hole are removed.

Table 1. Summary of recent studies on laser-enhanced chemical etching of solids by gases

Solid	Gas	Laser	Optical Configuration	Etch Rate or Etch Yield/Pulse	Spot Size or Resolution	References
Ge	Br_2	Ar (cw)	focused //	$\sim 10^{-3} \mu m/sec$	(NA)	(52)
GaAs InP	CH_3Br CH_3Cl CF_3I	Ar (cw)	focused $\perp$	$10^{-3} \mu m/sec$	$1.5 \mu m$	(7)
Si	Br_2	Ar (cw)	unfocused //	$\leq 10^{-4} \mu m/sec$	(NA)	(43)
Si	Cl_2 HCl	Ar (cw)	focused $\perp$	$0.02 \sim 10 \mu m/sec$	$5 \mu m$	(36)
Si	SF_6	CO_2 (pulsed)	unfocused $\perp$	$1.2 \text{Å}/pulse$	(NA)	(17)
Si	SF_6	CO_2 (pulsed)	focused //	$0.05 \text{Å}/pulse$	(NA)	(17)
Si	XeF_2	CO_2 (pulsed)	unfocused $\perp$	$0.6 \text{Å}/pulse$	(NA)	(31)
Si	XeF_2	Ar (cw)	unfocused $\perp$	$6 \times 10^{-4} \mu m/sec$	(NA)	(32)
SiO_2	HF	CO_2 (cw)	focused $\perp$	$0.05 \mu m/sec$	$\sim 100 \mu m$	(42)
SiO_2	CF_3Br CDF_3	CO_2 (pulsed)	focused //	$0.3 \text{Å}/pulse$	$\sim 200 \mu m$	(8)(46)
SiO_2	Cl_2	Ar (cw)	focused $\perp$	$3 \times 10^{-4} \mu m/sec$	$50 \sim 80 \mu m$	(15)
Ta	SF_6	CO_2 (pulsed)	unfocused $\perp$	$2.6 \text{Å}/pulse$	(NA)	(18)
Ta	XeF_2	CO_2 (pulsed)	unfocused $\perp$	$0.4 \text{Å}/pulse$	(NA)	(18)
Te	XeF_2	CO_2 (pulsed)	unfocused $\perp$	$10 \text{Å}/pulse$	(NA)	(15)
MnZn Ferrites	CCl_4 CF_4, SF_6 CF_3Cl	Ar (cw)	focused $\perp$	$10 \mu m/sec$	$5 \sim 100 \mu m$	(37)
Ni(80%) Fe(20%)	SF_6, CF_4 CCl_4, Cl_2	Ar (cw)	focused $\perp$	$0.1 \mu m/sec$	$80 \mu m$	(*)
TiC- Al_2O_3	CCl_4 SF_6	Ar (cw) Nd:YAG (pulsed)	focused $\perp$ focused $\perp$	$0.1 \mu m/sec$ $5 \times 10^{-3} \mu m/pulse$	10-$100 \mu m$ 10-$100 \mu m$	(*) (*)
W	I_2	(NA)	focused $\perp$	(NA)	(NA)	(53)
Polyester (Mylar)	O_2 air	Ar (cw)	focused $\perp$	$50 \mu m/sec$	$10 \sim 70 \mu m$	(*)
Polyester (Mylar)	air	ArF (pulsed)	unfocused $\perp$	$0.12 \mu m/pulse$	$< 1 \mu m$	(50)

Notes: (1) // and $\perp$, the laser beam incident either parallel (//) or perpendicular ($\perp$) to the solid surfaces. (2) NA, data either not available or unspecified. (*) Present work.

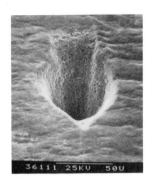 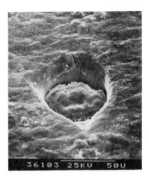

Figure 4. SEM micrographs showing the etched features on Ni(80%)-Fe(20%) alloy etched by (a) Cl_2 at 100 Torr and focused Ar laser at 6.3W-60 sec and (b) CCl_4 at 100 Torr and focused Ar laser 6.3W-120 sec.

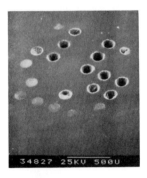 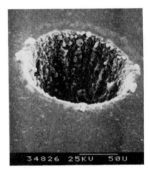

Figure 5. SEM micrograph of a pattern of holes on TiC-Al_2O_3 etched by CCl_4 at 2.5 Torr induced by a pulsed Nd:YAG laser. A molybdenum pattern mask with 100 μm holes is set on the solid in a reaction cell according to Figure 1d.

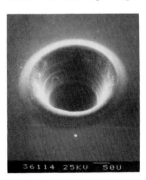 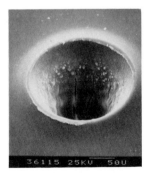

Figure 6. SEM micrographs of via holes on polyester films of 0.38 mm thickness produced by photoetching in air with a focused Ar laser at 515 nm; (left side): Ar laser 4W-60 sec and (right side): Ar laser 5W-15 sec.

focused Ar laser. Figure 3 shows the hole chemically etched with CF_4 gas. It is further observed that the metal fluorides produced from the etching reaction tend to deposit on the wall and on the outer edge of the etched hole (Figure 3a). After cleaning in a ultrasonic bath with simple organic solvents such as acetone, ether and alcohol, practically all the debris is removed (Figure 3b). Figure 4 shows the scanning electron micrographs (SEM) of the holes produced in Cl_2 and CCl_4 gases. Among the four gases that we have tested, Cl_2 gas can produce the highest etch rate. It also appears that chlorine-containing gases generate less debris accumulated around the etched features than the fluorine-containing gases, maybe because the chloride products are more volatile than fluoride compounds. Likewise, solid materials such as MnZn ferrites and $TiC-Al_2O_3$ can be etched only slowly by plasma technique. Using CCl_4 and CF_4 gases, we are able to etch the ferrites at a rate approaching 10 μm/sec or greater [37]. For $TiC-Al_2O_3$, the corresponding etch rates are substantially lower. Figure 5 shows the hole pattern generated by irradiation of the sample with a pulsed Nd:YAG laser through a molybdenum pattern mask set on the solid surface in CCl_4 ambiance, according to the optical arrangement shown in Figure 1d. The optical mask has a pattern of 100 μm diameter holes which are reproduced as an etching pattern on the solid. The depths of the etched holes vary from less than 0.1 μm to greater than 10 μm because of the inhomogeneous intensity distribution of the laser beam which has a multimode structure. It is expected when a more uniform beam is used, the variation in etching depth would be reduced.

In general, the radiation-enhanced metal etching behavior is not easily predictable because the chemical reactivity of a given gas to the metal and the volatility of reaction products are largely unknown. The reaction mechanisms under the highly nonequilibratory etching conditions are not well understood and remain to be further elucidated.

4.3 Organic polymers

Polymers such as polymethyl methacrylate (PMMA) have been widely used as photoresists in photolithography, an essential technique for microfabrications. Photoetching of PMMA with a KrF excimer laser was demonstrated by Kawamura et al. [48]. Recently we [38] and others [49,50] have observed that a complete dry-etching process on a similar polymer, i.e., polyethylene terephthalate (PET), can be accomplished by irradiating the polyester film (Mylar by Du Pont) in air or O_2 environment with an Ar laser or an ArF excimer laser. Some of our results are shown in Figure 6. As can be seen from the SEM micrograph, rather smooth via holes can be easily produced by focusing a cw Ar laser into the polyester film (0.38 nm thickness). If the laser intensity is too high, the etched structure becomes much rougher and small cracks can develop along the wall of the etched features (also shown in Figure 6). Srinivason et al. [49,50] have used a far-uv laser which can be much more effectively absorbed by the material and presumably can induce more efficient etching than the visible laser. An etch rate of about 0.12 μm per pulse by a pulsed ArF laser is reported with the spatial resolution in the submicron region [50]. In contrast, etch rates in 10-50 μm/sec range are readily obtainable with a cw Ar laser. The spot sizes are usually greater than 10 μm. The photoetching is probably caused by the combination effects of photolysis, oxidation reaction and physical ablation. Details of the reaction mechanisms are being further studied by Srinivason et al. [51].

V. SUMMARY

In this paper, major aspects of the laser-enhanced chemical etching have been outlined. It is shown that the laser technique not only can be applied to study basic processes involved in chemical etching of solids, but also can be utilized as an efficient tool for processing electronic materials. In the basic area, the fundamental processes that are believed to play important roles in the radiation-enhanced gas-solid interactions are discussed. Attempts are also made to relate the resulting concepts to the experimentally observed phenomena. SF_6 interactions with several solids have been used extensively as examples to illustrate the concepts which have evolved from these studies. The gas which may not be unique in causing chemical etching does possess some exceptionally good characteristics that allow us to examine the many facets of the laser induced surface processes. In the more applied area, experimental results on some materials of importance to microelectronics are presented. Considerations are given to the selection of laser systems and certain possible optical configurations are suggested. Comparisons with the plasma technique whenever pertinent are also made. From practical point of view, the laser chemical approach is still slow in most cases particularly in terms of total throughput. Nevertheless, the method has many advantages such as the ease of manipulating the laser beams and the relatively noncorrosive gases that can often be used for chemical etching. The technique can be particularly useful for three-dimensional material processing and personalized applications. It is quite conceivable that fabrications of certain materials on a wafer by wafer basis can be accomplished with commonly available laser systems in the near future.

ACKNOWLEDGMENTS

The author wish to thank J. Goitia for this assistance with the experiments, and F. A. Houle and L. Chen for their contributions to some of the work presented here. The author is also grateful to P. S. Bagus, H. F. Winters, J. W. Coburn, F. A. Houle, E. Kay, L. Chen and G. S. Mathad for many helpful discussions throughout this work.

REFERENCES

1. L. Holland, *J. Vac. Sci. Technol.* **14**, 5 (1977).
2. (a) J. W. Coburn and H. F. Winters, *J. Vac. Sci. Technol.* **16**, 391 (1979); (b) *ibid.*, *J. Appl. Phys.* **50**, 3189 (1979); (c) U. Gerlach-Meyer, J. W. Coburn and E. Kay, *Surf. Sci.* **103**, 177 (1981).
3. Y. Y. Tu, T. J. Chuang and H. F. Winters, *Phys. Rev.* **B23**, 823 (1981).
4. D. J. Ehrlich, R. M. Osgood, Jr. and T. F. Deutsch, *IEEE J. Quantum Electron.* **QE-16**, 1233 (1980).
5. T. J. Chuang, *J. Vac. Sci. Technol.* **21**, 798 (1982).
6. T. J. Chuang, *J. Chem. Phys.* **72**, 6303 (1980).
7. D. J. Ehrlich, R. M. Osgood, Jr. and T. F. Deutsch, *Appl. Phys. Lett.* **36**, 698 (1980).
8. J. I. Steinfeld, T. G. Anderson, C. Reiser, D. R. Denison, L. D. Hartsough and J. R. Hollahan, *J. Electrochem. Soc.* **127**, 514 (1980).
9. R. J. von Gutfeld, E. E. Tynam, R. L. Melcher and S. E. Blum, *Appl. Phys. Lett.* **35**, 651 (1979).
10. R. J. von Gutfeld and J.-Cl. Puippe, *Oberflache-Surface* **22**, 294 (1981).
11. R. M. Osgood, Jr., A. Sanchez-Rubio, D. J. Ehrlich and V. Daneu, *Appl. Phys. Lett.* **40**, 391 (1982).
12. H. F. Winters, J. W. Coburn and T. J. Chuang, *J. Vac. Sci. Technol.* (in press).
13. D. L. Flamm, V. M. Donnelly and J. A. Mucha, *J. Appl. Phys.* **52**, 3633 (1981).
14. J. A. Mucha, V. M. Donnelly, D. L. Flamm and L. M. Webb, *J. Phys. Chem.* **85**, 3529 (1981).
15. T. J. Chuang, *IBM J. Res. Develop.* **26**, 145 (1982).
16. C. J. Mogab and H. J. Levinstein, *J. Vac. Sci. Technol.* **17**, 721 (1980).
17. T. J. Chuang, *J. Chem. Phys.* **74**, 1453 (1981).
18. T. J. Chuang, *J. Vac. Sci. Technol.* **18**, 638 (1981).
19. T. L. Cottrell, *The Strengths of Chemical Bonds* (Butterworths, London, 1958), 2nd edition, p. 252.
20. P. Rai-Choudbury, *J. Electrochem. Soc.* **118**, 266 (1971).
21. L. J. Stinson, J. A. Howard and R. C. Neville, *J. Electrochem. Soc.* **123**, 551 (1976).

22. T. J. Chuang, *J. Appl. Phys.* **51**, 2614 (1980).
23. R. V. Ambartsumyan and V. S. Letokhov, in *Chemical and Biochemical Applications of Lasers*, ed. C. B. Moore (Academic, New York, 1977), Vol. 3, p. 167.
24. N. Bloembergen and E. Yablonovitch, *Physics Today* **31**(5), 23 (1978); P. A. Schulz, Aa. S. Sudbo, D. J. Krajnovich, H. S. Kwok, Y. R. Shen and Y. T. Lee, *Ann. Rev. Phys. Chem.* **30**, 379 (1979).
25. J. J. Wagner and W. W. Brandt, in *Proceedings of the 4th International Symposium on Plasma Chemistry*, ed. by S. Veprek and J. Hertz (University of Zurich, Switzerland, 1979), Vol. 1, p. 120.
26. T. J. Chuang, in *Proceedings of the 3rd International Conference on Vibrations at Surfaces* (Asilomar, California, September 1-4, 1982), ed. by C. R. Brundle (Elsevier, Amsterdam); also to be published in *J. Electr. Spectr. Relat. Phenom.*
27. V. M. Donnelly and D. L. Flamm, *J. Appl. Phys.* **51**, 5273 (1980).
28. M. von Allmen, in *Laser and Electron Beam Processing of Materials*, ed. by C. W. White and P. S. Pearcy (Academic, New York, 1980), p. 6; also, W. L. Brown, in the same book, p. 20.
29. S. A. Schafer and S. A. Lyon, *J. Vac. Sci. Technol.* **21**, 422 (1982); *ibid.*, **19**, 494 (1981).
30. W. G. Petro, I. Hino, S. Eglash, I. Lindau, C. Y. Su and W. E. Spicer, *J. Vac. Sci. Technol.* **21**, 405 (1982).
31. T. J. Chuang, *J. Chem. Phys.* **74**, 1461 (1981).
32. F. A. Houle, to be published.
33. M. Lax, *J. Appl. Phys.* **48**, 3919 (1977).
34. J. Mazumder and W. M. Steen, *J. Appl. Phys.* **51**, 941 (1980).
35. F. A. Houle and T. J. Chuang, to be published.
36. D. J. Ehrlich, R. M. Osgood, Jr. and T. F. Deutsch, *Appl. Phys. Lett.* **38**, 1018 (1981).
37. F. A. Houle and T. J. Chuang, to be published.
38. T. J. Chuang, cited in Ref. 5.
39. M. Chen and V. Marrello, *J. Vac. Sci. Technol.* **18**, 75 (1981).
40. J. F. Ready, *Effects of High-Power Laser Radiation* (Academic, New York, 1971).
41. G. Herzberg, *Spectra of Diatomic Molecules* (D. Van Nostrand, Princeton, New Jersey, 1950), 2nd edition.
42. K. Daree and W. Kaiser, *Glass Technol.* **18**, 19 (1977).
43. L. L. Sveshnikova, V. I. Donin and S. M. Repinskii, *Sov. Tech. Phys. Lett.* **3**, 223 (1977).
44. H. F. Winters and J. W. Coburn, *Appl. Phys. Lett.* **34**, 70 (1979).
45. M. Seel and P. S. Bagus, cited by P. S. Bagus, B. Liu, A. D. McLean and M. Yoshimine, in *Computational Methods in Chemistry*, ed. by J. Bargon (Plenum, New York, 1980), p. 229.
46. D. Harradine, F. R. McFeely, B. Roop, J. I. Steinfeld, L. Denison, L. Hartsough and J. R. Hollahan, SPIE, Vol. 270 *High Power Lasers and Applications* (1981), p. 52.
47. T. J. Chuang, to be published.
48. Y. Kawamura, K. Toyoda and S. Namba, *Appl. Phys. Lett.* **40**, 374 (1982).
49. R. Srinivason, *Polymers* (to be published).
50. R. Srinivason and V. Mayne-Banton, *Appl. Phys. Lett.* (to be published).
51. R. Srinivason, private communication.
52. I. M. Beterov, V. P. Chebotaev, N. I. Yurshina and B. Ya. Yurshin, *Sov. J. Quantum Electron.* **8**, 1310 (1978).
53. R. Solomon and L. F. Mueller, Jr., U.S. Patent 3,364,087 (1968).

HIGH RESOLUTION ETCHING OF GaAs AND CdS CRYSTALS*

D. V. PODLESNIK, H.H. GILGEN, R.M. OSGOOD
Department of Electrical Engineering, Columbia University, New York, NY 10027
A. SANCHEZ, V. DANEU
MIT Lincoln Laboratory, Lexington, MA 02173

ABSTRACT

Submicrometer gratings have been etched in GaAs and CdS crystals which have been immersed in an oxidizing etch and illuminated with interferring laser beams. A resolution of 170 nm was obtained. At high laser intensity and with prolonged etching time the surface properties of the material are degraded. The use of _in-situ_ optical measurements of grating parameters allows ready optimization of the grating fabrication process.

INTRODUCTION

Recent interest in guided wave optics [1] and distributed feedback lasers [2] has prompted the need for producing gratings with periods on the order of 100 nm on semiconductor materials. Other applications include surface acoustic wave devices [3] and negative-resistance electron devices [4]. Currently, there are two conventional methods for grating fabrication: holographic lithography [5] and electron-beam lithography [6]. With the former method, gratings with spacing as small as 110 nm have been produced; however, this technique is cumbersome, and grating periods are generally restricted to be greater than 180 nm. With electron-beam technique, gratings with the period less than 100 nm can be produced. But, this method is limited by the difficulties of producing uniform large-area structures and the long exposure times, which, for a 300 nm grating, can be as long as one hour per square millimeter [6]. Both methods involve multiple steps. In addition, for both methods, photoresist residues cause contamination problems, limiting their use in electro-optical applications.

In the present paper we describe a technique for producing submicrometer gratings by a holographic method with direct chemical etching in an oxidizing etch [7]. The resolution of this technique is comparable to those of other methods. Futhermore, this method is a single one-step process using very low laser intensity. Both uniform large-area gratings and special grating profiles (e.g. blazed) can be easily fabricated.

The anodic dissolution of a semiconductor in an oxidizing etch is generally influenced by the number of carriers present at the surface. Since light incident on the semiconductor surface produces electron-hole pairs, a pattern of light produces a corresponding pattern of available carriers. The photogenerated carriers, typically holes for n-type GaAs, control the etching rate of a semiconductor producing an engraved pattern in its surface. The resolution of the etching process may be shown to be a direct consequence of rapid surface recombination velocity, due to the etching reaction, and the surface-normal electric field, due to the semiconductor band bending at the interface. Our results show that 170 nm gratings are easily obtained and we anticipate that with an appropriate optical arrangement, a resolution below 100 nm is possible.

EXPERIMENT

The actual experimental arrangement used for the holographic exposure is shown in Fig. 1. A laser beam from an argon-ion laser emitting at 514.5, 488.0, or 457.9 nm passes through a spatial filter. The filtered beam is incident on a right angle corner on which are mounted a mirror and a semiconductor sample. The corner is inside an optical cell containing an etching solution. The interference pattern is produced by the superposition of the direct and the reflected beams inside the solution. The grating period, s, is given by

$$s = \frac{\lambda}{2 n \sin\theta_i} \qquad (1)$$

where λ is the free-space wavelength of incident light, n is the index of refraction of the solution and θ_i is the incident angle on the sample surface. The incident light is s-polarized. After passing through the spatial filter, the laser beam goes through the window of the optical cell, and it is, therefore, desirable to match as much as possible the indices of refraction of the solution and the window in order to reduce spurious interference patterns.

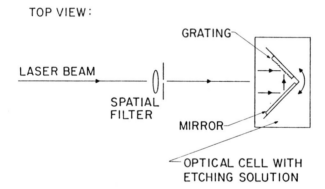

Fig. 1 Experimental arrangement for grating fabrication by direct chemical etching

The experiment was done on GaAs and CdS crystals. A comparison was made of etching gratings on $n(10^{18}$ cm$^{-7})$ and SI GaAs of (100) and (111) orientations. On all samples, good quality and small-period gratings were produced. Figure 2 shows a SEM photograph of 200-nm grating on n-type GaAs. Using 457.9 nm line we have recently obtained gratings with a 170-nm period. Successful gratings on CdS (undoped) were produced only on prismatic faces, parallel to the optical axes, as shown on Fig. 3. We failed to produce good quality gratings on A and B CdS faces.

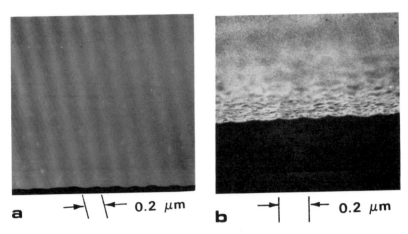

Fig. 2 The SEM photographs of a 200-nm grating on n-type GaAs. Fig. (a) shows the top view of the (100) surface and Fig. (b) shows the profile of the grating.

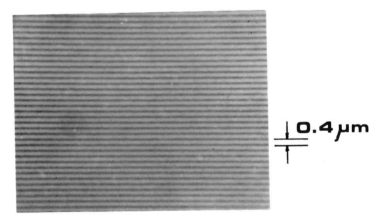

Fig. 3 The photograph of the grating formed on a prismatic face of CdS (undoped). The periodicity is about 400 nm.

Although several different etching solutions (e.g. NH_4OH, H_2O_2, and H_2O, or KCl, HCl, and H_2O) were used, most of the work was done with the following solution: H_2SO_4, H_2O_2 and H_2O [8]. Since we were primarily concerned with grating periods less than 400 nm, it was necessary to choose an etch composition with a sufficiently slow dark etching rate, so that the products of the etching reaction would not interfere with the development of the grating. Based on an initial measurement of the dark and light-enhanced etching rates for different compositions, we selected the following composition for our experiments: $H_2SO_4 : H_2O_2 : H_2O = 1:1:50$.

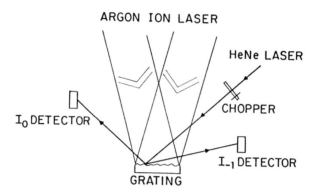

Fig. 4 Experimental arrangement for the <u>in-situ</u> measurement.

OPTICAL MEASUREMENT OF GRATING PARAMETERS

The in-situ measurement enabled us to observe the quality of the etched surface and determine grating parameters during the etching process. This provides a convenient means of studying the fabrication process and it has allowed the optimization of the process parameters. The in-situ measurement arrangement is represented in Fig. 4. The probe was a HeNe laser, operating at 633 nm. In order to minimize etching with the output from the HeNe laser, the beam was attenuated and chopped with a small duty cycle. The intensities of diffracted beams were measured with a power meter. For small period gratings, measured here, $\sim$ 400 nm, the relatively long wavelength of the probe-beam allowed only diffraction of the zero and the minus first order.

To determine the important parameters of the grating, the spacing, s, and the groove depth, d, we measured the angular position θ_{-1} and the relative intensity of the minus first diffraction order, I_{-1}/I_{00}, when the sample is irradiated with s-polarized light at the angle of incidence θ_i. The diffraction angle θ_{-1} is related to θ_i by

$$\sin \theta_{-1} = \frac{\lambda_p}{n \, s} - \sin \theta_i \tag{2}$$

where λ_p is the free-space wavelength of the probe beam. If I_{00} is the intensity of the beam reflected from the polished crystal surface (taken as 100%), the theoretical value [9] of the intensity of the minus first order as a function of the grating depth, d, is given by

$$\frac{I_{-1}}{I_{00}} = J_1^2 \left(\frac{2 \pi n \, d}{\lambda_p} (1 + \cos \theta_{-1}) \right) \tag{3}$$

where J_1 is the Bessel function of the first kind, order one. Here we assumed that the grating surface is purely sinusoidally corrugated. As one can see (Fig. 2), our gratings showed the deviation from the sinusoidal curvature, but we can use Eq. 3 as an approximation to estimate the grating depth. An exact calculation requires the Fourier expansion of the surface corrugation.

Figure 5 shows the dependence of the relative specular reflection intensity I_0/I_{00} on the exposure time (etching time). During the measurement we used only a single non-interfering argon-ion laser beam. As a result we obtained information about the scale of roughness that occurs when the sample is immersed in the solution. One can observe the surface degradation under different light intensities with prolonged etching time. The results indicate that the growth rate of the statistical surface roughness depends on the laser intensity.

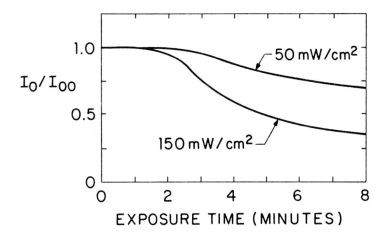

Fig. 5   The normalized intensity, I_0/I_{00}, of the reflected HeNe beam from the GaAs surface during the etching process as a function of the exposure time. Results for two different laser intensities are shown.

The relative intensity of the minus first diffraction order, I_{-1}/I_{00}, has been measured as a function of the exposure time. The results for two different incident laser powers are given in Fig. 6. We found that at the beginning of the grating growth the exposure time is proportional to the grating depth, assuming a constant etching rate. Thus, at the beginning, the growth of a good quality grating is observed, since the relative intensity I_{-1}/I_{00} follows the appropriate Bessel function. The later decrease of I_{-1}/I_{00} is related to the statistical roughness of the etched surface (see Fig. 5) and to a change of the etching rate. The proportionality of the exposure time and the grating depth is not valid in this region. In our example we found that the exposure time of 90 seconds was optimal, giving the grating depth of about 160 nm.

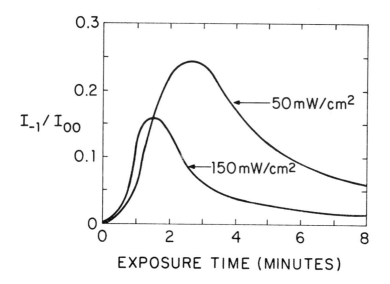

Fig. 6 Relative intensities of the minus first diffraction order vs the exposure time. The diffraction is from the n-type GaAs surface during the fabrication of a 400-nm grating.

From the Fig. 6, we can also observe the effect of laser-light intensity. At a higher intensity the etching rate is higher, but the surface degradation is faster and stronger. For the intensities above 1 W/cm^2 we even observed total distruction of gratings. For our experimental conditions the optimal laser intensities were between 10 and 50 mW/cm^2.

CONCLUSION

We have demonstrated a technique for producing a high-resolution periodic structure on compound semiconductors. Gratings with the spacing of 170 nm were produced. The method is distinguished by simplicity and efficiency. Optical measurements of grating parameters during the etching make the process optimization possible.

ACKNOWLEDGEMENTS

We would like to thank Professors G.W. Flynn and S.P. Schlesinger for their encouragement and support. In addition, we benefited from discussions with Dr. A. Szöke and Professor E.S. Yang.

*This work was supported by the Defense Advanced Research Projects Agency and the Air Force Office of Scientific Research.

REFERENCES

1. P.K. Tien, Rev. Mod Phys., <u>49</u>, 361 (1977).

2. A. Yariv and H. Nakamura, IEEE J. Quantum Electron, <u>QE-13</u>, 233 (1977).

3. R.C. Williams, H. I. Smith, Elect. Lett. <u>8</u>, 401 (1972).

4. H. Sakaki, K. Wagatsuma, J. Hamasaki, and S. Saito, Thin Solid Films, <u>36</u>, 497 (1976).

5. C.V. Shank and R.V. Schmidt, Appl. Phys. Lett. <u>23</u>, 154 (1973).

6. H.I. Smith, Proc. of the IEEE, 1361 (October 1974).

7. R.M. Osgood, A. Sanchez-Rubio, D.J. Ehrlich, and V. Daneu, Appl. Phys. Lett. <u>40</u>, 391 (1982).

8. S. Ida and K. Ito, J. Electrochem. Soc. <u>118</u>, 768 (1971).

9. I. Poekrand and H. Raether, Opt. Commun. <u>18</u>, 395 (1976).

LIGHT INDUCED ETCHING OF GaAs IN A ZINC ATMOSPHERE

R.P. SALATHE AND G. BASKHARA RAO[*]
Institute of Applied Physics, University of Berne, Sidlerstr.5,
3012 Berne, Switzerland

ABSTRACT

N-type GaAs substrates have been exposed to zinc atmospheres at 600 - 800 deg.C and focused light from a Kr-ion laser at 647.1 nm. Etch pits are generated at optical densities of 0.2 - 10 KW/cm^2 and exposure times of 5 - 60 minutes. They are characterized by a smooth profile with typical diameters of 50 - 80 μm and depths of 0.1 - 50 μm. The etch depth depends strongly on the laser power and on the zinc and arsenic vapor concentrations. The onset of etching is characterized by an increase in surface reflectivity of up to 10 per cent which is probably due to the formation of a thin liquid metal film. The growth of this film is initiated by optically generated holes at the semiconductor surface. The film is not saturated and dissolves GaAs from the substrate. In addition to etching, thermal diffusion of zinc can be observed in samples subjected to long exposure times or high temperatures.

INTRODUCTION

In III-V compound semiconductors zinc is frequently used as acceptor type impurity. Its interstitial-substitutional diffusion mechanism has been the subject of many investigations [1-3]. Diffusion experiments carried out with GaAs in a pure zinc atmosphere often result in a damaged substrate surface, particularly for diffusion temperatures above 700 deg.C [3,4]. In the experiments reported here, we demonstrate, that visible light accelerates considerably the attack of the surface under typical zinc diffusion conditions. The light enhanced etching is observed at temperatures of ∼ 600 deg.C and at light intensities as low as 200 W/cm^2. It can be explained by the formation of a liquid metal film, which does not attain thermodynamical equilibrium with the substrate.

EXPERIMENTAL ARRANGEMENT

The experimental arrangement is shown schematically in Fig.1. A Kr-ion laser operated at 647.1 nm has been used in the experiments. The laser light is focused through a slit in a furnace onto a GaAs substrate which is located

---

[*] permanent address: Laser Laboratory, Department of Mechanical Engineering, Indian Institute of Science, Bangalore-560012, India

within an evacuated quartz ampoule. A lens L with 100 mm focal length has been used for focusing. The intensity profile in the laser focus has a FWHM of 24 μm at room temperature. This value is increased if the furnace is heated because of Schlieren effects and turbulences in the light path: At 625 deg.C intensity profiles with halfwidths of 35 μm have been measured on the substrate surface. A beamsplitter has been inserted sometimes into the parallel laser beam in order to measure the laser light reflected from the surface with a Si-photodiode. This allowed to monitor the reflection changes of the surface during irradiation.

Tellurium doped substrates ($4 \cdot 10^{17}$cm^{-3}) with chemically polished surfaces of optical quality have been used in most cases. They have been deoxidized in 1-n KOH immediately before inserting them into the quartz ampoules. The ampoules had a volume of about 20 cm^3. They have been cleaned by a short etch in diluted HF followed by rinsing in deionized water and methyl alcohol. Then source material consisting of 50 mg elemental Zn (6-9er) and the GaAs substrate have been inserted. In some cases GaAs powder (~70 mg) was added or ZnAs$_2$ has been used as source material in order to increase the As pressure within the ampoule.

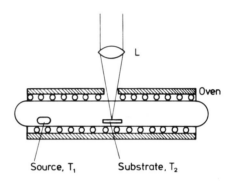

Fig.1: Experimental Arrangement

After loading the ampoules have been heated to 400 deg.C under vacuum for a few minutes and then sealed at typical pressures of $5 \cdot 10^{-7}$ Torr. A two zone furnace was used in order of beeing able to maintain the source and substrate at different temperatures. The furnace had a low thermal mass which allowed to reach processing temperatures of 600-800 deg.C within 3-4 minutes.

RESULTS

Fig.2 shows Nomarski photographs of the surface (2a) and cross-section (2b) of a GaAs substrate which had been exposed for 45 min. to a Zn-atmosphere and focused laser radiation. Source (elemental zinc) and substrate were held at temperatures of 600 deg.C and 625 deg.C, respectively, yielding a zinc concentration of approximately $4 \cdot 10^{17}$cm^{-3} at the substrate surface. The laser power impinging on the substrate was 32 mW. The sample has been cleaned in diluted HCl (1 HCl:5 H$_2$O) after the experiment and then cleaved along a (110)-plane perpendicular to the surface crossing the center of the irradiated zone. The corresponding micrograph of the cleavage plane is shown in Fig.2b. The zone damaged by light enhanced etching is clearly visible in Figs.2a,b. It has a diameter of 50 μm FWHM and a depth of about 30 μm. In comparison to the halfwidth of the optical beam profile the diameter is increased by 40 per cent. The increase can be explained by an etching process which is nonuniform in time, as will be discussed below. In such a case the averaged FWHM measured for the optical profile does not fully account for the beam pointing instability at 625 deg.C. The shape of the etched hole is slightly asymmetric and reflects a corresponding asymmetry of the optical beam.

No etching is observed under the same conditions if the arsenic pressure in the ampoule is increased by adding GaAs powder to the zinc source or if $ZnAs_2$ is used as source material. This indicates that the As vapor pressure within the irradiated zone is an important parameter for this etching process. However, at higher temperatures and considerably higher laser powers etching can also be observed with $ZnAs_2$. Fig. 3 shows the cross-section of a sample which had been subjected to a temperature of 845 deg.C and a laser power of 120 mW for 15 minutes, using 70 mg of $ZnAs_2$ as source material. The diameter of the etched zone is again 100 µm, the depth ~ 4 µm. Here, the etching can be due to a local increase in temperature induced by absorbed radiation. With an absorbed laser power of 80 mW, a laser spot diameter of 35 µm and a thermal conductivity of 0.122 deg.C·cm/Watt for GaAs at 850 deg.C [5], we estimate a temperature rise ΔT on the order of 100 deg.C. This local increase in temperature can lead to considerable changes in the thermodynamical equilibrium. It should be noted here, that no etching could be observed under the same conditions for incident laser powers below 70 mW ($\Delta T < 60$ deg.C).

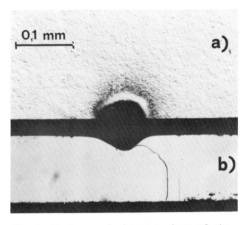

Fig.2: Surface and cleavage plane of the GaAs substrate after irradiation.

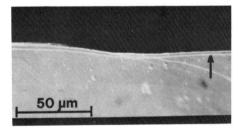

Fig.3: Cleaved and etched plane of GaAs substrate processed at 850 deg.C. Arrow indicates the p-n junction.

A solution of $H_2O:H_2O_2:HF$ (10:1:1) has been used to delineate the p-n junction in the cleavage plane. As shown in Fig.3, the zinc diffusion front is located 2.7 µm underneath the surface. From this value a thermal diffusion coefficient of $2 \cdot 10^{-11}$ cm^2/s is evaluated . This is in agreement to data reported by Rupprecht and LeMay [6] if a surface concentration of $2 \cdot 10^{19}$cm^{-3} of the Zn atoms is assumed. The diffusion depth in the etched zone is slightly reduced (2.2 µm). The presence of diffusion underneath the etched zone indicates that the etching is probably nonuniform in time. Though not shown in Fig.2, a shallow diffusion (~0.5 µm) has also taken place in the irradiated zone of the 625 deg.C experiment with elemental zinc as source material. This combination of laser induced etching and thermal diffusion demonstrates a new technological possibility, i.e. the laser induced displacement of p-n junctions. No attempts have been made so far to optimize this process with respect to resolution or to apply it to device fabrication.

The laser light reflected from the substrate and the substrate temperature have been measured as a function of exposure time. Fig.4 shows the corresponding result for the first 25 minutes of an irradiation experiment. Elemental zinc was used as source material here. The laser power impinging on the n-type GaAs substrate was 8 mW. At the beginning the reflectivity increases slowly with increasing temperature. This increase is attributed to an increase in refractive index due to the decreasing band gap energy. The onset of irreversible surface changes is characterized by a rapid increase in reflectivity at a time t = 4 min. followed by a pronounced decrease between t = 4 and 10 minutes. These characteristic changes cannot be observed if zinc is not present in the ampoule. We therefore attribute the increase at T ~ 420 deg.C to the formation of a liquid metal film consisting of zinc and/or gallium on the GaAs surface. The thickness of the film can be roughly evaluated from the measured peak reflectivity of 45 per cent [7]. With the optical constants for zinc, gallium [8] and GaAs [9,10] at 647 nm we estimate a film thickness on the order of 5 nm. The film is not in thermodynamical equilibrium with the substrate [11]. This leads to dissolution of GaAs. The changes in film composition and surface geometry result in the pronounced decrease of reflecti-

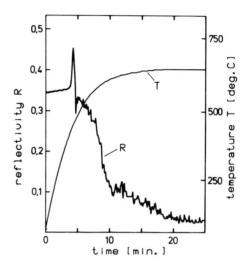

Fig.4: Substrate reflectivity R and temperature T vs. processing time.

vity observed between t = 4 and 10 minutes. Substrates which had been irradiated under such conditions for a total time of 45 minutes exhibited 2.7 μm deep etch pits. In order to check the uniformity of etch rate with time we interrupted the processing for one substrate by immersing the ampoule into water shortly after the rapid decrease in reflectivity at t = 4 minutes. The depth of the etch pits was 2 μm in this case. This indicates that most of the etching occurs at the beginning if the growing metal film is not in equilibrium with the substrate. Etch rates of > 1 μm/min. are measured here. The metal film cannot reach complete thermodynamical equilibrium because of arsenic evaporating from the film surface. Thus etching continues at a considerably reduced rate which is controlled by the As evaporation rate.

The influence of the zinc vapor pressure on the etch depth has been investigated at a constant substrate temperature of 625 deg.C by varying the source temperature from 580 to 620 deg.C. Elemental Zn and n-type GaAs have been used as source and substrate materials, respectively. The substrates have been irradiated with 8 mW for 45 minutes. Fig.5 shows the maximum etch depth measured as a function of zinc concentration N_{Zn} over the substrate. The zinc concentration has been evaluated from the measured temperatures with the vapor pressure data reported by Barrow et al.[12]. The measurement shows that the etch depth is increasing with the third power of the zinc vapor concentration.

This strong increase indicates that the etching is not caused by zinc dissolved in GaAs, since according to Casey and Panish [13], the zinc concentration in GaAs should increase only with $\sqrt{N_{Zn}}$. From the ternary phase diagram of Ga-As-Zn [11] we would expect the occurence of Zn_3As_2, if a liquid zinc film is formed at 625 deg.C on GaAs. We therefore speculate that the etching could be controlled by reactions between zinc, gallium and Zn_3As_2 according to:

$$3\ Zn + 2\ GaAs + 2\ h\nu \rightleftharpoons Zn_3As_2 + 2\ Ga \qquad (1)$$

The observed increase in reflectivity could originate from Zinc adsorbed on the GaAs surface (in the liquid state under processing conditions) or from liquid gallium which is formed together with Zn_3As_2. The N_{Zn}^3-dependency of the etch depth is also explained with equation (1). The equilibrium arsenic vapor pressure over Zn_3As_2 is $2 \cdot 10^{-4}$ atm.[14]., i.e. about six orders of magnitude higher than the As vapor pressure over GaAs [15]. This could explain the slow etching due to evaporating arsenic since only a small amount of As can be dissolved in the Ga-Zn melt [11]. Increasing the arsenic pressure in the ampoule would drive the equilibrium to the GaAs side and thus decrease the etch rate.

The participation of two photons in the initial stage is supported by measurements on the influence of laser power on the etch rate. Fig. 6 shows the maximum depth of the etch pits as a function of absorbed laser power. Source and substrate temperatures of 600 and 625 deg.C, respectively, and exposure times of 45 min. have been used for these measurements. The etch depth increases approximately quadratically with laser intensity. A laser induced temperature rise of 18 deg.C is estimated [6] for these experimental conditions at the maximum laser power used. This is much lower than the temperature rise of up to 190 deg.C created in corresponding experiments performed in a zinc and arsenic atmosphere at 850 deg.C. In these latter experiments controlled by the laser induced temperature we found a sublinear increase of etch depth with laser power ($d \propto P^{0.2}$). We therefore exclude the laser induced temperature rise as possible

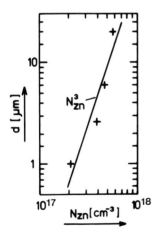

Fig.5: Etch depth d vs. zinc concentration N_{Zn} obtained with 8 mW at 625 deg.C.

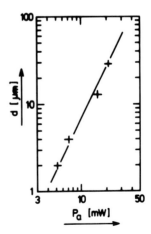

Fig.6: Etch depth d vs. absorbed laser power P_a obtained at a substrate temperature of 625 deg.C.

explanation for the quadratic dependency shown in Fig. 6. The lowest power density which induced etching at 625 deg.C substrate and 600 deg.C source temperature was 200 W/cm^2. Based on a carrier lifetime of ~1 ns and a laser spot diameter of 24 µm, we calculate a hole density of ~ $2\cdot10^{15}$cm^{-3}, or a separation of the quasifermi niveaus on the order of 0.5 meV for the onset of etching. No attempt has been made so far to further increase this sensitivity by, e.g., optimizing substrate and source temperatures.

Similar etching and diffusion results have been obtained with GaAs substrates covered by a 4 µm thick $Al_{0.3}Ga_{0.7}As$ epitaxial layer. However, no etching could be observed if samples were used with a layer of $Al_{0.6}Ga_{0.4}As$ on top. This layer does not absorb the Kr-ion laser radiation. Optically generated carriers in the GaAs substrate cannot diffuse to the surface because of the potential barrier at the hetero-interface. The absence of etching in this case indicates that the deposition of zinc in the initial stage of film formation is due to the local increase in carrier concentration at the surface.

P-type GaAs (Zn, $5\cdot10^{17}$cm^{-3}) subjected to a pure zinc atmosphere at 625 deg.C did not show laser induced etching at typical powers of 8 mW though in some cases the characteristic increase in reflectivity could be observed. However, the optically polished surface of these samples showed a rectangular shaped corrugation over the whole surface after exposure. Nomarski microscope and SEM investigations showed that a film with a thickness of about 20 µm has been formed on the surface. X ray spectroscopy indicated that this film consisted of zinc and arsenic with a ratio of 0.57:0.43. This corresponds to the atomic weight ratio for Zn_2As_3. The experiment indicates clearly that the film growth is initialized by holes present at the semiconductor surface.

In conclusion we have observed light induced etching of n-type GaAs exposed to a zinc atmosphere at 600 deg.C. We attribute the etching to the formation of an unsaturated metal film on the GaAs substrate. The growth of this film is induced by optically generated holes at the semiconductor surface.

ACKNOWLEDGEMENTS

The authors would like to thank Prof. H.P. Weber for the opportunity to perform this work. They also acknowledge the technical assistance of B. Wicki. and the SEM and X-ray investigations of R. Flueck.

REFERENCES

[1] F.A. Cunnel and C.H. Gooch, J. Phys. Chem. Solids 15, 127 (1960)

[2] L.R. Weisberg and J. Blanc, Phys. Rev. 131, 1548 (1963)

[3] H.C. Casey Jr., M.B. Panish, and L.L. Chang, Phys. Rev. 162, 660 (1967)

[4] J.F. Black and E.D. Jungbluth, J. Electrochem. Soc. 114, 181 (1967)

[5] A.B. Timberlake, P.W. Davies, and T.S. Shilliday,
     J. Appl. Phys. 33, 765 (1968)

[6] H. Rupprecht and C.Z. Le May, J. Appl. Phys. $\underline{35}$, 1970 (1964)

[7] O.S. Heavens, <u>Optical properties of thin solid films</u> (Dover Publ. Inc., New York 1965) pp. 76

[8] Landolt-Boernstein vol II/8, <u>Optische Konstanten</u> (Springer Verlag Berlin 1962) pp.I-13

[9] D.D. Sell, H.C. Casey Jr., and K.W. Wecht, J. Appl. Phys. $\underline{45}$, 2650 (1962)

[10] M.D. Sturge, Phys. Rev. $\underline{127}$, 768 (1962)

[11] M.B. Panish, J. Phys. Chem. Solids $\underline{27}$, 291 (1966)

[12] R.F. Barrow, P.G. Dodsworth, A.R. Downie, E.A.N.S. Jeffries, A.C.P. Pugh, F.J. Smitter, and J.M. Swinestead, Trans. Faraday Soc. $\underline{51}$, 1354 (1955)

[13] H.C. Casey Jr. and M.B. Panish, Trans. AIME $\underline{242}$, 406 (1968)

[14] R.C. Schoonmaker and K.J. Lemmerman, J. Chem. Eng. Data $\underline{17}$, 139 (1972)

[15] C. Pupp, JJ. Murray, and R.F. Pottie, J. Chem. Thermodyn. $\underline{6}$, 123 (1974)

LASER-CONTROLLED ETCHING OF CHROMIUM-DOPED AND n-DOPED <100> GaAs*

GARY C. TISONE AND A. WAYNE JOHNSON
Sandia National Laboratories, Division 1126, Albuquerque, NM 87185, USA

ABSTRACT

The photochemical etching of chromium-doped and n-doped <100> GaAs in HNO_3 and KOH is examined in the wavelength region of 334 to 514 nm from an argon-ion laser. The etching process is found to be not thermally controlled. The etch rates of chromium-doped GaAs agree with a diffusion-controlled model of the photochemically produced holes. For both types of GaAs, HNO_3 is found to produce morphologically superior results.

The use of GaAs as the semiconductor material in integrated circuits is growing. This semiconductor is being used in microwave integrated circuits, in the developing fields of very-high-speed integrated circuits, and in the fabrication of strained-layer superlattice devices. One of the inherent problems with wet chemical etching in fabricating microelectronic circuits is the isotropic property of the wet etching process. The usual chemical and electrochemical processes for etching of GaAs are reviewed in reference 1. Lasers are developing into useful tools for the controlling of etching. They offer three important advantages over conventional etching techniques. First, they produce high spatial resolution without using photolithography. Next, they produce an etching process with a very high differential rate between the irradiated and the nonirradiated areas. Finally, the laser process produces highly directional or anisotropic etching. Laser techniques not only would be useful for general etching problems but also could be developed into new fabrication techniques for customized circuits.
There have been a number of reports of electrochemical etching of GaAs where the etching process was assisted by the production of photogenerated minority carriers [2-9]. Photogenerated holes have been used to assist in the electrochemical etching of n-type III-V compounds by oxidative decomposition [2-4,7,8]. The decomposition of GaAs by oxidation is thought [9] to be due to the surface reaction

$$GaAs + 6h+ \rightarrow Ga(3+) + As(3+).$$

Photogenerated electrons have also been used to etch p-type III-V compounds by reductive decomposition. The reaction for the reductive decomposition of GaAs is suggested [9] to be

$$GaAs + 3e \rightarrow Ga + As(3-).$$

This process has the complication that the Ga remains and stabilizes on the surface, inhibiting the etching process [9]. Laser-controlled liquid etching of GaAs substrates has been studied both where the laser interacts with the reactants in the solvent to produce etching [10] and where the laser interacts with the surface of the substrate in the solvent to produce the etching [11].

---

*This work performed at Sandia National Laboratories supported by the U.S. Department of Energy under contract number DE-AC04-76DP00789, for the Office of Basic Energy Science.

We report studies of laser-assisted photochemical etching of Cr-doped and n-doped GaAs with laser intensities up to 80 kW/cm^2. The n-doped substrates contained Si at a density of about 2×10^{18}/cm^3. The semi-insulating GaAs was Cr-doped to yield a resistivity of 6×10^7 Ω cm. The etching solutions that were used were 5 and 10% HNO$_3$ and KOH. All measurements were made on the <100> crystal plane. We have systematically studied etching in the wavelength region of 334 to 514 nm. For Cr-doped GaAs, we have developed a model for the measured wavelength dependence of the etch rate. For the n-doped GaAs, we present the experimental results only.

For this experiment the GaAs substrate was placed vertically in a UV quartz cell that was filled with the etching solution. The laser beam was then focussed onto the sample with a 10-cm-focal-length lens. The minimum spot size that could be obtained with this lens was approximately 20 μ. The GaAs substrate was scanned perpendicular to the axis of the laser beam and maintained at the focus of the lens. Mesurements of the etch rates induced by the Ar-ion laser were made using lines from the visible (514 nm) to the UV (334 nm). In the visible the laser was operated on a single line with up to 8 watts of power in the strongest line at 514 nm. In the UV a multiline power of 3 watts could be obtained. The UV radiation was distributed in the following manner: 10% at 334 nm, 50% at 351 nm, and 40% at 364 nm. The etch rates for the individual UV lines were also measured in order to compare with the rates that were measured with the three UV lines simultaneously.

Etching with the laser was effected by scanning the substrate at a rate from 4 to 18×10^{-3} cm/sec. The total power from the laser was varied to determine the etch rate as a function of intensity at the substrate. A step profiling device was used to measure the shape and the depth of the etched lines. The intensity profile of the laser beam in the focal plane for the various etching conditions was estimated from these measurements. This estimate of the shape of the laser beam is based on the assumption that the depth of the etched line at any point is proportional to the time-integrated light intensity and that there is no threshold for the etching process.

The etching of Cr-doped GaAs by an HNO$_3$ solution exhibited a systematic wavelength dependence. (No measurable etching was produced in the KOH solutions.) The etch rates as a function of intensity for the combined UV lines and for the 514-nm radiation from the argon ion laser are shown in Figure 1 for 10-percent HNO$_3$ solutions. The results of etching in 5% HNO$_3$ were found to be identical to the results using 10% HNO$_3$ solutions. As can be seen in this Figure, the etch rate for the UV lines was found to be the most rapid. A monotonic decrease of the etch rates with increasing wavelength was observed (see R in Fig. 2). The etching by the UV produced a very smooth etched line while the etched line produced by radiation in the visible was rough and uneven. The etch rates at a given laser intensity for each of the individual UV lines were found to agree with the combined UV etch rates shown in Figure 1. The profile of the beam at the focus for the 334 nm line, which has the strongest absorption in the HNO$_3$ solutions, was found to change drastically at high laser intensity. This thermal distortion of the beam by absorption in the solution ws found for only the 334 nm line. Without the 334 nm line, the combined UV radiation from the laser is not thermally distorted.

The decrease of the etch rate with increasing wavelength for Cr-doped GaAs does not appear to be due to any difference in the heating of the substrate that results from the absorption of the laser. In Figure 2, the fraction of incident light that is absorbed in the substrate (I/I_o) is shown as a function of the wavelength. This intensity ratio and the absorption coefficient, α, were calculated from the equations

$$\frac{I}{I_o} = \frac{4 n_o n_1}{(n_o + n_1)^2 + k_1^2}$$

and

$$\alpha = 4\pi k_1 / \lambda$$

where I_o is the incident laser intensity on the substrate, I is the laser intensity transmitted into the substrate, n_o is the index of refraction in water, and n_1 and k_1 are the real and imaginary part, respectively, of the index of refraction in GaAs. [12-15]

As can be seen in Figure 2, the fraction of incident light (I/I_o) that is absorbed in the substrate does not depend strongly on the wavelength. Therefore a thermal process would not have a strong wavelength dependence. We have also measured the etch rate for HNO_3 solutions near the boiling point and have found that the etch rate (0.05 μ/s) is much less than the observed laser induced etch rates. Our estimation of the surface temperature during laser illumination in this experiment was always less than 100°C. The small etch rates observed for boiling HNO_3 solution is another indication that our laser-induced etch rates are not a thermal process.

Photochemical etching of GaAs is controlled by the number of holes, produced in the bulk material by the absorption of photons, that diffuse to the surface. The flux is determined by the balance between the diffusion of the holes and the recombination of the holes. The number of holes can be represented by the differential equation:

$$\frac{\partial n}{\partial t} = D \frac{\partial^2 n}{\partial x^2} - \frac{n}{\tau} + S$$

where D is the diffusion coefficient, τ is the lifetime of the holes and S is the source function for the production of holes by the incident photons. The variable X is the distance from the surface of the GaAs sample. Using the time independent solution to the above equation and our etch rate data, we estimate an effective diffusion length, $d = \sqrt{D\tau}$, to be 100 Å. In Figure 2 the published absorption coefficient, α, in units of μm^{-1} and the measured etch rate per unit of intensity, R, as a function of wavelength are shown. The strong onset of absorption near 460 nm results from the E_1 and $E_1 + \Delta_1$ absorption edge.

The results of the etching of n-doped GaAs for HNO_3 and KOH are shown in Figures 3 and 4 respectively. The etch rates for the two visible lines in Figure 3 are 5 times faster than any of the rates for the semi-insulating GaAs. In the UV the etching rate saturates at intensities above 1 to 2 kW/cm^2. There also appears to be a slight saturation of the visible etch rates.

The etching results for the KOH solution shown in Figure 4 have a strong saturation effect for all of the wavelengths. This saturation is most likely due to the production of the nonsoluable products at the surface of the substrate. Thermodynamic equilibrium studies [16] of the reactions possible at the interface predict that $Ga(OH)_3$ should be formed in KOH. Also a scanning Auger electron spectrometer showed a buildup of carbon, silicon and oxygen on the etched surface. At the highest etch rates the surface became very rough and developed columnar structures. Apparently, etching by KOH is limited by the formation of nonsoluable products at the surface.

The results of this experiment have demonstrated that etching by uv and visible laser irradiation can be induced on semi-insulating Cr-doped GaAs and on n-doped GaAs. The photon-enhanced etching mechanism is not due to heating of the substrate. The etch rates for the <Cr> GaAs were found to have a strong dependence on the wavelength of the laser, with the rate increasing toward lower wavelengths. We have found that a diffusion model can be used to describe the etching of Cr-doped GaAs by HNO_3. Etching of n-doped GaAs by HNO_3 is rapid and does not leave a surface residue while the etching of n-doped GaAs in KOH at high rates develops residues and columnar structures.

REFERENCES

1. Werner Kern and Cheryl A. deckert, "Chemical Etching", in *Thin Film Processes*, edited by John L. Vosen and Werner Kern, (Academic, New York, 1978), pp. 401-96.

2. F. Kuhn-Kuhnenfeld, J. Electrochem. Soc. *119*, 1063 (1972).

3. Akio Yamamoto and Soichi Yano, J. Electrochem. Soc. *122*, 260 (1975).

4. D. Lubzens, Electronics Letters *13* (7), 171 (1977).

5. Zh. Alferov, D. N. Goyrachev, S. A. Gurevich, M. N. Mizerov, E. L. Portnoi, and B. S. Ryvkin, Sov. Phy. Tech. Phys. *21*, 857 (1976).

6. Heinz Gerischer, J. Vac. Sci. Tchnol. *15* (14), 1422 (1978).

7. Ako Shimano, Hiromitsu Takagi and Gota Kano, IEEE Trans. Electron Devices, *ED-26* 8119, 1680 (1979).

8. H. J. Hoffmann, J. M. Woodall and T. I. Chappell, appl. Phys. Lett. *38* (7), 564 (1981).

9. F. W. Ostermaymer, Jr. and P. A. Kohl, Appl. Phys. Lett.

10. R. W. Haynes, G. M. Metze, V. G. Kreismanis, and L. F. Eastman, Appl. Phys. Lett. *37* (4), 344 (1980).

11. R. M. Osgood, Jr., a. Sanchez-Rubio, D. J. Ehrlinch and V. Daneu, Appl. Phys. Lett. *40* (5), 391 (1982).

12. H. Ehrenreich and H. R. Philipp, Phys. Rev. Lett. *8* (2), 59 (1962).

13. H. R. Philipp, and H. Ehrenreich, Phys. Rev. *129* (4), 1550 (1963).

14. Robert E. Morrison, Phys. Rev. *124* (5), 1314 (1961).

15. B. O. Seraphin and H. E. Bennett, "Optical Constants", in *Semiconductors and Semimetals*, edited by R. K. Willardson and Albert C. Beer (Academic, New York, 1967) pp. 499-545.

16. Su-Moon Park and Matthew E. Barber, J. Electroanal. Chem. *99*, 67 (1979).

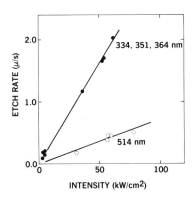

1. Etching rates of Cr-doped GaAs in 10 percent HNO_3 solution as a function of laser intensity. Results are shown for the combined UV lines and for the 514 nm line of the argon-ion laser.

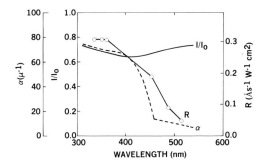

2. Comparison of the calculated wavelength dependence of the absorbed light (I/I_o), the calculated absorption coefficient, α, and the observed etching rate per unit intensity, R. Calculations and measurements are for Cr-doped GaAs in a 10 percent HNO_3 solution.

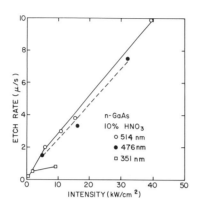

3. Etching rates for n-doped GaAs in 10 percent HNO_3 solution as a function of the laser intensity. Results are shown for the 514, 476 and 351 nm lines of the argon-ion laser.

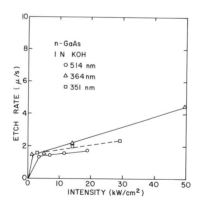

4. Etching rates for n-doped GaAs in 1N KOH solution as a function of the laser intensity. Results are shown for the 514, 476 and 351 nm lines of the argon-ion laser.

SECTION III
DIAGNOSTICS OF SEMICONDUCTOR STRUCTURES

OPTICAL MICROANALYSIS OF SMALL SEMICONDUCTOR STRUCTURES*

D. V. MURPHY AND S. R. J. BRUECK
Lincoln Laboratory, Massachusetts Institute of Technology
Lexington, Massachusetts 02173

ABSTRACT

Raman spectroscopy is a powerful tool for evaluating semiconductor crystal characteristics with a diffraction-limited spatial resolution of approximately 0.5 µm, comparable to device structure dimensions. Examples are presented of the use of Raman scattering to measure stress variations across Si-on-insulator and Si-on-sapphire stripes with dimensions down to 2 µm and, to probe the spatial variation in the effectiveness of annealing of a Si layer deposited over metal device structures. Detailed measurements of the variation in the Raman spectra of thin crystalline Si films, with thicknesses down to 3.0 nm, are discussed. Measurements made on roughened Si surfaces are presented which show that surface morphology on a submicron spatial scale results in enhanced Raman intensities.

INTRODUCTION

Optical diagnostic techniques have a number of features that make them attractive for probing solid-state material parameters on a small spatial scale. Foremost among these is that such techniques are generally nondestructive, requiring neither special sample preparation nor physical contact with the sample during the measurement. Additionally, many optical techniques are sufficiently sensitive that laser powers can be kept low enough to avoid perturbing the sample (through laser heating, for example), so that the techniques are nonintrusive as well. The spatial resolution achievable with optical techniques is determined by the incident laser wavelength and the absorption depth in the material being probed. For visible light incident on Si, for example, this means a laser spot diameter of ~ 0.5 µm and an absorption depth of < 1 µm. These techniques can be extended to the ultraviolet spectral region with an accompanying improvement in the transverse resolution because of the shorter wavelength, and in depth resolution because of the increased absorption coefficient above the direct band edge in semiconductors such as Si. This should be contrasted with more conventional techniques such as x-ray analysis which typically have a spatial resolution of several millimeters. An additional advantage of light scattering techniques is that alignment onto particular device structures using the visible pump-laser beam for illumination is straightforward.

Raman scattering from optical phonons in semiconductor materials provides a sensitive probe for a number of important material parameters, including:
- (1) Stress – An applied stress results in a lattice strain which affects the phonon energy and causes a shift in the position of the optical phonon line;
- (2) Defect density – Increased phonon scattering from lattice defects causes a shortened phonon lifetime which results in a broadened Raman linewidth;

---

*This work was supported by the Department of the Air Force, in part with specific funding from the Air Force Office of Scientific Research.

(3) Surface morphology - Scattering from a roughened surface is depolarized and in some cases is increased in intensity with respect to that observed from bulk Si;
(4) Crystallinity - The crystallite size and orientational texture in polycrystalline material affect the lineshape and linewidth of the phonon line as well as the polarization of the scattered radiation;
(5) Temperature - The lattice temperature is accessible through the phonon population which determines the ratio of intensity in the Stokes and anti-Stokes lines. The linewidth and position of the individual phonon lines are also sensitive functions of temperature.

The phonon Raman spectrum is relatively insensitive to the low concentration impurities that control many of the electrical characteristics of semiconductor devices. These can be probed, on a somewhat larger spatial scale because of carrier diffusion effects, by laser-excited luminescence techniques.

This paper presents several specific examples of the use of Raman scattering to probe the stress profiles in small structures fabricated from silicon-on-insulator materials and to probe the spatial variation in crystallite size in an annealed Si layer deposited over a 4-μm period tungsten grating. In addition, the results of a study of the effect of finite dimensions on the Raman spectra of semiconductors are also presented. Raman spectra of extremely thin (< 10 nm) crystalline Si films exhibit an asymmetric broadening due to the relaxation of momentum selection rules for these small dimensions. Finally, observations of enhancements in the Raman scattering intensity due to a submicron transverse surface morphology in Si are presented and discussed.

STRESS PROFILES IN SOI STRUCTURES

Device structures fabricated from high-quality silicon films deposited on insulating substrates are of great interest for VLSI applications due to improved isolation between densely packed devices as compared with bulk silicon material. Silicon-on-sapphire (SOS) material grown by vapor phase epitaxy is commercially available; a number of alternate growth techniques and material systems are currently under development [1,2].

For these heterogeneous material systems there is often an inherent two-dimensional stress on the Si film caused by the differential thermal contraction of the Si and the substrate material upon cooling from the growth temperature of 1000-1400 C to room temperature. This stress results in variations of the silicon energy-level structure and electronic transport properties which can affect device characteristics. Specifically, for the two-dimensional compressive stress characteristic of SOS the conduction band energy level structure is altered and the heavy-mass directions of the electronic structure are lowered relative to the light-mass directions [3,4]. This results in a higher effective mass and, consequently, a reduced electron mobility [4,5] compared to bulk Si. For other materials systems such as silicon-on-fused quartz (SOQ), the stress is tensile rather than compressive resulting in a higher effective electron mobility [5].

In addition to these changes in the electronic properties, the stress-induced strain modifies the lattice characteristics. For a two-dimensional stress, the triply-degenerate zone-center phonon modes in unstressed Si are split into a singlet and a doublet. The frequencies of both of these modes shift linearly with applied stress [6,7]. For the (100) wafers used for many device configurations, the singlet is Raman active and the Raman frequency can be used to monitor the local stress. Raman scattering has found wide application as a probe of the residual stress associated with laser annealing, both for SOS [8,9] and bulk Si [10] materials.

Previously, determinations of the inherent SOI stress have been limited to large-area wafers of the silicon-on-insulator material rather than to actual fabricated devices. Significant variations in the stress may be expected to occur near the edges of Si structures because of the thermal cycling involved in fabricating devices from these materials. In particular the effects of this cycling on the very small structures, with linear dimensions of less than 2 µm, currently being fabricated for VLSI applications have not been investigated. Different device processing technologies such as fabricating isolated Si islands on the sapphire substrate or isolating the devices by growing a local oxide layer through the unused Si areas to the substrate may be expected to yield different stress profiles. An initial report on this work has previously been presented [11].

The experimental arrangement used to probe the stress profiles in small structures fabricated from SOI materials is shown schematically in Fig. 1. The 5145-Å argon-ion pump laser beam was reflected from a dichroic mirror and focused onto the Si device with a 60X-microscope objective. A spot size of less than 1-µm diameter was inferred from the measured scattering intensity profiles. Typically, laser powers of less than 2 mW, corresponding to power densities of ~ 500 kW/cm^2, were used. The Raman spectra were insensitive to laser power at this level. The Raman scattered light was collected by the same objective, transmitted through the dichroic filter, analyzed with a 3/4-meter computer-controlled double monochrometer and detected with a small-area, S-20 surface, photomultiplier using photon-counting electronics. The spectral resolution was approximately 2 cm^{-1}. The computer also controlled a stepping motor which translated the sample across the laser beam focal position with steps as small as 0.25 µm; Raman spectra were obtained at each position. These spectra were then least-squares fitted to a Lorentzian lineshape to obtain the integrated Raman intensity, the Raman frequency, and the linewidth (FWHM) as a function of position. Typical RMS deviations of the data from the Lorentzian fit were less than 5%. Relative Raman frequency measurements were repeatable to within ± 0.05 cm^{-1}. Raman spectra of (100) bulk Si were taken following each spatial scan and served as a calibration standard.

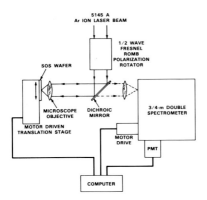

Fig. 1. Experimental setup for the measurement of Raman spectra with $\sim$ 1-µm spatial resolution.

The devices were fabricated on SOS and SOQ wafers with 0.5-µm thick Si layers. Devices with their active regions defined by both the CIE and coplanar techniques [12] were investigated. In both cases the active area oxidation cycle was performed at 1000 C in a dry O_2 ambient to produce 100 nm of SiO_2 on (100) Si. The device fabrication followed a standard self-aligned poly-Si gate process. The oxidation step was the highest temperature processing stage. Minimum active area widths were approximately 6 μm. The coplanar-defined widths were somewhat smaller since the oxidation process consumed approximately 0.5 μm of Si from each edge of the stripe.

Figure 2 shows the Raman parameters that were measured in a scan across a 6-μm wide stripe fabricated by the CIE technique. The penetration depth of the 5145 Å pump laser light is comparable to the 0.5-μm Si thickness so that the Raman scattering probes the entire Si film. The integrated intensity of the Raman scattering is shown in the upper curve; the rapid changes in intensity at the edges of the structure indicate that a spatial resolution of ~ 1 μm has been achieved. The enhanced scattering just at the edges of the device is a repeatable effect that becomes more pronounced as the laser beam spot size is decreased and seems to be associated with the rough Si edge. This enhancement will be discussed at greater length below. The corresponding Raman frequencies for the CIE defined structure are shown in the middle trace of Fig. 2. As a result of the compressive stress of SOS the Raman frequencies are shifted to a higher frequency than that of bulk Si. In the center of the 6-μm structure, only a very small relaxation from the frequency of a nearby 50-μm-wide structure is observed. At the edges of the structure, however, there is a significant shift of the Raman fre-

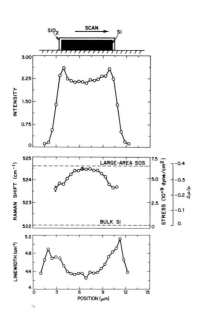
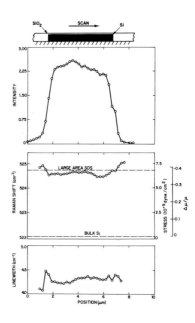

Fig. 2. Raman intensity, frequency shift, and linewidth as a function of position across a 6-μm-wide CIE-defined Si stripe on an Al_2O_3 substrate. The stress and relative electron mobility variations deduced from the measurement are also indicated. The CIE device structure is also shown.

Fig. 3. Raman intensity, frequency shift, and linewidth as a function of position across a 4.5-μm-wide coplanar-defined Si stripe on an Al_2O_3 substrate.

quency towards the frequency of bulk Si indicating that a substantial relaxation of the stress has occurred. The stress variation and the corresponding relative electron mobility variation [4,5] deduced from these Raman frequency shifts are also shown in the figure. The measured stress variation corresponds to a 20% stress-induced mobility variation across the stripe. The actual mobility variation may be different as a result of defect variations. The bottom trace shows the measured Raman linewidths. The linewidth of ~ 4.35 cm^{-1} obtained in the center of the stripe is significantly larger than the linewidth of ~ 3.1 cm^{-1} obtained for bulk Si. This difference may be due to the higher defect density commonly found in SOS materials [13]. At the edges of the stripe there is an increase in the linewidth which is due to the spatial inhomogeneity of the stress within the laser beam diameter. This is clear both from the variation of the stress-induced frequency shifts and from the asymmetry of the Raman lines in this region. When the laser beam is mainly to the side of the Si structure and only the very edges of the beam are scattering from the Si, the Raman linewidth is again ~ 4 cm^{-1} which suggests that the stress relaxation is not accompanied by a large increase in the local defect density.

Similar results were obtained for measurements made on device structures fabricated by the CIE technique from silicon-on-quartz. The stress in SOQ is tensile rather than compressive, resulting in a lower Raman frequency with respect to that of bulk Si; we observed relaxation of the stress at the edges of a 6-μm-wide stripe similar to that observed in the SOS devices fabricated by the same processing technique.

The results of similar measurements on the coplanar devices are shown in Fig. 3. The width of the active area is somewhat narrower in these devices due to the lateral oxidation of the active region during the fabrication. There was no significant variation of either the Raman frequency or the linewidth over the active region except for a slight increase in the Raman shift corresponding to an increase in the local stress just at the edges of the stripe. This may be the result of a lateral confinement due to the SiO_2 pushing in on the Si.

Raman parameters obtained for scans across 2-μm-wide SOS stripes fabricated by the CIE technique are displayed in Fig. 4. The noteworthy feature of these measurements is that the phonon frequency was nearly constant across the stripe and was strongly shifted from the large area SOS frequency of 524.6 cm^{-1} toward that of bulk Si at 522.1 cm^{-1} (the absolute calibration of the spectrometer was $\sim \pm 1$ cm^{-1}; however, the relative shifts in phonon frequency between bulk Si and the SOS material were accurate to ± 0.05 cm^{-1}). This corresponds to a 65% relaxation of the compressive SOS stress across the entire width of the structure. Raman frequencies and linewidths obtained in the regions between the 2-μm-wide stripes, where the small Raman intensity is due to scattering of the incident light in the wings of the focal spot from the sidewalls of the stripes, are not reliable because of the poor signal-to-noise ratios of the spectra recorded in those regions and because of the poorly defined scattering geometry.

The observation of local stress variations extending as far as 1.5 μm from the edges of 6-μm wide Si stripes in SOS and SOQ devices and of substantial stress relaxation throughout 2-μm-wide SOS stripes clearly indicates that the fabrication of silicon-on-insulator device structures with micrometer and submicrometer dimensions is accompanied by changes in material parameters. As shown in these measurements, variations are dependent on the techniques employed for device fabrication and must be characterized in order to optimize device designs. Raman scattering has been shown to be be a useful diagnostic tool for nondestructively probing these changes with micrometer resolution.

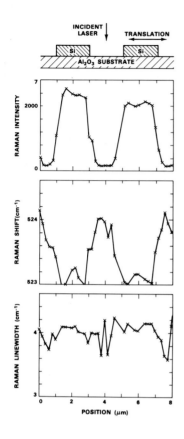

Fig. 4. Raman intensity, frequency shift and linewidth as a function of position across 2-μm-wide CIE-defined stripes on an Al_2O_3 substrate.

CHARACTERIZATION OF POLYCRYSTALLINE Si

Raman spectroscopy also provides information on the crystal morphology of semiconductors. The first order Raman spectrum of bulk, strain-free Si consists of a single Lorentzian line of full-width ~ 3 cm^{-1} centered at 521 cm^{-1} at room temperature. The spectrum of fine-grain polycrystalline material shows a much broader line with an asymmetric tail extending to the low frequency side. Completely amorphous material has a very broad first-order line centered at 480 cm^{-1}. In addition to this dependence of the linewidth and lineshape on the degree of crystallinity, the polarization of the scattered radiation also provides information about the material crystallinity because the polarization selection rules depend strongly on crystal orientation. According to the selection rules for backscattering from the (100) plane of Si, for example, the scattered light is polarized parallel to the incident light for incident polarization along a [110] direction, but is orthogonally polarized for incident polarization along a [100] direction. Polycrystalline material consists of small crystallites of random orientation so that the scattering is generally depolarized by an amount that depends on the crystallite size and orientational texture. Thus, the depolarization ratio of the scattered intensity provides qualitative information about sample crystallinity.

Raman spectroscopy has been frequently employed to characterize laser- and furnace-annealed polycrystalline Si films [14,15]. Unfortunately, a clear relationship between crystallite size and Raman lineshape and peak position has not been established either experimentally or theoretically. Although the majority of the experimental evidence indicates that the optical phonon line asymmetrically broadens and shifts to low frequency with decreasing crystallite size [16,18], there are also reports of broadening without a concomitant shift in peak position [19,20]. The discrepancies may be due to the widely different methods used to prepare the films used in the various studies. Several mechanisms have been proposed to explain the observed effects; some of these are: relaxation of wavevector selection rules due to the small crystallite size [17,21]; inhomogeneous stress distribution caused by laser annealing [20]; and lifetime broadening due to increased phonon scattering at grain boundaries and other defects, coupled with the growth of a low frequency ($\sim$ 500 cm^{-1}) mode due to scattering from Si atoms at the grain boundaries [19]. It is difficult to infer the relative importance of these effects in determining the spectra of polycrystalline films because the films are difficult to characterize with respect to crystallite size and orientation, defect density, and stress. In an effort to assess the relative importance of purely dimensional effects on the Raman spectrum, we have made a study of the effect of finite sample size on the Raman spectrum of the first order optical phonon in Si films that have long range crystalline order in two dimensions but are very thin in the third dimension (down to $\sim$ 3 nm). These films are free from the spatially inhomogeneous stress associated with laser annealed polycrystalline films, and the contribution of Si atoms at grain boundaries to which Sarott et al. [19] attribute a low frequency mode is negligible. Previous reports [22] of the Raman spectra of extremely thin Si films, obtained by a coherent Raman gain technique, did not have sufficient discrimination from extraneous nonlinear effects to resolve the details of the Raman lineshape.

Thin Si films were prepared from commercially obtained 0.5-μm-thick (100) Si epitaxially grown on 2" diameter polished sapphire substrates. The Si was uniformly oxidized until a thin Si layer remained under an SiO$_2$ cap. The individual layer thicknesses of the resulting Al$_2$O$_3$-Si-SiO$_2$ structure were determined by fitting experimental transmission spectra recorded over the 0.4 to 3.0-μm wavelength range. Good agreement between calculated and experimental transmission spectra was obtained down to Si thicknesses on the order of 5 nm using the optical constants of bulk Si. Because of the nonuniform thickness of the starting SOS material, the thickness of the Si layer used for the measurements varied from 0 to 65 nm with a linear wedge of 3.5 nm/mm across the wafer. It was therefore possible to investigate a wide range of Si film thickness using a single wafer.

The Raman spectra of the optical phonon were recorded in a backscattering geometry similar to that shown previously. Measurements were typically made with a spectrometer resolution of 3.2 or 6.4 cm^{-1} and an incident laser power of 30-40 mW. No broadening of the phonon line due to laser heating of the thin films could be observed at these power levels although thermal broadening was apparent in bulk Si and in 0.5-μm SOS for laser powers > 5 mW.

Experimental spectra of silicon films 40, 10, and $\sim$ 4 nm thick are shown in Fig. 5. A series of similar spectra recorded over the thickness range of 40 to 3 nm exhibit the following behavior with decreasing film thickness: (1) the optical phonon line broadens and develops a low frequency tail extending as far as 70 cm^{-1} from line center; and (2) the peak position of the phonon line shifts slightly ($\sim$ 2.5 cm^{-1} for the 3-nm film) to low frequency with respect to that of the 40-nm film. Dramatic broadening of the Raman line does not occur for film thicknesses greater than approximately 10 nm.

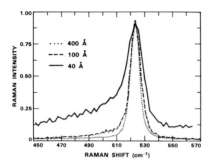

Fig. 5. Experimental Raman spectra of 40, 10 and 4-nm-thick crystalline films on an Al_2O_3 substrate.

Because the Si film is layered between the Al_2O_3 substrate and an oxide cap, it is important to consider the possible effects of the interfaces on the Raman spectrum of the thin Si. A thick transition region of disordered Si due to interface induced defects, for example, might cause a broadened and shifted phonon line that could mask the purely dimensional effects. However, this does not appear to be the case. Ellipsometric analysis of the $Si-SiO_2$ interface suggests a transition region of < 0.8 nm between the crystalline Si and SiO_2 [23]. This may have an effect on the spectra of the thinnest films, although spectra obtained after stripping the thick oxide cap are qualitatively similar to those obtained with the cap in place, except that they show somewhat broader lineshapes. The additional broadening is consistent with a slight thinning of the Si film due to the regrowth of a native oxide. The effect of the interface between the Si film and the substrate should also be minimal; recent TEM studies of the $Si-Al_2O_3$ interface indicate that the Si atoms are well ordered right up to the interface [24]. Additional evidence that the observed effects were not due to interface-induced disorder in the Si are the polarized nature of the scattering observed from even the 4-nm film and the lack of any peak at 480 cm^{-1} that would indicate the presence of amorphous Si.

The energy and momentum selection rules for Raman scattering from bulk crystalline material normally allow only zone center phonons to contribute to the Raman spectrum. For sufficiently small samples this picture is modified in two important respects: (1) the wavevector selection rule is relaxed in samples with dimensions less than the wavelength of light so that phonons with wavevectors extending out into the Brillouin zone contribute to the scattering; and (2) the vibrational spectrum of the crystal may be affected by the sample boundaries so that the bulk phonon dispersion curves are no longer appropriate. Sample size and shape are particularly important in determining the phonon spectra of small ionic crystals [25] due to long range coulombic forces that are not present in nonpolar materials such as Si. We have used a simple model which assumes the bulk phonon dispersion for even the thinnest Si slabs but includes the contributions to the scattering from non-zone center phonons to calculate Raman spectra for a range of film thickness. In qualitative agreement with the experiment, this simple model does indicate dramatic broadening to low frequency only for films < 10 nm thick, although we do not obtain good quantitative agreement with experimental lineshapes.

The fact that the finite sample thickness introduces significant perturbation to the Raman spectrum of Si only for dimensions less than ~ 10 nm is largely because of the flatness of the optical phonon bands near the zone center. This finding is consistent with the work of Iqbal et al. [17] who also observe broadening in films with grain sizes < 15 nm. However, Salathe et al. [16] observed significant broadening and shifting of the phonon line in polycrystalline Ge films for grain sizes > 1 μm. In addition, we do not observe the large shifts in peak position that are reported by some authors [14-18]. Clearly factors other than grain size, such as strain at crystallite boundaries and defects, must play a role in determining the Raman spectra of polycrystalline films; the relative importance of the different effects may depend on the exact method of film preparation.

Even without a quantitative calibration for the grain size in polycrystalline films, however, Raman scattering can yield useful qualitative information about annealed, polycrystalline material. In the application presented here, the spatial variation in crystallinity of thermally annealed CVD Si put down over a tungsten grating was investigated. The samples were prepared by reactive-ion-etching 2-μm-wide grooves on 4-μm centers 0.2-μm deep along the [110] direction in bulk (100) Si. A 50-nm-thick tungsten layer was then deposited in the bottom of the grooves, and a 0.3-μm Si layer was put down over the entire surface by chemical vapor deposition (CVD) (see Fig. 6). Samples were annealed under different conditions in an effort to obtain the best solid-phase epitaxial recrystallization of the CVD Si.

Raman spectra of the samples were recorded with an experimental arrangement similar to that used in the SOI measurements reported above. The integrated Raman intensities in the allowed (VV) and forbidden (VH) polarizations for scattering from (100) Si with incident polarization along the [110] direction were recorded as the sample was scanned in a direction normal to the buried tungsten fingers and are shown for two samples in Fig. 6. A spatial variation of the

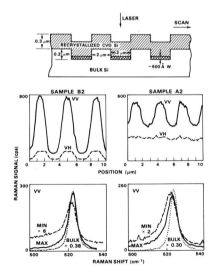

Fig. 6. Structure of sample with furnace annealed CVD Si over buried tungsten grating with 4-μm period shown at top. Spatial variation of integrated Raman intensity in allowed (VV) and forbidden (VH) polarizations is displayed for two samples prepared under different annealing conditions. Complete spectra recorded at maxima and minima of VV scans are shown along with spectra of bulk Si for comparison.

scattered intensity (VV) of approximately a factor of 2 is expected due to penetration of the probe light into the bulk Si substrate in the regions between the buried tungsten fingers. In these regions scattering is collected from an entire absorption depth (0.75 µm), while only the 0.3-µm-thick CVD layer contributes to the scattering from the regions over the tungsten. In addition to this effect, spatial variation in the orientational texture of the crystallites contributes to the spatial variation of the depolarization ratio, and spatial variation of the crystallite size contributes to the variation of both the depolarization and the overall signal intensity because the linewidth associated with small crystallites becomes broader than the 10-cm^{-1} spectrometer bandpass used in the measurements. The large ratio of allowed to forbidden scattering in the regions over the Si substrate for sample B2 indicates relatively complete recrystallization of the CVD Si. The ratio of allowed to forbidden scattering is greater at the peaks than at the valleys, indicating that the material over the deposited tungsten has a more polycrystalline texture than that over the Si. The small overall ratio of allowed to forbidden scattering for sample A2 indicates that the recrystallization to single crystal texture is not as complete as for B2 and, again, the material over the tungsten is less crystalline than that over the Si. These observations are supported by the spectra, displayed at the bottom of the figure, which show generally broader linewidths for sample A2 than for B2 and, in each case, broader linewidths over the buried tungsten fingers than over the Si substrate.

SURFACE MORPHOLOGY

The intensity of the Raman scattered radiation from a particular material is proportional to the Raman scattering cross section, the temperature dependent phonon population, the scattering volume, and the magnitude of the incident electric field within the medium. Changes in the scattered Raman intensity from a particular material are usually interpreted as due to changes in the temperature or volume of the scattering medium. However, we have observed anomalously large Raman signals from several Si samples that cannot be explained by changes in the volume or temperature of the Si. The enhanced scattering appears to be associated with a roughened surface morphology having a submicrometer spatial scale. This enhancement must be taken into account in interpreting the results of Raman studies of device structures.

One example of enhanced Raman intensity is the increase in the integrated intensity of the Raman scattered radiation observed at the edges of the structures in the SOS and SOQ devices, as seen for the SOS stripe in Fig. 2. Additional measurements have shown that the increased Raman intensity at the edges is accompanied by decreases in the incident laser radiation reflected from the sample and in that transmitted through the substrate. Observation of these effects in both the elastic and inelastic scattering at the edges of the SOI strips depends critically upon the focus adjustment of the microscope objective, which has a depth of field of < 2 µm. This finding is consistent with the enhancement being localized at the sharp edge of the structure, so that as the scattering area increases, the enhanced signal from the edge becomes less significant relative to the normal scattering from the bulk material of much greater volume. As can be seen in the SEM micrograph (Fig. 7) of a 6-µm-wide SOS stripe, the ion etch technique used to pattern the stripe resulted in a roughened Si edge.

Similar enhancements have been observed in a number of other samples which exhibit roughness on a spatial scale of 0.1 to 0.2 µm, comparable to that at the edges of the stripe in Fig. 7. The spectra from these samples were generally undistorted, i.e., the linewidth and shift of the optical phonon agree closely with that observed in bulk Si, but observed signals were as much as a factor of 10 greater than those observed from bulk Si under identical experimental conditions. Actual enhancements are larger, however, depending on the

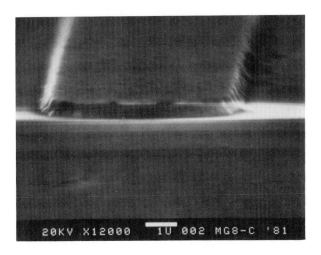

Fig. 7. SEM micrograph showing edge view of 6-μm-wide SOS stripe patterned by CIE technique.

volume of the roughened Si responsible for the increased scattering. For example, Fig. 8 shows a SEM micrograph of 0.1 to 0.2-μm diameter Si spheroids formed on a fused quartz substrate by strip-heater annealing a 50-nm thick CVD Si film. The signal observed from this sample was 10 times that from bulk Si in which the absorption depth is 0.75 μm, so the enhancement in Raman signal normalized to scattering volume is on the order of 100. The enhancements appear to be associated only with three-dimensional structures; no significant enhancements (> 2) were observed in the thin film measurements.

There are two major differences between this enhanced scattering and that observed in the case of surface enhanced Raman scattering (SERS) from molecules adsorbed on roughened metallic surfaces [26]. Firstly, Raman scattering from Si is a bulk effect so that the entire Si volume, not just a thin surface layer, contributes to the Raman signal; and secondly, Si exhibits dielectric optical properties in the visible. Therefore, the large field enhancements associated with localized dipolar plasmon resonances in metallic structures with dimensions much less than a wavelength are not a factor in the present measurements. Because of the high refractive index of Si, the 0.1-μm-diameter spheroids seen in Fig. 8 correspond to about a wavelength in the medium. Possibly, the observed enhancements are due to excitation of internal cavity-like resonances in the Si spheroids. Electromagnetic structure resonances of this type are well documented theoretically and experimentally for both elastic and inelastic scattering from low index dielectrics [27,28]. Detailed Mie scattering calculations are required to verify the possibility of similar resonances in a high index, lossy dielectric like Si.

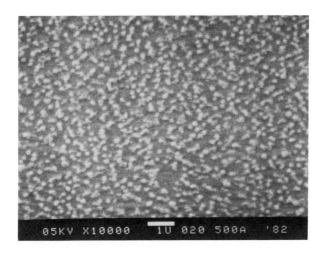

Fig. 8. SEM micrograph of Si spheroids of 0.1 to 0.2 µm diameter on a fused quartz substrate.

SUMMARY

Several applications of Raman scattering to the characterization of solid-state materials and devices have been presented. These examples demonstrate the utility of optical techniques in the non-destructive probing of local material properties such as strain and degree of crystallinity with a spatial resolution of ~ 1 µm. Quantitative information about the residual strain in the SOI materials can be obtained directly from the shift in optical phonon energy; no such quantitative connection has been clearly established between crystallite size and the position and shape of the phonon line observed in the Raman spectra of polycrystalline films. Results of measurements on thin Si films have been presented and suggest that the effect of finite crystallite size alone cannot adequately explain the observed effects. Nonetheless, Raman spectroscopy is still useful as a qualitative probe of crystallite size. Finally, examples have been presented of textured Si surfaces from which unusually large Raman signals have been observed. The enhancement appears to be associated with submicrometer roughness in the Si and may be due to electromagnetic structure resonances in the roughened Si. To our knowledge, this is the first observation of a morphology-induced enhancement of inelastic scattering from a semiconductor.

ACKNOWLEDGMENT

We wish to acknowledge M. W. Geis, D. D. Rathman, D. J. Silversmith, B-Y. Tsaur, J. C. C. Fan and T. F. Deutsch for supplying many of the samples used in these measurements, and for numerous helpful discussions. We also wish to acknowledge P. M. Nitishin for the SEM micrographs.

REFERENCES

1. J. C. C. Fan, M. W. Geis and B-Y. Tsaur, Appl. Phys. Lett. 38, 365 (1981).

2. E. W. Maby, M. W. Geis, Y.-L. LeCoz, D. J. Silversmith, R. W. Mountain and D. A. Antoniadis, IEEE Electron Device Lett. EDL-2, 241 (1981).

3. J. Hynecek, J. Appl. Phys. 45, 2631 (1974).

4. H. Schlotterer, Solid State Electron. 11, 947 (1968).

5. B-Y. Tsaur, J. C. C. Fan and M. W. Geis, Appl. Phys. Lett. 40, 322 (1982).

6. I. I. Novak, V. V. Baptizmanskii and L. V. Zhosa, Opt. Spectrosc. (USSR) 43, 145 (1977).

7. Th. Englert, G. Arbstreiter and J. Pontcharra, Solid State Electron. 23, 31 (1980).

8. G. A. Sai-Halasz, F. F. Fang, T. O. Sedgwick and A. Segmuller, Appl. Phys. Lett. 36, 419 (1980).

9. Y. Kobayashi, M. Nakamura and T. Suzuki, Appl. Phys. Lett. 40, 1040 (1982).

10. R. J. Nemanich and D. Haneman, Appl. Phys. Lett. 40, 785 (1982).

11. S. R. J. Brueck, B-Y. Tsaur, John C. C. Fan, D. V. Murphy, T. F. Deutsch and D. J. Silversmith, Appl. Phys. Lett. 40, 895 (1982).

12. In the coplanar process, active Si islands are masked with Si_3N_4 and the unutilized Si is oxidized, in steam, to the Al_2O_3 substrate. Subsequently, the exposed oxide is wet-etched to the level of the Si islands and the Si_3N_4 mask is stripped.

13. A. C. Ipri, in Silicon Integrated Circuits, Part A Supplement 2, Applied Solid State Science, D. Kahng, editor (Academic Press, New York, 1981), p. 253.

14. T. Kamiya, M. Kishi, A. Ushirokawa and T. Katoda, Appl. Phys. Lett. 38, 377 (1981).

15. Z. Iqbal, A. P. Webb and S. Veprek, Appl. Phys. Lett. 36, 163 (1980).

16. R. P. Salathe, H. P. Weber and G. Badertscher, Phys. Lett. 80A, 65 (1980).

17. Z. Iqbal, S. Veprek, A. P. Webb and P. Capezutto, Solid State Commun. 37, 993 (1981).

18. J. F. Morhange, G. Kanellis and M. Balkanski, Solid State Commun. 31, 805 (1979).

19. F.-A. Sarott, Z. Iqbal and S. Veprek, Solid State Commun. 42, 465 (1982).

20. S. Nakashima, S. Oima and A. Mitsuishi, Solid State Commun. 40, 765 (1981).

21. G. Kanellis, J. F. Morhange and M. Balkanski, Phys. Rev. B 21, 1543 (1980).

22. B. F. Levine, C. G. Bethea, A. R. Tretola and M. Korngor, Appl. Phys. Lett. 37, 595 (1980).

23. D. E. Aspnes and J. B. Theeten, Phys. Rev. Lett. 43, 1046 (1979).

24. F. A. Ponce, Appl. Phys. Lett. 41, 371 (1982).

25. R. Ruppin and R. Englman, Rep. Prog. Phys. 33, 149 (1970).

26. See, for example, Surface Enhanced Raman Scattering, edited by R. K. Chang and T. E. Furtak, (Plenum Press, New York, 1982).

27. A. Ashkin and J. M. Dziedzic, Phys. Rev. Lett. 38, 1351 (1977).

28. R. E. Benner, P. W. Barber, J. F. Owen and R. K. Chang, Phys. Rev. Lett. 44, 475 (1980).

RAMAN SCATTERING AS A TEMPERATURE PROBE FOR LASER HEATING OF Si

DIMITRY KIRILLOV AND JAMES L. MERZ
Department of Electrical & Computer Engineering, University of California, Santa Barbara, CA 93106

ABSTRACT

The frequency of the phonon line in the Raman scattering spectrum recorded during CW laser-beam heating of Si was used as a characteristic of the lattice temperature inside the laser spot. It is shown that Raman scattering is a good temperature probe up to the laser power approaching optical damage of Si.

INTRODUCTION

Laser beam processing and annealing of electronic materials has promising industrial applications. There is a number of works dedicated to calculations of the temperature at the surface of Si illuminated by a focused laser beam (see for example [1-5]), and the calculations are usually used for evaluation of the temperature in the region of the laser beam in experiments on laser annealing. These evaluations are in principle very approximate for a variety of reasons: the thermal conductivity of amorphous Si and its temperature dependence are unknown (consequently, calculations are done for the case of crystalline Si), the nonlinear optical properties of Si at high pumping are also unknown, as is the electronic contribution to the thermal conductivity within the laser spot due to photoexcited carriers [5]. As a result of these uncertainties, it is very important that actual measurements of the lattice temperature be made of the laser-heated material. However, experimental temperature measurements are difficult, due to the very small volume of heated material. Measurements of the lattice temperature utilizing the temperature dependence of the reflectivity (see for example [6]) have problems with accuracy because of the low sensitivity of reflectivity to temperature, the unknown dependence of the reflectivity on the concentration of photo-excited carriers (which may be large), and the complicated character of the processes occuring at the surface during laser beam heating. Ordinary pyrometric measurements of the temperature of semiconductors [7] are usually incorrect because of the difference between the ideal black-body radiation spectrum assumed and the actual spectrum of a heated and/or optically-excited semiconductor. On the other hand, spectroscopic measurement of the temperature of laser-heated semiconductors using laser-excited luminescence or Raman scattering is a more direct and more precise method, particularly for laser power below the damage threshold. The lattice temperature may be deduced from the spectra. In the present work we applied Raman spectroscopy to measure the temperature of Si heated by a CW laser beam. In contrast with earlier work [8], we used the position and linewidth of the optical phonon as a probe of lattice temperature, and believe that the Stokes-Antistokes ratio is a less-reliable temperature indicator. We studied the simple case of CW laser-beam heating, allowing us to study the spectrum in detail at different laser powers.

Raman scattering may be effectively used to probe the quality of material subjected to laser annealing not only during annealing but also before and after annealing. We have applied Raman scattering to characterize laser-beam annealed Si samples after implantation by As ions.

Laser Beam Heating and Raman Spectra of Si

When photon energies exceed the band-gap, laser heating consists of the following stages. (1) Absorption of electromagnetic radiation and excitation of electrons and holes with high kinetic energy in the conduction and valence bands. (2) Relaxation of electrons with a correspnding transformation of the carrier's kinetic energy into phonons and heat. This process of heat generation is very fast, in the range of 10^{-12}-10^{-13}s, and in the case of the CW laser heating of Si, it may be considered to be instantaneous [5,9]. (3) Thermalized carriers in the bands may recombine with the emission of photons and phonons, or by means of Auger-type mechanisms for which the energy released by carrier recombination is transformed into kinetic energy of a free carrier in one of the bands. Auger processes are the principal source of heat generation in our case, limiting the photoexcited carrier density [9].

For strong laser pumping, a large number of photoexcited carriers are present. In the case of CW argon-laser pumping, the number of carriers may be as high as 10^{17} to 10^{19} cm^{-3}. These carriers contribute to the thermal conductivity within the laser spot, resulting in a more uniform spatial temperature distribution in the spot [5] than might be otherwise expected. The presence of photoexcited carriers can influence the Raman spectra of Si. It has been shown experimentally [10] that free carriers interact with optical phonons in Si through the deformation potential, and that this anharmonic interaction causes broadening of phonon lines and a small frequency shift. The broadening due to this interaction is of the order 2-6 cm^{-1} for carrier concentrations obtained by doping in the range of 10^{19} cm^{-3}. The resulting frequency shift is less than 2 cm^{-1} [10]. Another effect which appears at higher carrier concentrations (up to 10^{20} cm^{-3}) is Fano-type interference between light scattering by optic phonons and free carriers [11]. This interference may produce asymmetry in the phonon lineshape, the type of asymmetry being dependent upon the type of carriers primarily responsible for the interference [12].

The main influence on the Raman spectra is, of course, the heating of the lattice. High lattice temperature corresponds to a large number of excited phonons. These phonons interact with each other through anharmonic processes which cause the shift and broadening of phonon lines [13]. Raman scattering in Si probes long wavelength optical phonons at the Γ-point of the Brillouin zone. The major phonon processes contributing to the frequency shift include three-phonon and four-phonon processes, which may be approximated in our case by the decay of an optical phonon into two or three acoustic phonons. The acoustic phonons participating in the process are selected according to the momentum and energy conservation laws. Frequency shifts of phonons due to anharmonic interactions may be experimentally divided into two cases: (1) a shift due to the lattice expansion, and (2) a shift resulting even though the lattice volume remains constant. When the temperature dependence of the phonon frequency is known experimentally, as is the case for Si [14], the phonon frequency may be a good standard for lattice-temperature determination.

The processes which contribute to the Raman linewidth of Si may be approximately represented by the decay of the Γ-point optical phonons into two acoustic phonons with energy equal to one-half of that of the optical phonon and with opposite directions of momenta [14].

Experimental Results and Their Discussion

Radiation from the Spectra Physics model 171 argon ion laser was used to heat the sample, and at the same time to excite the Raman spectrum. The laser was operating in a multiline regime in the TEM$_{00}$ mode. The Raman spectrum excited by the 4880A line was measured. The spectrum was analyzed by a 1m McPherson spectrometer with 600 grooves/mm grating, working in second order, using photon-counting electronics and a cooled RCA 8852 photomultiplier. The slit-width was 100μm. A small Bausch and Lomb grating monochromator with a bandpass

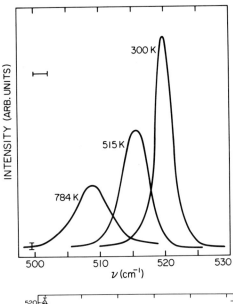

Fig. 1. Phonon lines in the Raman spectra of Si at different temperatures. Instrumental linewidth is shown. Low power excitation and oven heating were used.

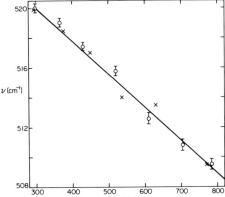

Fig. 2. Temperature dependence of the phonon frequency in Si. x: data of ref. [14], o: our data, continuous line: theory [15].

of ~200 cm^{-1} was used as a filter to isolate the spectral region including the Raman line from the background of elastic scattering. The Si sample was a Boron-doped plate of ~400μm thickness with (100) polished face and resistivity 10-20 ohm·cm. The radiation from the laser was focused on the surface of the sample at normal incidence; the focal length of the focussing lens was either 8.5 cm or 21 cm. Scattered light was collected at an angle of ~45° to the surface. In order to determine the dependence of the phonon frequency and linewidth on the lattice temperature we measured the Raman spectra using low power laser excitation (p~200mW) and heating the sample with an electrical oven. The resulting spectra are shown in Fig. 1 for three different temperatures. As can be seen, the phonon frequency decreases and the linewidth increases, as ex-

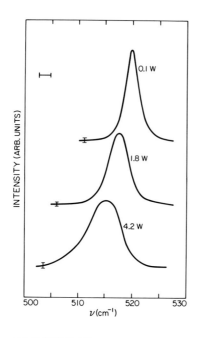

Fig. 3. Phonon lines in the Raman spectra of Si at different laser powers. The laser beam spot diameter at 1/e level is ~60μm.

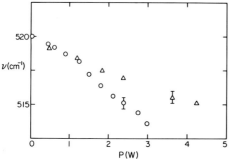

Fig. 4. Phonon frequency as a function of laser power. Δ: laser-beam spot diameter ~60μm. o: spot diameter ~34μm.

pected. The temperature dependence of the phonon frequency is given in Fig. 2. Theoretical dependence [15] and earlier experimental data [14] are shown together with our data. This figure represents our "calibration curve", and was used for determination of the lattice temperature from the value of the phonon frequency determined during laser heating. Phonon spectra for several values of laser power are shown in Fig. 3. In this case, a 21 cm focal-length lens was used to produce a ~60μm diameter spot (measured at the 1/e intensity level). The shift and broadening of the spectral lines caused by laser heating is clearly seen. The dependence of the phonon frequency as a function of incident laser power is shown in Fig. 4, for laser spot diameters 60μm (f = 21 cm lens) and 34μm (f = 8.5 cm lens). Corrections for the reflection coefficient of Si are not included. Measurements using the 60μm spot were limited by the avail-

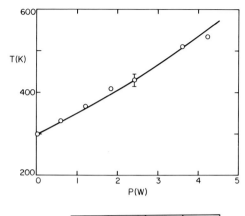

Fig. 5. Temperature in the central part of the laser spot as a function of laser power. Spot diameter ~60μ, at 1/e intensity level. o: experimental data, continuous line: dependence based on calculations [4].

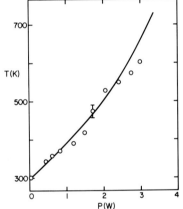

Fig. 6. Temperature in the central part of the laser spot as a function of laser power. Spot diameter ~34μm at 1/e intensity level. o: experimental data, continuous line: dependence based on calculations [4].

able laser power; in the case of the 34μm spot, optical damage occurs in the sample above 3W.

As we can see from Figs. 1 and 3, and from the data of Hart et al. [14], the linewidth of phonons observed during laser heating is slightly larger (~2-3 cm^{-1} at high temperature) than the linewidth produced by oven heating. Two possible mechanisms may be responsible for this extra broadening: non-uniform heating of the sample by the beam, and broadening due to phonon interactions with photo-excited carriers. In order to separate these contributions we compared spectral results obtained when (a) only the enlarged central region of the laser spot was projected onto the spectrometer entrance slit (Raman intensity reduced by factor ¼), or (b) the peripheral "colder" part of the spot, excluding the central part, was projected. We found no differences in the spectra, suggesting a rather uniform temperature profile across the laser spot. The strongest Raman scattering comes from the central (hottest) region of the beam. Furthermore, the phonon contribution to the thermal conductivity, and diffusion of photo-excited carriers, also contribute to the spreading of the heated region within the laser spot. Therefore, it is reasonable to assume that the phonon frequencies measured here allow us to determine temperatures which are close to the

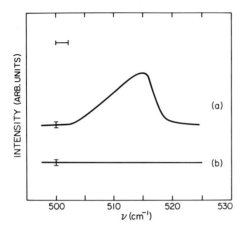

Fig. 7. Raman spectrum at laser power level close to the optical damage threshold (a) allowed $X(XY)\bar{Z}$ configuration (b) prohibited $Z(XX)\bar{Z}$ configuration.

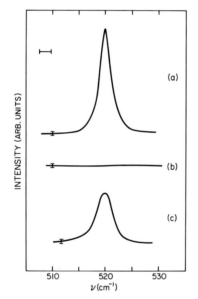

Fig. 8. Raman spectra of (a) virgin Si, (b) ion-implanted and unannealed Si and (c) ion-implanted and laser-annealed Si.

maximum temperatures in the spot, and that the extra broadening is caused by the high concentration of photoexcited carriers (of the order of 10^{18} cm^{-3}) [10].

The temperature in the central part of the laser spot were determined using the data of Fig. 2 and Fig. 4. The temperatures in the central part of the spot are given in Fig. 5 and Fig. 6 as functions of laser power, for two different spot diameters. Theoretical results are also shown, based on calculations of Ref. [4]. These results are similar to others [1-3], with the exception that they include both the temperature dependence of the thermal conductivity and the temperature dependence of the reflectivity of Si. There is good agreement between the calculated and experimental values, despite the fact that the electronic contribution to the thermal conductivity is not taken into account in references [1-4]. Because of the very small illuminated volume, and the low thermal conductivity outside of the spot, we believe that the photoexcited carriers are more effective in smoothing out the temperature distribution in the illuminated, highly-conductive spot than in decreasing the maximum temperature.

In the case of the 34μm diameter spot, optical damage occured for laser power ~3W. This power level (~1.9 kW/cm) corresponded to a temperature ~620K. It was impossible to record Raman spectra after the threshold for optical damage, due to a very high level of elastic scattering. More sophisticated experimental techniques are required to record Raman spectrum when the surface is damaged and/or unstable. The changes in the surface structure could be seen by changes in the interference pattern formed by elastically scattered light.

The determination of the temperature in the laser spot from the Raman spectra at a power level close to the damage threshold becomes difficult because of the highly nonlinear character of the processes taking place. The Raman spectrum of Si close to the optical damage threshold is shown in Fig. 7. Large bandwidth and strong asymmetry are characteristic for this spectrum. The strong asymmetry develops only at the power level close to the damage threshold. As can be seen from Fig. 7, selection rules for light scattering by optical phonons with F2g-type symmetry are well satisfied (e.g., the phonon line in the $Z(XX)\bar{Z}$ configuration is absent) which indicates that non-uniform thermal stresses distorting the crystalline symmetry in the central part of the spot are small. The origins of the line asymmetry are not clear at present. A possible explanation may be a Fano-type interference between light scattering by optically-excited free carriers and optical phonons [11,12]. The sharper cut off towards higher phonon energy probably corresponds to electron effects rather than hole effects.

In addition to these temperature measurements, we also used Raman spectroscopy to characterize CW laser-annealed Si samples. Boron doped Si (100) wafers with a resistivity of 10-20 Ωcm were implanted with As^+ ions at 100 keV to a dose of 4×10^{15} cm^{-2}, and subsequently annealed using a CW argon laser with ~60μm beam diameter, 6μm steps, and substrate temperature of 250°C [16]. The spectrum (a) in Fig. 8 corresponds to virgin Si. The absence of the Γ-point phonon in spectrum (b) shows that the ion-implanted and unannealed sample is completely amorphous. The spectrum of the laser-annealed sample (c) has a noticeably larger (by ~2 cm^{-1}) linewidth than the spectrum of the undoped sample (a). This increase in the linewidth may be explained by the increase in the free carrier concentration induced by implant-doping and subsequent laser annealing.

CONCLUSIONS

We have shown that the scattering of light by optical phonons may be successfully used as a temperature probe during the CW laser heating of Si. Spectra obtained at power levels close to the damage threshold require further study, but they may contain interesting information on the nature of the damage. Raman spectroscopy may in principle be used for studies of laser-beam heating of amorphous Si, although the spectrum of amorphous Si is more difficult to obtain.

ACKNOWLEDGEMENTS

The authors wish to thank Don Zak for technical assistance. This work was performed under Air Force Contract No. F19628-82-K-0006, ROME/RADC, Hanscom AFB, Mass.

REFERENCES

1. M. Lax, J. Appl. Phys. $\underline{48}$, 3919 (1977).
2. M. Lax, Appl. Phys. Lett. $\underline{33}$, 786 (1978).
3. Y.I. Nissim, A. Lietoila, R.B. Gold and J.F. Gibbons, J. Appl. Phys. $\underline{51}$, 274 (1980).
4. J.E. Moody and R.H. Hendel, J. Appl. Phys. $\underline{53}$, 4365 (1982).
5. J.Z. Wilcox, J. Appl. Phys. $\underline{51}$, 2866 (1980).
6. S.A. Kokorowski, G.L. Olson, J.A. Roth and L.D. Hess, in Laser and Electron-Beam Interactions with Solids, v. 4, ed. by B.R. Appleton and G.K. Celler (North-Holland, 1982), p. 195.
7. T.O. Sedgwick, in Laser and Electron-Beam Solid Interactions and Materials Processing, v. 1, ed. by J.F. Gibbons, L.D. Hess and T.W. Sigmon (North-Holland, 1981), p. 147.
8. A. Compaan, A. Aydinli, M.C. Lee and H.W. Lo, in Laser and Electron-Beam Interactions with Solids, v. 4, ed. by B.R. Appleton and G.K. Celler (North-Holland, 1982), p. 43. H.W. Lo and A. Compaan, Phys. Rev. Lett. $\underline{44}$, 1604 (1980).
9. W.P. Dumke, Phys. Lett. $\underline{78A}$, 477 (1980).
10. F. Cerdeira and M. Cardona, Phys. Rev. $\underline{B5}$, 1440 (1972).
11. F. Cerdeira, T.A. Fjeldly and M. Cardona, Phys. Rev. $\underline{B8}$, 4734 (1973).
12. M. Jouanne, R. Beserman, I. Ipatova and A. Subashiev, Solid State Comm. $\underline{16}$, 1047 (1975).
13. W. Cochran and R.A. Cowley, Handbook der Physik, XXV/2a (Spinger-Verlag, 1967).
14. T.R. Hart, R.L. Aggarwal and B. Lax, Phys. Rev. $\underline{B1}$, 638 (1970).
15. R.A. Cowley, J. Phys. (Paris) $\underline{26}$, 659 (1965).
16. N.H. Sheng and J.L. Merz, in Laser and Electron Beam Interactions with Solids, v. 4, ed. by B.R. Appleton and G.K. Celler (North-Holland, 1982), p. 313.

MEASUREMENT OF GRAIN BOUNDARY PARAMETERS BY LASER-SPOT PHOTOCONDUCTIVITY

E. POON, H.L. EVANS, W. HWANG, R.M. OSGOOD, JR. AND E.S. YANG
Department of Electrical Engineering, Columbia University, New York, NY 10027

ABSTRACT

An experimental technique has been developed to study the electrical properties of semiconductor grain boundaries (GBs) by a focused laser beam. The laser beam is trained on a GB while the photoconductivity of the sample is measured. Both the steady-state and transient signals are recorded as functions of temperature. From these data, we obtain well-defined GB parameters, including the barrier height, interface charge density, trap energy and thermal capture cross-section. This technique allows us to examine localized regions of individual GBs in a semiconductor with multiple grains.

INTRODUCTION

Electronic properties of polycrystalline silicon have been recently studied extensively because of their importance in the development of photovoltaic devices and integrated circuit technology. It appears that the grain boundary plays a key role in determining the operating characteristics of polycrystalline silicon devices.

Because of the changing structural properties along the GB between two adjacent grains [1], accurate measurement of GB parameters has not been possible. Present techniques such as capacitance and conductance measurement methods require large contact areas and can only yield average electrical parameters over the entire cross-sectional area. LBIC and EBIC methods require formation of p-n junctions, which is not desirable because high temperature process alters GB properties by causing segregation of oxygen impurity at the GB [2-3]. Here we introduce a method that allows convenient local probing of small regions in polycrystalline semiconductor, with only evaporation of ohmic contacts required for sample preparation. With this method, the influence on the GB of various steps in the device processing can be determined.

MATERIAL AND METHOD

The schematic diagram of the experimental setup is shown in Fig. 1. The chopped He-Ne laser beam is focused on a GB of a p-type Wacker polycrystalline silicon sample which rests on the x-y stage. The sample, with a doping concentration (N_a) of 2×10^{15} cm^{-3} and a dark resistance (R_S) of about 2 KΩ, is approximately 2 mm x 10 mm x 0.2 mm and contains two electrically active GBs that run across the whole width. The external d.c. bias (V_B) is kept constant throughout the experiment. A very large series load resistor ($R_L \gg R_S$) is used and V_B is adjusted so that the sample bias (V_S) is small compared with kT/q.

In the dark, those GB traps above the Fermi level are stripped of electrons. The positively charge GB repels holes in the neighboring grains, forming depletion layers around the GB and a potential barrier that impedes the flow of majority carriers.

Under illumination, the photogenerated electrons are captured by the GB traps. The GB becomes less positive and the barrier height is reduced, resulting in a decrease in sample resistance. Consequently, the voltage across the load resistor rises. When the laser beam is shut off, the process is reversed. Captured electrons are emitted to the conduction band by the GB traps and the signal decays. The chopping of the laser beam thus gives rise to a periodic photoconductance transient signal which is measured by a boxcar average in real time.

If the laser intensity is high enough to reach the flat-band condition, the amplitude of the signal (V_m) is given by [4]

$$V_m = \frac{V_B}{R_L} \cdot \frac{k}{qAA^*T} e^{\phi_b/kT} \qquad (1)$$

using a thermionic emission model.[5] Since the pre-exponential factor is not sensitive to the temperature in the logarithmic scale, the barrier height (ϕ_b) can be obtained from the slope of the semilog plot of V_m vs $1/T$. The density of the traps above the Fermi level is related to the diffusion potential (V_{do}) by

$$N_t = (8 \varepsilon N_a V_{do}/q)^{\frac{1}{2}} \qquad (2)$$

where

$$V_{do} = \phi_b - (kT/q)\ln(N_v/N_a) \qquad (3)$$

Using Shockley-Read-Hall statistics, the decay time constant (τ_d) is related to the electron emission rate (e_n) by

$$\tau_d = \frac{1}{e_n} = \frac{1}{\sigma_n V_{th} N_c} e^{(E_c-E_t)/kT} \qquad (4)$$

The energy of the trap (E_t) can be obtained from the slope of semilog plot of τ_d vs $1/T$. The electron thermal capture cross-section (σ_n) can then be deduced using Eq.(4).

RESULTS AND DISCUSSION

The position on the grain boundary is chosen such that the largest signal is obtained. R_L is 150 kΩ and V_B is set at 1.5 V. The laser intensity is estimated to be 12.7×10^2 mW/cm^2 (4×10^{18} photons/cm^2 - s) with a spot size of about 50 μm. The flat band condition is believed to be established at this intensity since the signal saturates.

Figure 2 shows the plot of the signal amplitude at peak intensity vs $1/T$. The barrier height of 0.37 eV is obtained. This is in the range determined by earlier experiments [6-7]. Using Eq.(2), the interface charge density above the Fermi level is found to be 1.25×10^{11} cm^{-2}.

Figure 3 shows a typical example of the decay. The line with shorter time constant is obtained by subtracting the line with longer time constant from the data. Since our present setup has limited resolution, our decay analysis is based on a dominant trap which has longer decay time constant. Figure 4 shows the plot of this decay time constant vs $1/T$. It gives a trap energy of 0.5 eV below the conduction band. This value is in remarkable agreement with the known energy level of oxygen impurity in silicon [8]. From Eq.(4), the electron thermal capture cross-section is found to be

2×10^{-16} cm^{-2} using $N_c = 10^{19}$ cm^{-3} and $V_{th} = 10^7$ cm/s.

CONCLUSION

The laser-spot photoconductivity experiment has been employed as a GB diagnostic tool. Under steady-state conditions, the GB barrier height has been determined from the temperature dependence of the photoconductance. From the photoconductivity transient response, we have obtained a trap energy of 0.5 eV and a capture cross-section of 2×10^{-16} cm^2. These preliminary data tend to support the model of oxygen segregation at the GB.

The method is simple and has good spatial resolution which is limited by the region activated by the focused laser beam. By observing the steady-state and transient response, we show for the first time that the photoconductance can be used to calculate some grain-boundary trapping states parameters in an unambiguous way.

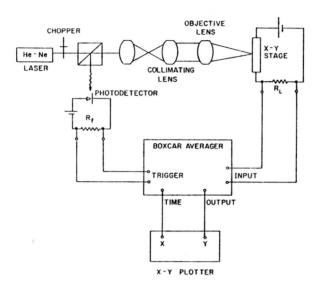

Fig. 1 Laser-spot photoconductivity experiment

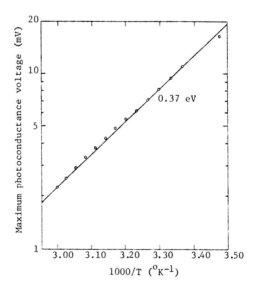

Fig. 2 Photoconductance signal amplitude vs temperature

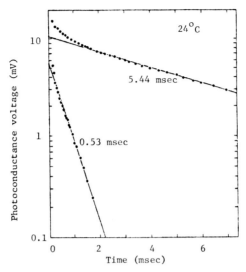

Fig. 3 Typical example of the decay

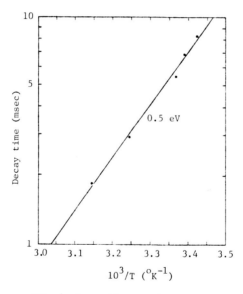

Fig. 4 Decay time constant vs temperature

ACKNOWLEDGEMENTS

The research is supported by SERI Contract #XW-1-1272-1 and JSEP Contract DAAG 29-79-C-0079.

REFERENCES

1. B. Cunningham and D.G. Ast in "Grain Boundaries in Semiconductors", Eds. H.J. Leamy, G.E. Pike and C.H. Seager, North-Holland, NY (1982).

2. D. Redfield, Appl. Phys. Lett. $\underline{40}$ 163 (1982).

3. K. Nagasawa, Y. Matsushita and Kishino, Appl. Phys. Lett. $\underline{37}$ 622 (1980).

4. E. Poon, E.S. Yang, H.L. Evans, W. Hwang and R.M. Osgood Jr., to be published.

5. M.L. Tarng, J. Appl. Phys. $\underline{49}$ 4069 (1978).

6. C.H. Seager, G.E. Pike and D.S. Ginley, Phys. Rev. Lett. $\underline{43}$ 532 (1979).

7. E.S. Yang, E.K. Poon, C.M. Wu, W. Hwang and H.C. Card, IEEE Trans. $\underline{ED-28}$ 1131 (1981).

8. J.W. Chen and A.G. Milnes, Ann. Rev. Material Sci. $\underline{10}$ 157 (1980).

HIGH RESOLUTION LASER DIAGNOSTICS FOR DIRECT GAP SEMICONDUCTOR MATERIALS

R.P. SALATHE and H.H. GILGEN,
Institute of Applied Physics, University of Berne, Sidlerstr. 5,
3012 Berne, Switzerland

ABSTRACT

The laser-induced luminescence of direct gap semiconductors can be measured with high spatial (1 μm) and temporal (< 1 ns) resolution. A profiling technique is described for in-situ measurements during laser processing. It allows the evaluation of temperature, carrier density and band gap energy within the focal zone. The technique has been applied to (Al,Ga)As heterostructure material subjected to highly focused cw-Kr-ion laser radiation. The measurements reveal low temperature rises (<200 deg.C) at high excitation densities (>1MW/cm^2) and an inhomogeneous distribution of optically excited carriers for concentrations above $2 \cdot 10^{17}$ cm^{-3}.

INTRODUCTION

Most direct gap semiconductors exhibit efficient radiative transitions between states located near the conduction and valence band edges. This luminescence property can be used to diagnose defects and material modifications introduced during material processing. Photoluminescence [1,2] or cathodoluminescence [3] mapping techniques allow spatial localization of defects and from spectroscopic investigations [4] the energy levels involved can be evaluated. Here, we discuss the possibilities of measuring the laser induced luminescence during processing of direct gap semiconductors. In contrast to Raman measurements [5,6], in-situ luminescence measurements do not require photon counting techniques, because of the much higher transition probabilities involved. The band gap energy and the temperature within the laser heated zone can be evaluated from luminescence spectra. The distribution of the optically excited carriers is obtained from luminescence profiles. The techniques have been applied to well focused Kr-ion laser radiation in (Al,Ga)As. The results indicate a surprisingly low temperature rise and a nonuniform carrier distribution at high excitation densities.

EXPERIMENTAL ARRANGEMENT

A treelayer structure of $Al_xGa_{1-x}As$ grown by liquid phase epitaxy on GaAs [7] has been used in the experiments. Fig. 1 shows schematically a cross-section (top) and the energy diagram of the conduction band edge (bottom). The 647.1 nm laser light is absorbed in the $Al_{0.22}Ga_{0.78}As$ layer (no 2) and to some extend also in the GaAs substrate. The absorbing layer is sandwiched between two transparent $Al_{0.6}Ga_{0.4}As$ layers. It has a thickness of 1 μm. This value is much smaller than typical carrier or thermal diffusion lengths [8,9]. Temperature variations along the optical axis can be neglected within this layer. The layers were doped with Ge at a concentration of $3 \cdot 10^{17}$ cm^{-3}. The top layer (no 1) protects the absorbing layer and eliminates nonradiative carrier recombination at the surface. This improves the luminescence efficiency of the second layer. A microscope objective with a numerical aperture of 0.95 has been used for focusing. The resulting diameter of the laser focus is below 1 μm. Such small focal diameters are essential if high carrier concentrations have to be generated under cw excitation. In large excitation zones the carrier concentration would be limited to $1-2 \cdot 10^{18}$ cm^{-3} because of a reduction in carrier lifetime due to stimulated emission.

The experimental arrangement is shown schematically in Fig. 2. A Kr-ion laser (Spectra Physics Model 171-7) operating at 647 nm in the TEM$_{00}$ mode with an electrooptical feedback system for noise reduction was used in the experiments. The laser beam is focused by means of a microscope objective L1 (100x, f = 2.09 mm) into the second layer of the sample S. A beamsplitter (BS) and a lens L2 are used to direct the photoluminescence collected by the microscope objective onto an infrared sensitive vidicon camera (VC)(Philips XQ 1176) and on a 1/2 m double monochromator (DM). The luminescence mapping system is protected from reflected laser light by an IR transmission filters F1 (Schott RG 715). The mapping system is used to control the focal length by minimizing the radius of the luminescence pattern. A slit of 25 μm at the entrance of the spectrometer discriminates spatially against the luminescence from less heated regions. A diffraction limited resolution of 0.6 μm within the second layer was obtained with the spectral system. The lens L2 was mounted on a translation stage. Profiles of luminescence light were recorded by moving L2 perpendicularly to the optical axis and the slit of the spectrometer. The light was detected at the exit of the spectro-

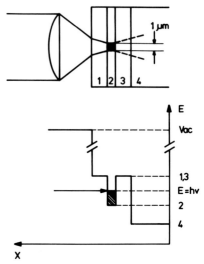

Fig.1: Schematic cross-section of (Al,Ga)As sample (top) and bandgap energy E vs. distance x (bottom). The layers are:
1: 3 μm Al$_{0.6}$Ga$_{0.4}$As
2: 1 μm Al$_{0.22}$Ga$_{0.78}$As
3: 3 μm Al$_{0.6}$Ga$_{0.4}$As
4: ~100 μm GaAs (substrate).

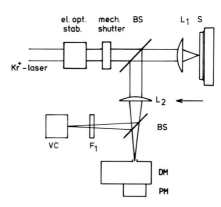

Fig.2: Experimental Arrangement. S:sample; L1,2:lenses; BS:beamsplitters; F1:IR-filter; VC:vidicon; DM:double monochromator PM:photomultiplier.

RESULTS AND DISCUSSION

Fig. 3 shows two luminescence spectra on a logarithmic intensity scale. The spectra have been recorded at laser powers of 0.5 and 15 mW. The corresponding power densities impinging on the sample are 50 kW/cm^2 and 1.5 MW/cm^2, respectively. As indicated in the 0.5 mW spectra, the band-to-band recombination and the band-to-acceptor level recombination peaks cannot be separated. A pronounced band tailing is observed on the low energy side. The intensity on the high energy side is $I(E) \propto E^2 \exp((E-E_g)/kT_e)$, with T_e the temperature of the electrons [10]. Evaluation of the electron temperature from the slope on the high energy side results in temperatures of 300°K at 0.5 mW and 470°K at 15 mW irradiation power. An average energy relaxation time of $\sim 4 \cdot 10^{-14}$ s is estimated from Hall mobility measurements performed at 300-400°K in identically doped samples with similar composition [12]. This is two orders of magnitude lower than measured relaxation times in GaAs at 80°K [13]. We therefore assume that the electron temperature does not deviate significantly from the lattice temperature T_ℓ for our experimental conditions. If this assumption would be invalid our temperature measurement can be interpreted as an upper limit of the actual lattice temperature. The temperature of 170°C for the high

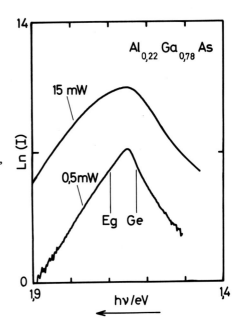

Fig.3: Luminescence spectra recorded at 0.5 and 15 mW excitation power. Position of bandgap E_g at 300°K and Ge-acceptor level is also shown.

excitation condition is 40 per cent below the temperature rise estimated with the approximation of Lax [14]. The discrepancy is due to neglection of carrier diffusion out of the laser focus. This effect becomes important for very small focal radii [15]. The temperature induced shift of the band gap ΔE_{th} can be calculated with the Varshini equation [16]. A value of $\Delta E_{th} = -70$ meV is expected for the focal zone. A much larger shift of $\Delta E \approx -130$ meV is seen on the low energy side of the spectra in Fig. 3. The additional shift, $\Delta E_{pl} \approx -60$ meV, is attributed to a band gap shrinkage introduced by the high carrier density. Values of $\Delta E_{pl} = 28 - 35$ meV at $n = p = 10^{18}$ cm^{-3} have been reported for GaAs excited under pulsed conditions at T = 2°K [17,18]. Since this shrinkage scales with $n^{1/3}$ a carrier density of $8 \cdot 10^{18}$ cm^{-3} would be expected in our case. As discussed below such densities can be expected from the luminescence profile and decay time measurements.

Fig. 4 shows the luminescence measured at various wavelengths as a function of position x on the substrate. The spectral resolution is ~ 0.5 Å. A laser power density of 50 kW/cm^2, corresponding to the "low" excitation conditions in Fig. 3, has been used for excitation. The profiles have been normalized to approximately the same peak intensity. The 1/e-width of these profiles is indicated by slim lines. The average width is 5.3 μm. Deviations from this value are less than 5 %. The corresponding width of the laser focus (0.9 μm) has been evaluated from the measured beam divergency and is shown for comparison. The increased width of the luminescence profiles is due to carrier diffusion. As shown in Fig. 4, the diffusion does not depend on the energy of the optically excited carriers. The recombination time of the carriers has been measured with a mode-locked Dye laser system as a function of excitation density. At 50 kW/cm^2 we measured 2 ns on a sample with identic composition and doping conditions. Based on these luminescence profile and decay time measurement, we evaluate a carrier density of $1.4 \cdot 10^{17}$ cm^{-3}. This is a factor of 2 below the p-type carrier concentration.

Normalized luminescence profiles obtained at an excitation density of 1.5 MW/cm^2 are shown in Fig. 5. Compared to the low excitation measurement, the 1/e-widths are considerably reduced. This decrease can be explained by a reduced

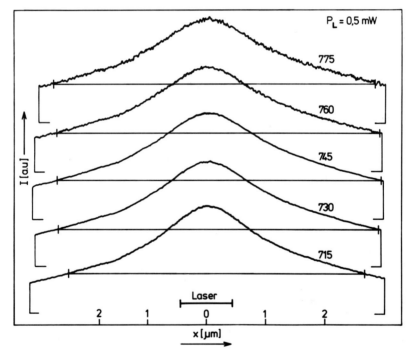

Fig.4: Normalized luminescence profiles recorded within the focal zone at an excitation density of 50 kW/cm^2. Number indicates wavelenghts in nm.

diffusion length due to a reduction in carrier liefetime (c.f. below) and to the transition from minority carrier diffusion to ambipolar diffusion. In Fig.5, different 1/e-widths of the profiles are measured at different wavelengths. This indicates that the spatial distribution of electrons and holes depend on the carrier energy. The largest extension (3.6 μm) is measured at wavelengths of 735 - 755 nm, i.e. for carriers in the vicinity of the parabolic band edges. At the high and low energy side of the luminescence spectrum the widths decrease monotonically to 1.5 μm at 1.9 eV (655 nm) and to 1.7 μm on the low energy side (1.64 eV, 775 nm). We attribute these additional decreases to two different mechanisms: At the high energy side intraband scattering into the L band minima plays an important role. The L band minima in $Al_{0.22}Ga_{0.78}As$ are located at 1.773 eV (700 nm) at 470 °K [19]. we estimate that 50 per cent of the carriers with an energy of 1.9 eV are within the L-band minima. The mobility here, μ_L, is decreased with respect to μ_Γ by a factor of 7 at 470°K [19,20]. This yields a reduction factor in diffusion lengths of $(0.5+3.5)^{1/2} = 2$. The decrease on the low energy side can be explained by the temperature and carrier induced shrinkage of the band gap. This effect is most pronounced in the center of the focus and decreases with increasing distance from the center. The band edges form depressions which tend to confine the carriers with low energy. The luminescence decay time measurements described before yielded a decay time of ~ 1 nsec for this high excitation conditions. With an averaged width of 3.3 μm from the profiles with the highest intensity we evaluate carrier densities of $n = p = 6 \cdot 10^{18}$ cm^{-3}. As discussed, such densities can only be achieved under cw conditions in very small focal diameters.

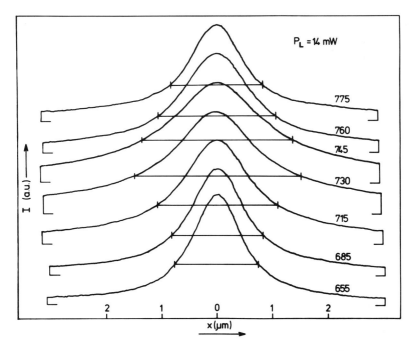

Fig.5: Same as Fig.4 but for a excitation density of 1.5 MW/cm².

Irreversible material modifications are observed if the layers are exposed to irradiation densities >0.5 MW/cm^2 [20, 21]. They are characterized by a sudden decrease in luminescence efficiency which indicate the appearance of recombination centers. These centers are nonradiative under laser processing conditions. They exhibit, however, efficient radiative transitions below the band gap at low excitation densities. Fig. 6 shows a micrograph of the photoluminescence of the second layer measured after proprocessing with the IR-vidicon camera. An excitation density of ~1 kW/cm^2 has been used for this measurement. The radiative recombination centers created in the focal zone increase the total luminescence efficiency and the irradiated zone appears as bright spot.

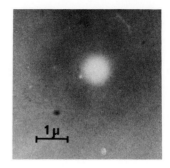

Fig.6: Photoluminescence micrograph of processed zone.

The new recombination center cause local changes in the carrier density. Fig. 7 shows two luminescence profiles recorded at λ = 785 nm under the same condition as with Fig. 4. The profile a) has been recorded before, b) after exposure to 1.6 MW/cm^2 for ~30 seconds. The generation of efficient recombination center within the laser focus is manifested by a decrease in halfwidths from 4.2 to 0.6 μm. The halfwidth measured after processing corresponds to the resolution limit of the optical system. SEM measurements on cleaved and etched (110) planes indicate that the processed zone is ~ 0.5 μm wide. The

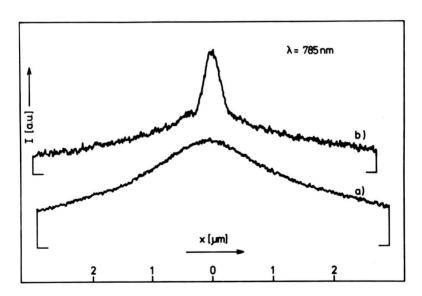

Fig.7: Luminescence profile recorded before (a) and after (b) processing.

luminescence emitted from these centers can be described by a configuration-coordinate model. From an analysis of the luminescence data, it has been speculated that the centers consist of an Al vacany complex comprising more than two lattice sites [22]. Time resolved luminescence measurement indicate that the formation of these centers occurs in two steps involving the formation of nonradiative centers by recombination or stress enhanced diffusion mechanisms at the beginning of irradiation and the generation of the luminescence center with a nonlinear process after a "latent" time of several seconds [23]. The second mechanism is related to the high carrier density generated within the laser focus. Speculations on the nature of this nonthermal process, e.g. mechanical stress [24], carrier instability or phonon assisted mechanisms [23], could not yet been confirmed experimentally.

ACKNOWLEDGEMENTS

The authors are grateful to Prof. H.P. Weber for the opportunity to perform this work and to Drs. F.K. Reinhart and R.A. Logan, Bell Telephone Laboratories, Murray Hill N.J., for providing the (Al,Ga)As double heterostructure material. They also acknowledge B. Zysset for supplying computer programs and B. Wicki for technical assistance.

REFERENCES

[1] W.D. Johnston and R.A. Logan,
Appl. Phys. Lett. 28(3), 140 (1976)

[2] C.H. Henry and R.A. Logan,
J. Appl. Phys. 48(9), 3962 (1977)

[3] P.M. Petroff, D.V. Lang, J.L. Strudel, and R.A. Logan,
in "Scanning Electron Microscopy" (SEM Inc. AMF, O'Mare,
IL, 1978), Vol. 1, p. 235

[4] see, e.g., E.W. Williams and H.B. Bebb,
in "Semiconductors and Semimetals ", edited by
R.K. Willardson and A.C. Beer (Academic Press, New York,
1972) Vol. 8, Chap. 5

[5] R.F. Wood and C.E. Giles,
Phys. Rev., B 23, 2923 (1981)

[6] D. Kirillov and J.L. Merz,
paper I3.2, this conference

[7] R.A. Logan and F.K. Reinhart,
J. Appl. Phys., Vol. 44, pp. 4172 - 4176, 1973

[8] See, e.g., A.M. Sekala, D.L. Feucht, and A.G. Milnes, in
GaAs and Related Compounds, 1976, London: Institute of
Physics Conf. Series no. 33a, 1977, p. 245

[9] M.A. Afromowitz, J. Appl. Phys., Vol. 44, pp. 1292 - 1294, 1973

[10] A. Mooradian and H.Y. Fan,
Phys. Rev. 148, 873 (1966)

[11] A. Chandra and L.F. Eastman,
J. Appl. Phys. 51, 2669, 1980

[12] S. Zukotynski, S. Sumski, M.B. Panish, and H.C. Casey, Jr., J. Appl. Phys. 50, 5795 (1979)

[13] C.V. Shank, R.L. Fork, R.F. Leheny, and J. Shah,
Phys. Rev. Lett 42, 112, 1979

[14] M. Lax, J. Appl. Phys. 48, 3919, 1977

[15] To be published

[16] Y.P. Varshini, Physica (Utrecht) 34, 149 (1967)

[17] O. Hildebrand, E.O. Goebel, K.M. Romanek, H. Weber, and G. Mahler,
Phys. Rev. B17, 4775 (1978)

[18] J. Shah, R.F. Leheny, and W. Wiegmann,
Phys. Rev. B16, 1577 (1977)

[19] H.J. Lee, L.Y. Juravel, and J.C. Wolley,
Phys. Rev. B21, 659 (1981)

[20] H.H. Gilgen, R.P. Salathé, and Y. Rytz-Froidevaux,
Appl. Phys. Lett. 38, 241 (1981)

[21] R.P. Salathé, H.H. Gilgen, and Y. Rytz-Froidevaux,
IEEE J. Quant. Electron, QE-17, 1989 (1981)

[22] B. Zysset, R.P. Salathé, and H.H. Gilgen
To be publ. Appl. Phys. Lett. 42, Jan 83

[23] R.P. Salathé, H.H. Gilgen, and B. Zysset,
in Proc. of the 12th Int. Conf. on Defects in Semiconductor, Amsterdam 1982 to be publ. in Physica B, North Holland 1982

[24] J.A. Van Vechten, ibid.

SECTION IV
PHOTOFORMATION OF INSULATORS

LASER PHOTOLYTIC DEPOSITION OF THIN FILMS[†]

P. K. BOYER, C. A. MOORE, R. SOLANKI,[*] W. K. RITCHIE,[+] G. A. ROCHE[**] AND GEORGE J. COLLINS
Department of Electrical Engineering, Colorado State University, Fort Collins, CO 80523

ABSTRACT

An excimer laser is used to photochemically deposit thin films of silicon dioxide, silicon nitride, aluminum oxide, and zinc oxide at low temperatures (100-350°C). Deposition rates in excess of 3000 Å/min and conformal coverage over vertical walled steps were demonstrated. The films exhibit low defect density and high breakdown voltage and have been characterized using IR spectrophotometry, AES, and C-V analysis. Device compatibility has been studied by using photodeposited films as interlayer dielectrics, diffusion masks, and passivation layers in production CMOS devices.

Additionally, we have deposited metallic films of Al, Mo, W, and Cr over large (>5 cm^2) areas using UV photodissociation of trimethylaluminum and the refractory metal hexacarbonyls. Both shiny metallic films as well as black particulate films were obtained depending on the deposition geometry. The black films are shown to grow in columnar grains. The depositions were made at room temperature over pyrex and quartz plates as well as silicon wafers. We have examined the resistivity, adhesion, stress and step coverage of these films. The films exhibited resistivities at most $\sim$20 times that of the bulk materials and tensile stress no higher than 7×10^9 dynes/cm^2

INTRODUCTION

There exists a need for low-temperature semiconductor fabrication processes to minimize wafer warpage, dopant redistribution, and defect generation and propagation [1]. Moreover, film deposition over photoresist for applications such as tri-level resists for high-resolution lithography and direct patterning via lift-off is desired at temperatures below $\sim$200°C (above which resist degradation occurs) [2]. In this work we discuss a new low temperature, high deposition rate (up to 5000 Å/min) film growth technique which uses a excimer laser to photolyze gas-phase reactants whose products condense and form the desired film. This technique has been used to deposit dielectric films of SiO_2, Si_3N_4, Al_2O_3 and ZnO, and conducting films of Al, Cr, Mo, and W. The properties of these films are reviewed and compared to conventional deposition techniques.

[†]This work supported by the Office of Naval Research.
[+]NCR Microelectronics, Fort Collins, CO 80526
[*]Present Address: Johns Hopkins University, Department of Physics, Baltimore, MD 21218.
[**]Present address: Thermco Inc., Orange, CA 92668.

EXPERIMENTAL APPARATUS

A Lumonics 860T excimer laser provides ultraviolet photons in a beam of rectangular cross-section which is down-collimated to a cross-sectional area of 12 x 1.5 mm for parallel deposition, as shown in Figure 1, or is expanded

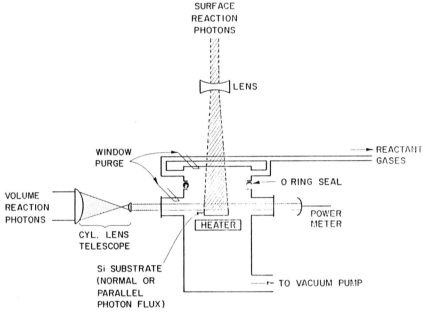

Fig. 1. Experimental Set-up.

using a negative lens to deposit over large areas during normal irradiation. The insulating films in this work were deposited using a wavelength of 193 nm (ArF* transition) while the metallic films were deposited using either a 193 nm or the 248 nm (KrF*) wavelength; repetition rate for each wavelength was 90-100 Hz. UV transmitting windows were purged with a rare gas to prevent deposition on them. Surface reaction photons, whose role is described herein, were provided by a low pressure mercury lamp or by folding back the portion of the beam transmitted through the cell. A substrate heater capable of heating up to 500°C was used during the deposition of dielectric films.

A major advantage of this experimental scheme is the ability to vary laser power, wavelength, and spatial location independently while not affecting the deposition process. This is in direct contrast to plasma-enhanced CVD where process parameters are strongly interrelated and one is limited to pressure regimes where a discharge can be started and maintained. The only pressure constraint on the laser CVD technique is that the gases used for a given deposition must be at optically thin concentrations. Thus beam attenuation across a sample is minimized and thickness uniformity is preserved. For example, deposition of SiO_2 is possible at total pressures up to 8 Torr since the beam intensity will vary by less than 10% across a 3 inch wafer at this pressure.

Additionally, conformal step coverage is possible by this technique due to the photodissociation volume being an "infinite plane source" with respect to topographical features on the sample. This is demonstrated herein.

DEPOSITION OF OXIDE AND NITRIDE FILMS

Films of SiO_2, Si_3N_4, Al_2O_3 and ZnO have been deposited via the following reactions, respectively:

$$SiH_4 + N_2O + h\nu(193 \text{ nm}) \rightarrow SiO_2 + \text{products} \qquad (1)$$

$$SiH_4 + NH_3 + h\nu(193 \text{ nm}) \rightarrow Si_xN_y + \text{products} \qquad (2)$$

$$Al(CH_3)_3 + N_2O + h\nu(193 \text{ nm}) \rightarrow Al_2O_3 + \text{products} \qquad (3)$$

$$Zn(CH_3)_2 + NO_2 + h\nu(193 \text{ nm}) \rightarrow ZnO + \text{products} \qquad (4)$$

The silicon-compound insulator films are compared to the competitive low-temperature deposition schemes of plasma-enhanced and mercury photosensitized CVD, while the metal oxides are discussed on the basis of their properties alone.

Typical deposition conditions for deposition of SiO_2 are shown in Table Ia. A relatively high reactant gas ratio N_2O/SiH_4 was used in this work.

TABLE I
Typical Deposition Conditions

	Laser	RF Plasma[1]	Hg Photox
a) SiO_2			
Substrate temperature	150–400°C	380°F	100–200°C
Cell pressure	6 Torr	1.1 Torr	0.3–1 Torr
N_2O/SiH_4	73	33	25
Deposition rate	600 Å/min (He buffer)	300 Å/min	120 Å/min
	800 Å/min (N_2 buffer)		
b) Si_3N_4	Laser	RF Plasma[1]	Hg Photride
Substrate temperature	200–425°C	380°C	150–200°C
Cell pressure	2 Torr	2 Torr	4 Torr
NH_3/SiH_4	1	7	30
	10 SCCM NH_3		
	10 SCCM SiH_4		
	50 SCCM N_2		
Deposition rate	700 Å/min	350 Å/min	65 Å/min
c) Al_2O_3	Laser	RF Planar Magnetron[2]	
Substrate temperature	100–400°C	150–400°C	
Cell pressure	1 Torr	10^{-2} Torr	
Deposition rate	1500 Å/min	350 Å/min	
	(up to 1μ/min)		

[1] Reactor manufactured by ASM, Phoenix, AZ.
[2] R. S. Nowicki, J. Vac. Sci. Tech. **14**(1), 127 (1977).

Deposition rates (which are for films of area $\sim$20 cm^2) could be increased using a higher silane density since this reactant is optically transparent at 193 nm. Deposition rates of $\sim$5000 Å/min have been observed over areas of $\sim$3 cm^2.

The electrical, chemical and physical properties of the laser CVD SiO_2 films have been measured. The films are comparable to plasma and photosensitized CVD films with respect to adhesion, stress, index of refraction stoichiometry, and hydrogen incorporation as shown in Table II. The laser deposited films are

TABLE II
Comparison of Deposited SiO_2 Films

	Laser CVD	Plasma	Hg Photox
Breakdown voltage (MV/cm)	6.5-8 (1000 Å film)	10 (2000 Å)	4-8 (1000-10,000 Å)
Resistivity (Ω-cm) at 5 MV/cm	up to 6.7×10^{13}	10^{16}	2×10^{12}
Stoichiometry	SiO_2	SiO_2	$SiO_{1.9}$
H content (by IR) as Si-H (at.%) as Si-OH	1-4 <1	<4 <1	None None
Etch Rate in 5:1 BHF	>55	22 (7:1 BHF)	140
Refractive index	1.48	1.49	1.46
Stress on Si (10^9 dyne/cm^2) (all compressive)	1.5	3.6	2

inferior compared to plasma-enhanced CVD films in terms of electrical resistivity (∼100 times lower), dielectric strength (20% lower breakdown voltage), and etch rate in a buffered oxide etch (∼2 x faster). Laser CVD films exhibited the lowest internal stress and pinhole densities. A 1000 Å SiO_2 film photodeposited at 400°C had no pinholes in 5 cm^2, while a 2000 Å plasma CVD film showed <1/cm^2 and a 10,000 Å photox SiO_2 film had 5 to 10 per square centimeter. In the laser CVD approach conformal step coverage is achieved over a wide range of deposition conditions. Figure 2 shows SiO_2 (∼5000 Å thick) photodeposited over a 4000 Å polysilicon step which was formed on a oxidized silicon wafer. It should be noted the rough surface atop the step is due to the underlying poly-Si while the even morphology of the oxide is retained below the step, over smooth oxidized Si wafer.

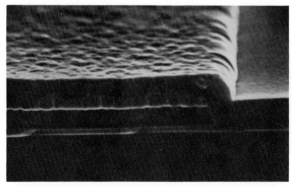

Fig. 2. Step Coverage of SiO_2 over 4000 Å Polysilicon Step.

Silicon nitride has also been deposited using laser-induced CVD using the reaction in equation (2). The conditions for deposition are similar to the two techniques under comparison and to those of the SiO_2 deposition process discussed above (Table Ib). A notable difference is that lower concentrations of ammonia are required since its absorption cross-section is $\sim 10^3$ higher than nitrous oxide at 193 nm [3]. Deposition rate is still much higher than that of plasma or mercury sensitized reactions.

Again the photodeposited films have comparable physical properties (i.e. adhesion, compressive stress, refractive index, step coverage and stoichiometry) as shown in Table III. Pinhole densities are comparable to plasma CVD films

TABLE III
Comparison of Deposited Silicon Nitride Films

	Laser CVD	Plasma	Hg Photride
Stoichiometry	<SiN	>SiN	Variable
Impurities (at. %)			
H by IR-as Si-H	12	12-16	-----
as N-H	11-20	2-7	<"typical plasma"
O by ESCA	<5	----	-----
Etch rate (Å/sec) in 5:1 BOE	15 (dep. at 425°C)	1.7 (7:1 BOE)	12
No surface photons	44 (dep. at 380°C)	----	-----
254 nm photons	27	----	-----
193 nm photons	8	----	-----

but superior to photride films. The laser CVD films lack in terms of etch rates; they etch approximately ten times faster than plasma deposited nitrides. However, at the bottom of Table III the effect of low level surface irradiation can be seen. As deposited at 380°C, the laser CVD silicon nitride films etched at 44 Å/sec in 5:1 buffered oxide etch, indicative of a porous or low density film. Illumination during deposition with 254 nm photons from a low pressure mercury discharge lamp reduced this etch rate to 27 Å/sec. This etch rate was reduced further to 8 Å/sec by folding back the transmitted portion of the 193 nm dissociating laser beam. The power density of both on the substrate surface was weak so as not to cause surface heating. Clearly, a surface reaction is occuring but has not been modeled at this time.

Using this technique, oxides of aluminim and zinc have been deposited but are not as fully characterized at this time. Conditions for Al_2O_3 growth are tabulated in Table Ic. As compared to films obtained by RF plasma deposition, the laser CVD Al_2O_3 films shown comparable adhesion, stress, stoichiometry, and refractive index. As with the silicon compounds discussed previously, the photodeposited films show higher etch rate (x 10) but have a low pinhole density (none in 5 cm^2 for an 1100 Å laser CVD film versus 36/cm^2 for a 2500 Å plasma deposited film). The only other major difference known presently is that the photodeposited films have shown up to 1% carbon contamination, probably due to dissociation of methyls in the aluminum donor gas. The effect of this impurity on the electrical properties is not known at this time.

To obtain ZnO, an oxygen donor, either NO_2 or N_2O was introduced into the cell together with dimethylzinc (DMZ). At 248 nm laser wavelength (KrF) and using N_2O as the oxygen donor, clear films of ZnO were obtained but at a very slow deposition rate (5000 Å/min) was obtained with NO_2 irradiated at 193 nm. Best results with respect to both the deposition rate and stoichiometry of the films were obtained with NO_2 flow rate of 34 sccm and DMZ pressure of 30 mTorr. The He window purge flow rate was 100 sccm. An automatic throttling valve maintained the total cell pressure at 2 Torr. The substrate temperatures ranged from room temperature to a maximum of 220°C.

The deposited ZnO films appeared clear. Uniform films over 2 cm x 5 cm area were obtained at deposition rates of over 5000 Å/min. The difference in thickness over 5 cm (end to end) was less than 5%. It should be pointed out that the uniformity of the deposited ZnO films is important for fabrication of surface acoustic wave (SAW) devices [4]. At higher deposition rates ($\sim$1 μ/min) the films had a tendency to peel when exposed to atmospheric pressure and were nonuniform.

The stoichiometry of the deposited film, by ESAC, showed the films to be composed of 49% Zn and 51% oxygen. Carbon was less than 1% and there was no measureable trace of N. By increasing the ratios of DMZ to NO_2 flows, ZnO stoichiometry was easily changed causing the measured sheet resistivities to range from 10^3 to 10^{-1} ohms/square for 0.5μ thick films. The refractive index of the stoichiometric film, deposited at 200°C was measured on an ellipsometer to be 1.86. The index of refraction increased with the abundance of Zn in the film and with higher deposition temperatures as expected.

When the film adhesion was measured, in all cases the Si substrates cracked ($\sim 10^7$ dynes/cm^2) before the ZnO films could be detached. The stress of the photodeposited ZnO film was determined by the x-ray technique. The stress of a 2000 Å thick ZnO film on a Si wafer was $7 \times 10^{+9}$ dynes/cm^2, tensile. The etch rate in 5:1 buffered oxide etch (BOE) of ZnO deposited at 200°C was found to be <20 Å/min. The pinhole density of 1000 Å thick film of ZnO deposited at 180°C was measured on a Gasonics pinhole monitor to be <1 cm^2.

DEPOSITION OF METALS

We have previously reported laser-induced deposition of refractory metals over small areas (10^{-4} cm^2) [5]. As an extension of our earlier work we have investigated large area (>5 cm^2) photodeposition of Al, Mo, W and Cr. Uniform films of these metals were deposited on pyrex and quartz substrates as well as silicon wafers at room temperature. We have examined the resistivity, adhesion, stress, and step coverage of these films.

Plasma assisted CVD of refractory metals occurs as low as 350°C (nm/min deposition rates) for refractory halides [6] but plasma parameters such as rf power and frequency, gas flow, electrode spacing, total pressure and substrate heating are all interrelated and difficult to control individually. Photodissociation occurs only along the path of the laser beam, unlike plasma excitation, therefore there is less impurity generation from the walls due to plasma ion bombardment. Moreover, the cracking pattern is less complex in photodissociation and hence we have better control and repeatibility of deposition conditions.

Our experimental arrangement is shown in Figure 1. All substrates were precleaned in HF and deionized water prior to deposition. The substrates were held either parallel or normal to the incident laser beam. Either a reservoir containing the carbonyl or a flask of trimethylaluminum (TMA) was connected to the cell. For the carbonyls, both the reservoir and the pyrex connecting tube were heated with a heater tape to about 50°C.

The substrate was first placed into its holder and the cell pumped down with a roughing pump to a few microns. The laser then irradiated the substrate to preclean the surface with the UV radiation; this improves the adhesion of the deposited films. The vacuum pump was then throttled to reduce the cell throughput and the donor gas introduced into the cell. The deposited films appeared as bright silvery films. When the beam was parallel to the substrate, black particulate films of columnar growth resulted, as shown in Figure 3. For this reason, all the films characterized were obtained at

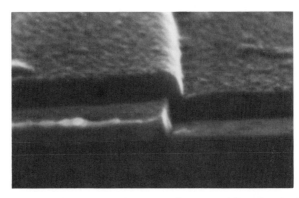

Fig. 3. Columnar Grain Growth of Chromium Film. Magnification is 20,000X.

normal incidence. Thick (>1 μ) Cr and Mo films deposited at room temperature had a tendency to peel when exposed to air. This could be avoided by heating the substrate to about 150°C during deposition or prior to removal from the cell. All the photodeposited films discussed below were obtained at room temperature.

The purity of the photodeposited films was examined by Auger and ESCA analysis. The major impurity in all the films was oxygen (<7%) probably due to the relatively poor vacuum obtained with a roughing pump. We hope to reduce this impurity by using a improved deposition cell and a better vacuum system. A surprising result was the relatively low concentration of carbon in these films (Table IV). The most carbon-free films and the highest deposition rates were obtained using a laser wavelength of 248 nm; 0.25, 0.17, 0.10 and 0.2 μ/min deposition rates were measured for Mo, W, Al and Cr, respectively, over 2.5 x 2.5 cm area. But even this low contamination by carbon can limit the obtainable film resistivity [7]. These rates will vary with the laser power, the cell pressure, and the size of the area over which the film is deposited. The film over the 2.5 x 2.5 cm area was uniform to ±15%. It should be pointed out that the area of deposition can be varied by changing the divergence of the laser beam with a lens; with tight focusing and substrate or beam translation, patterned lines can be deposited.

The adhesion of the photodeposited films was measured. In the case of W, the machine reached its upper limit without detaching the films, while in the case of Al, Mo and Cr, the quartz substrates chipped off before the films were detached. Of the four metals, Cr films were the least adhesive while W were the best, which remained intact even when placed in an ultrasonic cleaner. The most adhesive films were deposited using the 193 nm laser wavelength for photodissociation. The reasons for the change of carbon content and adhesion with the laser wavelength are not fully understood at this time. Stress measurements of the photodeposited films were made by the substrate bending technique. The metal films were deposited on microscope cover slips and the bowing caused by the films was measured. All the films had tensile stress and none was higher than 7×10^9 dynes/cm^2).

The electrical resistivities of the deposited metal films were measured with a four-point probe. These resistivities are tabulated along with the bulk values in Table IV. These resistivities are at most about a factor of 20 higher than bulk resistivity values, while the aluminum had, even with its high carbon content, a resistivity approaching the bulk value.

TABLE IV
Summary of the Physical Properties of the Laser Deposited Al, Mo, W and Cr Films

	Deposition Rate (Å/min)	Resistivity ($\mu\Omega$-cm) bulk	film	Percent Carbon in Film	Adhesion, on quartz (dynes/cm^2)	Tensile Stress (dynes/cm^2)
Mo	2500	5.2	36	<0.9	>5.5 x 10^8	<3 x 10^9
W	1700	5.65	135	<0.7	>6.5 x 10^8	<2 x 10^9
Cr	2000	12.9	210	<0.8	>5.4 x 10^8	<7 x 10^9
Al	1000	2.66	3.0	<4.0	>5.5 x 10^8	<1 x 10^9

One important quality of a film deposition technique is the ability of the deposited film to cover vertical-walled steps. Step coverage patterns used to check our deposited refractory films were the same as those used to examine SiO$_2$ step coverage. The photodeposited refractory metal thicknesses were varied between 0.2 and 0.6μ. After deposition, the metal coated wafers were chilled in liquid nitrogen and then cleaved. The step coverage was examined with a SEM An ∼5000 Å Al film is shown in Figure 4. It can be seen that the film is of

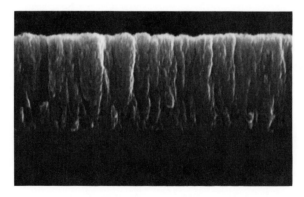

Fig. 4. Step Coverage of 5000 Å Aluminum Film Over 4000 Å Polysilicon Step.

even thickness over the flat, as well as the vertical walls, and clearly demonstrates conformal step coverage. The vertical striations in the films are due to wafer cleaving. It is interesting to note that SEM examination of all our films showed absence of microstructures similar to those seen in laser photodeposited Cd and Zn films [8].

SUMMARY

We have described a technique to deposit oxide, nitride, and metal films via ultraviolet photolysis of gas-phase donor molecules. All films are deposited at fast rates (up to 5000 Å/min) and demonstrate conformal step coverage over vertical steps. The insulating films exhibit low pinhole densities but are inferior in terms of etch rate and electrical resistivity. Surface photon impingement during film deposition is shown to drastically reduce silicon nitride etch rate. Future work will focus in this area. Metallic films have been deposited and exhibit good physical properties. The refractory metals show high resistivities which may be limited by carbon incorporation. The effect of annealing these films has not been studied yet.

REFERENCES

1. S. Su, Solid State Technology 24, 72 (1981).

2. M. P. Lepselter and W. T. Lynch, in VLSI Electronics Microstructure Science, edited by N.G. Einspruch (Academic, New York, 1971) p. 87.

3. J. Zavelovich, M. Rothschild, W. Gornik, and C. K. Rhodes, J. Chem. Phys. 74(12), 15 June 1981, and M. Ashford, M. T. Macpherson, and J. P. Simons, in Topics in Current Chemistry, Vol. 86, (Springer-Verlag, Berlin, 1979) p. 22.

4. J. E. Bowers, R. L. Thornton, B. T. Khuri-Yakub, R. L. Junemian, and G. S. Kino, Appl. Phys. Lett. 41, 805 (1982).

5. R. Solanki, P. K. Boyer, J. E. Mahan, and G. J. Collins, Appl. Phys. Lett. 38, 572 (1981).

6. J. K. Chu, C. C. Tang, and D. W. Hess, Appl. Phys. Lett. 41, 75 (1982).

7. L. H. Kaplan and F. M. D'Heurle, J. Electrochem. Soc. 117, 693, (1970).

8. R. M. Osgood and D. J. Ehrlich, Opt. Lett. 7, 385 (1982).

UV LASER-INITIATED FORMATION OF Si_3N_4*

T. F. DEUTSCH, D. J. SILVERSMITH, AND R. W. MOUNTAIN
Lincoln Laboratory, Massachusetts Institute of Technology
Lexington, Massachusetts 02173

ABSTRACT

Si_3N_4 films have been deposited on Si by using 193 nm ArF excimer laser radiation to initiate the reaction of SiH_4 and NH_3 at substrate temperatures between 200–600°C. Stoichiometric films having physical and optical properties comparable to those produced using low-pressure chemical vapor deposition (LPCVD) have been produced. The dielectric properties of the films are at present inferior to those of LPCVD material.

INTRODUCTION

The use of UV radiation to initiate photolytic reactions which deposit compound films at lower substrate temperatures than used with conventional chemical vapor deposition (CVD) has recently been investigated. Lamp sources have been used to deposit SiO_2, Si_3N_4 and other compounds on a variety of substrates [1,2]. More recently ArF excimer laser radiation has been used to deposit SiO_2 and Si_3N_4 on Si substrates [3,4]. The ArF laser source is able to provide several watts of power at 193 nm and thus makes possible higher growth rates than can be obtained with lamp sources.

Such low-temperature deposition has several advantages for semiconductor processing. It reduces unwanted diffusion or chemical reactions on a semiconductor wafer. Furthermore, it can make it possible to deposit films on compound semiconductors, such as GaAs and InP, that would dissociate at the temperatures required for conventional CVD.

This work is concerned with evaluating the physical and electrical properties of silicon nitride grown by UV laser-initiated deposition. An ArF excimer laser was used to initiate the reaction of SiH_4 and N_2O to form Si_3N_4.

While SiH_4 has negligible linear absorption at 193 nm, it can be dissociated by multiphoton processes at relatively low powers (< 10 MW/cm^2) [5]. NH_3 is strongly absorbing at 193 nm; we have measured an absorption coefficient of 0.32 cm^{-1} $Torr^{-1}$. The 193 nm photodissociation of NH_3 has been examined and the primary photoproduct is ground state NH_2, formed with nearly unit efficiency [6]. The chemistry of the laser deposition process remains to be examined.

EXPERIMENTAL

Figure 1 shows a schematic diagram of the deposition system. The ArF excimer laser was operated at 4 Hz and produced 10-nsec-long pulses of ~ 60 mJ energy. A 40-cm focal length BaF_2 cylindrical lens was used to focus the beam to a slit image ~ 2 cm wide and ~ 1 mm high. The beam passed less than 1 mm above the substrate used for deposition. The deposition chamber was a stainless-steel cross capable of accepting 2" diameter Si wafers and heating them to 600°C. The Si wafers were mounted on a stainless-steel pedestal, which also served to keep the heater element outside the deposition chamber. The gases used in

---

*This work was sponsored by the Department of the Air Force, in part under a specific program sponsored by the Air Force Office of Scientific Research, by the Defense Advanced Research Projects Agency, and by the Army Research Office.

Mat. Res. Soc. Symp. Proc. Vol. 17 (1983) ©Elsevier Science Publishing Co., Inc.

the deposition were introduced into the chamber by an injector ring located above the sample; a similar ring served as a pump-out port. In addition, an Ar gas purge was directed at the entrance and exit windows to minimize deposition upon them. Electronic grade NH_3 and SiH_4 (10% SiH_4 in Ar) were used as reagent gases. Ultrapure, carrier grade, Ar (> 99.999% pure) was used for the window purge. Mass flow controllers were used to obtain typical gas flows of 11 SCCM NH_3, 8 SCCM 10% SiH_4 in Ar, and 50 - 100 SCCM Ar purge gas. A mechanical pump was used to maintain a chamber pressure ~ 7 Torr.

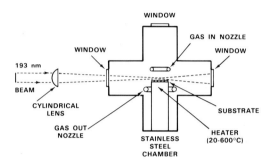

Fig. 1. Schematic diagram of UV laser-induced film deposition system.

Measurements of film thickness and refractive index were made using an automatic ellipsometer. Composition profiles were obtained using both Auger electron spectroscopy (AES) and secondary ion mass spectroscopy (SIMS), the latter technique being useful for the detection of minor impurities. Infrared transmission measurements were made on films deposited on ZnSe substrates which are essentially free of absorption in the region 2.5-20 µm. The dielectric properties of the nitride were evaluated by performing capacitance-voltage (C-V) measurements on capacitors made by evaporating an Al film onto nitride films deposited on n-Si (n = 3 x 10^{15} cm^{-3}) substrates and photolithographically patterning it into dots (A = 9.1 x 10^{-3} cm^2). The Al film was subsequently sintered at 400°C (15 min in N_2). The high-frequency C-V measurements were made using an HP 4061A automated test system. Films of silicon nitride grown by low-pressure chemical vapor deposition (LPCVD) at 780°C using SiH_2Cl_2:NH_3 (1:3) were used as comparison standards for measurements of etch rate, refractive index, and dielectric properties.

RESULTS

Depositions were generally made on 2" diamter Si wafers at temperatures between 200 and 600°C. The deposition rate using an average 193 nm laser power of 0.2 W was ~ 50 Å/min over ~ 7.5 cm^2 and was independent of temperature in the range 200 - 600°C. Since the rate is proportional to laser power, a more significant figure of merit is the efficiency of the process. We define this as the number of Si_3N_4 molecules deposited on the substrate, obtained from measurements of film area and thickness, per incident photon. The measured efficiency is ~ 4 x 10^{-3}; since the gas mixture is chosen to be optically thin in order to obtain uniform films, the efficiency in terms of photons absorbed is of the order of 1%.

Figure 2 shows a scanning electron microscope (SEM) micrograph of a nitride film ~ 1000 Å thick deposited on a Si substrate which had a 5000 Å high SiO_2 line pattern on the surface. The deposition is conformal over the steps; the surface morphology is somewhat textured. By contrast, a sample of material deposited by plasma-enhanced CVD showed no surface texture at all when examined under similar conditions. Note that the surface texture is not present in the underlying SiO_2 steps.

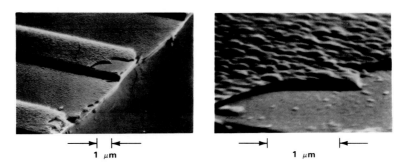

Fig. 2. SEM micrographs of laser-deposited Si_3N_4 (600°C) over 5000 Å SiO_2 steps.

Table I shows the dependence of refractive index and etch rate on $SiH_4:NH_3$ ratio and substrate temperature. $SiH_4:NH_3$ ratios from 1:3 to 1:14 were examined; at a deposition temperature of 600°C the refractive index varied from ~ 2.2 for the 1:3 mixes to 1.97 for the 1:14 ones. At lower deposition temperatures the refractive index decreased. The etch rate in 1:1 $BHF:H_2O$ for 600°C depositions compares favorably with the etch rate of 12 Å/min obtained on 780°C LPCVD material. For lower deposition temperatures the etch rate increases rapidly. The increase in etch rate is due to at least two factors, a decreased density, as indicated by the lower index, and increased chemical impurities in the low-temperature material.

Recent measurements of the hydrogen content of a variety of plasma-deposited and LPCVD nitrides using nuclear reaction analysis have shown a correlation of etch rate with hydrogen content for etch rates varying over three orders of magnitude [7]. This study also showed a systematic increase in hydrogen content with decreasing deposition temperature for plasma-deposited nitride. In addition, SIMS analysis of the hydrogen content of LPCVD material and 600°C laser-deposited material showed approximately 5 to 10 times more hydrogen in the laser-deposited material. This suggests that at least part of the reason for the increase in etch rate with decreased deposition temperature is increased hydrogen incorporation.

Infrared absorption spectra were obtained for films deposited at 300 and 600°C. The 600°C deposition (950 Å thick) showed only the broad absorption band at 850 cm^{-1} characteristic of pure Si_3N_4 [8]. The 300°C deposition (2100 Å thick) showed the same 850 cm^{-1} band, but in addition showed absorption bands at 1150, 2130, and 3330 cm^{-1}. The latter two absorption bands can be assigned to Si-H and N-H bonds respectively [9]. The 1150 cm^{-1} absorption band has not been assigned. It should be pointed out that the 1080 cm^{-1} band characteristic of Si-O bonds is not observed.

TABLE I
Properties of laser-deposited Si_3N_4 films as a function of substrate temperature and $SiH_4:NH_3$ ratio

Substrate Temperature (°C)	$SiH_4:NH_3$ Ratio	Refractive Index	Etch Rate (Å/min) 1:1 BHF*:H_2O
600	1:4	2.21	50
500	1:4	2.10	130
400	1:4	1.9-2.2	3200
780 (LPCVD)		2.003	12
600	1:14	2.00	90
505	1:14	1.93	380
400	1:14	1.94	5500
310	1:14	1.90	----

*1 vol. HF (49%) - 5 vol. NH_4F (40%)

Figure 3 shows compositional profiles for both LPCVD and 600°C laser nitride films as obtained by AES. The LPCVD material shows some oxygen at the interface. This was somewhat unexpected, since the native oxide is stripped from the Si by an HF etch before deposition. On examination of the LPCVD process, however, we found that the wafer is loaded into a hot furnace under normal atmospheric conditions, allowing the reformation of surface oxide. Subsequent ellipsometric measurements indicated that the oxide was ~ 15 Å thick. The laser nitride composition profile is similar, except that some oxygen is found throughout the material.

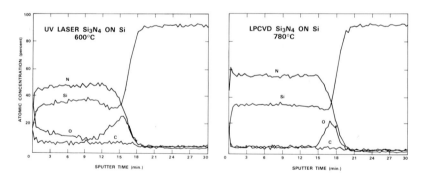

Fig. 3. Composition profiles of Si_3N_4 films prepared by laser-induced depositions and LPCVD as obtained by Auger electron spectroscopy.

The results of C-V measurements on nitride deposited at 305 and 600°C are shown in Table II. In order to determine the role of the initial surface conditions on the dielectric properties of the material, two different treatments were used. In one case the native oxide was removed by an HF etch just before loading the sample into the deposition chamber; in the other ~ 15 Å of oxide were grown on the wafer. The latter condition simulated the surface oxide grown on wafers during the initial portion of the LPCVD process, as discussed above. As the table shows, there is no correlation between either flatband voltage, V_{FB}, or interface state density, Q_s, and either substrate temperature or initial surface condition. For comparison, C-V measurements on LPCVD material show $V_{FB} = 0 - 1$ V and $Qs = 1 - 5 \times 10^{11}$ cm^{-2}. The large flatband voltage indicates a high density of fixed charge in the dielectric [10,11].

TABLE II
Dielectric properties of laser-deposited Si_3N_4 films as a function of substrate temperature and surface condition

Substrate Temperature (°C)	Surface Condition	V_{FB} (V)	Q_s (cm^{-2})
305	15 Å SiO_2	-28.0	5.5×10^{12}
305	SiO_2 Stripped	-27.0	5.5×10^{12}
600	15 Å SiO_2	-24.5	7.1×10^{12}
600	SiO_2 Stripped	-29.7	6.7×10^{12}

The effect of a 900°C, 15 min anneal in H_2 was also examined by fabricating capacitors on both annealed and unannealed halves of the same wafer; no effect was found. In order to examine the possibility that the large flatband voltage shift might be due to traps generated by scattered UV light, a number of LPCVD nitride films were placed in the deposition chamber and exposed to the same conditions as during a normal deposition, except that the reagent gases were not present. Capacitors were then fabricated from the films and C-V measurements performed. No difference between the C-V characteristics of these capacitors and those fabricated from unirradiated material was found. The SIMS measurements, in addition to showing a higher level of hydrogen in the laser-deposited nitride than in LPCVD material, also indicated a mass 23 (Na) level in the 600° laser film at least ten times that in LPCVD material. The Na was concentrated at the $Si-Si_3N_4$ interface. These results suggest that impurities such as Na may be responsible for the high levels of fixed charge observed in the material.

Measurements of breakdown strength, made using an I-V curve tracer, gave breakdown values of 3.5 - 5 MV/cm for deposition temperatures of 500 and 600 °C.

CONCLUSIONS

UV laser-initiated deposition of Si_3N_4 films has a quantum efficiency of ~ 0.4% and can be used to produce films at temperatures lower than those used in LPCVD. The stoichiometry and physical properties of films can be comparable to those of LPCVD films; the dielectric properties of the material are not adequate for device purposes. The films may be useful for low-temperature encapsulation of devices.

ACKNOWLEDGMENTS

We would like to thank J. Burke for his careful experimental work, S. Bailey for the C-V measurements, M. Finn for many AES spectra, P. Nitishin for SEM photos and G. Ramseyer of Cornell University for SIMS measurements. We gratefully acknowledge helpful discussions with D. Rathman and A. Strauss.

REFERENCES

1. H. M. Kim, S. S. Tai, S. L. Groves, and K. L. Schuegraf, in Proceedings of the Eighth International Conference on Chemical Vapor Deposition, (Electrochemical Society, Pennington, New Jersey, 1981), Vol. 81-7 p. 258.

2. J. W. Peters, in Technical Digest of the International Electron Devices Meeting 1981, (Institute of Electrical and Electronics Engineers, New York, New York, 1981), p. 240.

3. P. K. Boyer, G. A. Roche, W. H. Ritchie, and G. J. Collins, Appl. Phys. Lett. 40, 716 (1982).

4. G. A. Roche, P. K. Boyer, and G. J. Collins, Technical Digest of the Conference on Laser and Electro-Optics, CLEO '82, (Optical Society of America, Washington, D.C., 1982), p. 20, paper WE-2.

5. R. W. Andreatta, C. C. Abele, J. F. Osmundsen, J. G. Eden, D. Lubben, and J. E. Greene, Appl. Phys. Lett. 40, 183 (1982).

6. V. M. Donnelly, A. P. Baronauski, and J. R. McDonald, Chem. Phys. 43, 271 (1979).

7. R. Chow, W. A. Lanford, W. Ke-Ming, and R. S. Rosler, J. Appl. Phys. 53, 5630 (1982).

8. J. Wong, J. Electron. Mater. 5, 113 (1975).

9. W. A. Pliskin, J. Vac. Sci. Technol. 14, 1064 (1977).

10. P. V. Grey, Proc. IEEE 57, 1543 (1969).

11. E. H. Nicollian and J. R. Brews, MOS (Metal Oxide Semiconductor) Physics and Technology (John Wiley & Sons, New York, 1982).

EVIDENCE FOR LASER INDUCED SURFACE SILANOL FORMATION

D. F. MULLER,[+] M. ROTHSCHILD,[++] AND C. K. RHODES
Department of Physics, University of Illinois at Chicago, Chicago, Illinois 60680

ABSTRACT

Evidence for the selective formation of surface silanol induced by ultraviolet irradiation in the intensity range between 3×10^7 W/cm^2 and 10^8 W/cm^2 is presented. Enhanced metallic deposition (Ti) on appropriately prepared samples is also reported.

INTRODUCTION

Photolithography is an attractive process for the fabrication of submicron architectures on condensed matter substrates. Nevertheless, a major problem in photolithographic patterning arises from the lack of adequate control of the properties of adhesion of most common photoresists. Although line definition on the submicron scale can be achieved, considerable damage to the pattern, especially in the case of submicron islands, often occurs upon separation of the substrate and the resist. Blurring and even complete removal of the desired pattern can result.

It has been suggested [1] that this problem of pattern degradation could be substantially reduced by the use of an appropriate photoresist in combination with silicon prepared with a high density of surface silanol (SiOH). The photoresist would be designed in such a manner as to make it chemically reactive with the silanol, the net result being a chemical bond between the resist and the silicon surface. After processing, the silanol surface can be easily removed, enabling a simple separation of the pattern and resist faithfully preserving the detail of the pattern.

The present study was undertaken to determine the feasibility of selective laser controlled formation of surface silanol. In addition, an attempt was made to determine the reactivity of the silanol using several hygroscopic organometallic reagents. In the performance of these studies a possible alternative method for site selective metal vapor deposition has been demonstrated.

EXPERIMENTAL PROCEDURES

The silicon used was single crystal (100) Cz-silicon $\sim$ 2 mil thick and irradiation of the samples was accomplished with a focussed excimer laser (Lambda Physik EMG-101) operating in the unstable resonator configuration. The laser intensity was varied over the range of 3×10^7 W/cm^2 to 1×10^8 W/cm^2 in a pulse of $\sim$ 10-15 nsec duration through adjustment of the focus of the laser beam. Although irradiation was performed at 353 nm (XeF*), 248 nm (KrF*),

---

[+]Present address: Western Research Corporation, 8616 Commerce Avenue, San Diego, California 92121.
[++]Present address: Center for Laser Studies, University Park, University of Southern California, Los Angeles, California 90007.

and 193 nm (ArF*) in several preliminary experiments, the results reported herein pertain exclusively to the 193 nm wavelength.

Samples were exposed to ultraviolet radiation under different conditions of preparation. Some of the samples were irradiated in air with water droplets placed directly on the Si surface. In other cases, an evacuable cell constructed of a stainless steel cross was used to more precisely control the environment of the sample. All chemicals were admitted through an evacuable sidearm which was put through several freeze-pump-thaw cycles at LN_2 to remove noncondensable impurities. The chemical materials, H_2O (Burdick & Jackson Spec Grade), Ta $(EtO)_2$ (Alfa Chem.), $TiCl_4$ (Aldrich Chem.), and Al $(CH_3)_3$, 2 M in Toluene (Aldrich Chem.), were used as received from the suppliers. In all cases, the cell was filled to the vapor pressure ($\sim$ 28°C) of the chemical being used. ESCA analysis was performed to determine the quantity of oxygen bonded to non-oxidized silicon. SEM was performed using an ISI DS 130 Dual Stage scanning electron microscope.

Si which was covered with H_2O and irradiated in air was found to selectively deposit large quantities of tantalum oxide when treated with a concentrated solution of Ta $(EtO)_2$ and EtOH. No quantitative determinations were made, but the SEM (Fig. 1) of the laser treated spot clearly demonstrates the nature of this result.

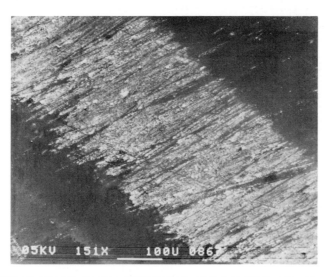

Fig. 1. SEM of silicon showing preferential tantalum oxide adhesion on laser treated area.

Silicon samples which were irradiated in the presence of several torr of H_2O were analyzed by ESCA both directly on the center of the laser spot as well as on the perimeter of the irradiated region. The results, contained in Table I, indicate that a large amount of oxygen was bonded to metallic (non-oxidized) silicon. The O_2/Si_O value represents the ratio of oxygen to oxidized silicon and is corrected for oxygen bonded to any carbon impurities in the sample. Therefore, the value shown specifically indicates oxygen bonded to metallic silicon. A sample of this same material, which had been exposed to a vapor of $TiCl_4$, exhibited a 4:1 enhancement of titanium deposition on the laser irradiated spot and had very little surface silicon remaining.

TABLE I
Results of ESCA analysis performed on laser treated samples as described in the text.

	$O_2/Si_{Oxidized}$	Ti/Si
Reference sample	1.56-1.91	0
Laser + H_2O	2.16-2.29	0
Laser + H_2O + $TiCl_4$	—	4.4
H_2O + $TiCl_4$	—	1.04

Figure 2 allows comparison of the surface morphology of samples exposed to $TiCl_4$ with or without laser/H_2O treatment. Samples which were placed under vacuum ($\sim 10^{-5}$ torr) for several hours prior to metal vapor treatment showed very little metal enhancement, but nevertheless indicated that a large quantity of oxygen was bonded to non-oxidized Si, as shown in Table II.

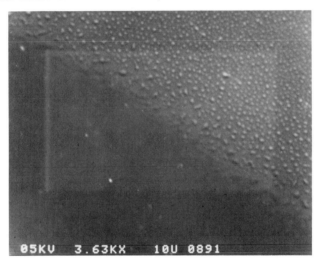

Fig. 2. SEM of the edge of a laser treated spot after exposure to $TiCl_4$. Note that the surface relief is only on the laser treated area.

TABLE II
Results of ESCA analysis performed on laser treated samples which were placed under vacuum prior to $TiCl_4$ exposure.

	$O_2/Si_{Oxidized}$	Ti/Si
Reference sample	1.6-1.9	0
Laser + H_2O + $TiCl_4$	2.3-2.6	0.07
H_2O + $TiCl_4$	1.8-2.1	0.05

DISCUSSION

The most significant aspect of these experimental findings is the evidence that a high density of surface silanol may be selectively formed. The ratio of the total amount of bonded oxygen to the amount present as SiO_2 clearly shows the presence of an -Si-O- moiety. In addition, the ESCA elemental analysis does not disclose the presence of other species for which proper account cannot be made. The principal uncertainties in these measurements arise from having a small spot size for ESCA analysis and a large intrinsic carbon concentration in the sample. The small spot size conspires to diminish the ability to determine the effect of the laser irradiation, since inaccurate location of the ESCA probe beam results in averaging data from the laser irradiated area with data from virgin material. With this uncertainty, the evidence for silanol formation can be interpreted as a lower limit for its formation.

Several methods were used to determine if the irradiated surface contained active -OH sites. Initially, as a preliminary test, a concentrated solution of $Ta(EtO)_2/EtOH$ was applied to the laser irradiated sample and subsequently removed by absorption with a tissue. As shown in Fig. 1, tantalum oxide was formed preferentially on the area defined by the laser spot.

This procedure was followed by a quantitative study comparing samples prepared under more accurately controlled conditions. Identical silicon samples were irradiated at the same intensity in an evacuated cell or in a cell filled with H_2O vapor. These samples were then exposed to $TiCl_4$ vapor. In the presence of H_2O the following reaction ensues: $TiCl_4 + 2H_2O \rightarrow TiO_2 + 4HCl$. Although -Si-OH should not be as reactive as H_2O, a similar tendency is anticipated. The results for these experiments are given in Table I. From these data it can be seen that an enhancement of titanium on the laser irradiated spot is present for both cases, namely, with and without the H_2O present. The significant information is the relative abundance of Ti present in the two cases which, according to observation, represents approximately a 4:1 enhancement when the Si is treated with the laser and H_2O.

In order to determine the influence on these results of any absorbed material loosely bound on the surface, several samples were placed in an evacuable chamber for several hours after exposure to the laser, but prior to exposure to the metal donors. These results are contained in Table II. In this case, the enhancement of metallic deposition is no longer seen, but the presence of -Si-O- is still clearly observable. This evidence raises the possibility that the enhancement of Ti deposition is actually caused by the reaction of $TiCl_4$ with H_2O which is hydrogen bonded preferentially to the area covered by -Si-OH. Although there would be H_2O covering the whole surface, it is expected to be considerably more dense in the region of a hydrogen bonding partner such as silanol.

CONCLUSION

Experimental observations indicate the selective formation of surface silanol induced by ultraviolet irradiation. Because the laser radiation does not directly interact with the H_2O present, the silanol formation is attributed to a thermal reaction between the laser produced molten surface silicon and the water vapor. The lack of titanium enhancement in the samples which were conditioned under vacuum appears to be a measure of the poor reactivity of silanol with $TiCl_4$, as these samples also showed the definite presence of an -Si-O- moiety.

SUPPORT STATEMENT

Support for these studies was provided by the Air Force Office of Scientific Research.

ACKNOWLEDGEMENTS

The authors wish to thank Dr. Robert Linden of Surface Sciences, Inc., Mountain View, California for performing the ESCA analysis, Ronald G. Wibel for performing the SEM analysis, and Jim Wright and Steve Vendetta for technical assistance.

REFERENCE

1. C. G. Wilson and W. M. Moreau, Tutorial Session, Fundamentals of Polymeric Resist Materials, SPIE Conference on Microlithography, Santa Clara, Calif., March 28, 1982.

SELECTIVE Mn DOPING of THIN FILM ZnS:Mn ELECTROLUMINESCENT DEVICES by LASER PHOTOCHEMICAL VAPOR DEPOSITION*

A. KITAI and G.J. WOLGA
School of Electrical Engineering and National Research and Resource Facility for Submicron Structures, Cornell University, Ithaca, NY 14853

ABSTRACT

U.V. laser radiation from a krypton ion laser was used to dissociate manganese carbonyl [$Mn_2(CO)_{10}$] at the surface of a ZnS thin film. The resulting Mn deposit was thermally diffused into the film to form a ZnS:Mn thin film electroluminescent (TFEL) device with spatially selective Mn doping. Process parameters and techniques are described as well as electroluminescence measurements on display elements. Finally we suggest applications of this process to future TFEL displays.

INTRODUCTION

TFEL devices have been fabricated for several years using co-evaporated ZnS:Mn films [1]. The resulting displays exhibit long life, high brightness, broadband yellow emission centered at 580 nm. A major shortcoming of the co-evaporation process is that both constituents are distributed over the film area and therefore spatial patterning of the Mn is not possible. We demonstrate laser chemical vapor deposition (LCVD) as a means of patterning Mn on a ZnS film that offers excellent resolution and has the advantage of being maskless. Only the laser processed areas of the completed TFEL device emit light.

LCVD has recently been used to deposit several metals on substrates with good spatial definition [2,3]. It has been shown that $Mn_2(CO)_{10}$ dissociates into $2[Mn(CO)_5]$ under UV irradiation with photons of wavelength ~ 337 nm [4,5]. The $Mn(CO)_5$ molecule is an unstable intermediate that will thermally or photolytically break up into $Mn + 5(CO)$. We are not aware of any previous attempts to utilize this mechanism for Mn deposition.

FABRICATION

The structure of the TFEL device is shown in fig. 1. The doping concentration of Mn for maximizing the electroluminescence efficiency is approximately 1 mole % [6]. Tin oxide coated 7059 glass was purchased from Corning. Layer 2 was e-beam evaporated and layer 3 thermally evaporated using a baffle boat containing ZnS powder. No Mn was introduced with the ZnS.

The sample was then placed in a cell fitted with a quartz window, a loading port and a vacuum pump as shown in fig. 2. The cell walls may be heated to over 100°C. A small quantity of $Mn_2(CO)_{10}$ powder was placed inside the cell through the loading port. The cell was evacuated and backfilled with N_2 several times to drive out remaining oxygen. Finally, the cell was again evacuated to 0.1 torr and sealed off from the pump. As the cell was heated, the pressure rose due to sublimation of the $Mn_2(CO)_{10}$. At a pressure of 2 torr,

---

*Work supported by the National Science Foundation under Grant ECS-8200312 to the National Research and Resource Facility for Submicron Structures.

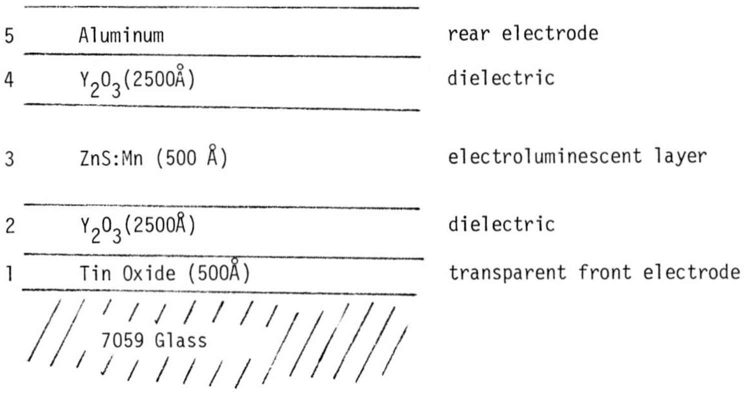

5	Aluminum	rear electrode
4	Y_2O_3 (2500Å)	dielectric
3	ZnS:Mn (500 Å)	electroluminescent layer
2	Y_2O_3 (2500Å)	dielectric
1	Tin Oxide (500Å)	transparent front electrode
	7059 Glass	

FIG. 1   Thin Film Electroluminescent Device Structure

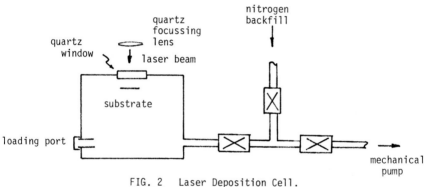

FIG. 2   Laser Deposition Cell.

The lens focusses the laser beam onto the substrate.
The laser beam and lens may be translated relative to the cell.

the focused laser beam scanned the substrate where Mn was to be deposited; in our case we scanned a straight line. The beam power was 10mW in the 337.4-356.4 nm multi-line range of a Spectra Physics Model 171 krypton ion laser. The focused beam intensity was approximately 3×10^4 W/cm^2 and the scan rate was 0.042mm/sec.

Subsequently, the cell was allowed to cool to room temperature and was backfilled to 1 atm. The sample was removed, washed carefully with acetone to dissolve any condensed $Mn_2(CO)_{10}$, and heated in vacuum to 450°C for 2 hours to diffuse Mn into the ZnS film. Finally, layers 4 and 5 were grown.

MEASUREMENTS

An A.C. drive was applied across electrodes 1 and 5. Characteristic yellow electroluminescence was observed in a stripe along the path of the laser deposition. See Fig. 3.

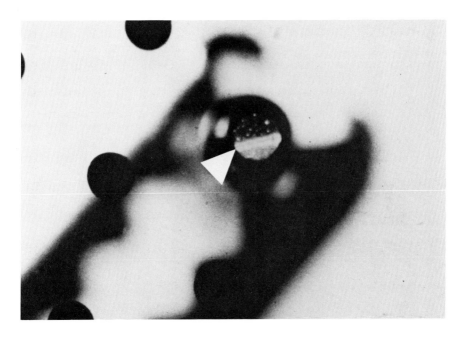

Fig. 3   Photograph of the laser deposited stripe showing observed electroluminescence. The circles are 0.05" diameter aluminum rear electrodes. Only the area of the active electrode is being driven. The arrow points to the stripe.

Measurements of intensity versus position were made using a scanning optical fiber and lens, coupled to a photomultiplier tube. The scan was perpendicular to the E.L. stripe. Due to the finite dimensions of the optical fiber, a deconvolution was necessary to calculate the actual E.L. emission profile. See Fig. 4.

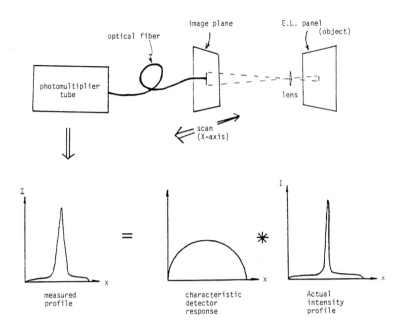

Fig. 4   Electroluminescent Intensity Measurement

Fig. 5 shows the results of the measurements. A contrast ratio of greater than 10 is observed. Preliminary brightness measurements using a United Detector model 40 A photometer indicate approximately 40 foot lamberts in the stripe, with an A.C. drive consisting of alternating polarity 160 volt pulses at 1 KHz.

Using our diffusion temperature of 450°C and time of 2 hours, the diffusion coefficient may be calculated [6] from

$$D = D_0 \exp\left(\frac{-E_A}{kT}\right) \qquad (1)$$

With E_A = 1.2eV and D_0 = 8 × 10^{-7} cm²/sec, D = 3.47 × 10^{-15} cm²/sec. Now, the characteristic diffusion length is given by

$$L_D = \sqrt{Dt} \qquad (2)$$

which yields 500 Å for our data, equal to the ZnS thickness. One may therefore expect a substantially uniform Mn concentration with depth.

Since the width of the E.L. stripe is ~25μm, (see Fig. 5) we can conclude that the stripe width is determined by the laser deposition process and/or surface rather than bulk diffusion of Mn. On the other hand, the electroluminescent spot size we have already achieved is entirely adequate for display applications.

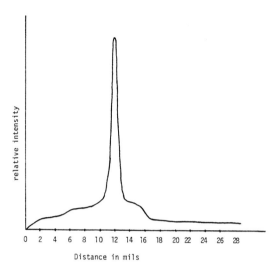

FIG. 5a) Electroluminescent Intensity Measurements showing relative intensity as a function of distance along a line in the plane of the substrate and perpendicular to the stripe in fig. 3. A contrast ratio of 10:1 or better is achieved. The peak is approximately gaussian, with a width at half power of 1 mil or 25μ. The plot is a deconvolution of the actual data taken.

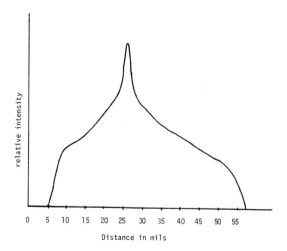

FIG. 5b) Same as 5a) but showing a sample where the acetone wash before diffusion was omitted. Note the high background electroluminescence. The intensity falls to zero at the edges of the sample.

CHARACTERIZATION

The laser deposited material was characterized by Auger analysis. The manganese was deposited on a Si substrate using the laser process with conditions identical to those described above. The Auger spectrum in Fig. 6 shows only Mn and O_2 peaks.

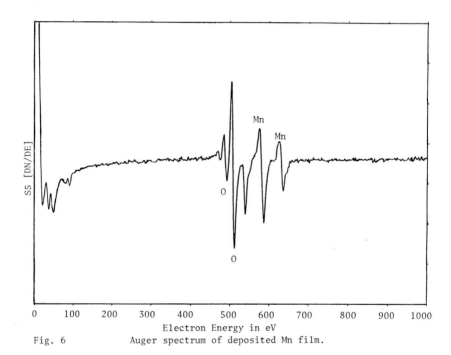

Fig. 6   Auger spectrum of deposited Mn film.

The deposition thickness versus laser power was measured. The results are shown in Table 1.

TABLE 1
Thickness of Mn deposition versus laser power

LASER POWER	POWER DENSITY	THICKNESS
1mW	$3 \times 10^3 \text{W/cm}^2$	300 Å
10mW	$3 \times 10^4 \text{W/cm}^2$	900 Å
50mW	$1.5 \times 10^5 \text{W/cm}^2$	8000 Å

To validate that photodissociation rather than thermal deposition takes place in our laser process, we used a focussed 50 mW laser beam in the red (6471 Å) and obtained no observable deposition on a Si substrate.

CONCLUSIONS

A laser processing technique for patterning E.L. displays has been demonstrated. Using this technique, fixed-format alphanumerics can be permanently patterned using a modulated laser and a two-dimensional scanning system. The laser-written message will not be visible until the drive voltage is applied to excite the electroluminescent panel.

Since the Mn is localized, a two color thin film display can be produced using a background doping for one color and the Mn deposition for the other, or two separate LCVD processes, one for each dopant. In the latter case, spatially selective laser heating could diffuse each dopant individually into the ZnS and thereby allow the use of dopants with widely varying diffusion rates.

It should be noted that ZnS:Mn is also an efficient phosphor for cathodoluminescence. Laser deposited activators such as Mn could offer spatial control not previously available in situations where masking is difficult, such as for CRT faceplates that are curved and/or already attached to tube necks.

Further investigation is required to improve laser deposition throughput, to optimize brightness, and to demonstrate multi-color displays.

ACKNOWLEDGMENTS

The authors would like to thank Michael Miller for his valuable suggestions concerning photochemistry, and Brian Whitehead for vacuum deposition work.

This work was supported by the National Science Foundation under Grant ECS-8200312 to the National Research and Resource Facility for Submicron Structures (NRRFSS). The Auger analysis as well as oxide layer deposition were performed at the facilities of the NRRFSS.

REFERENCES

1. Inoguchi et al., in 1974 SID Int. Symp. Dig., p. 84, 1974

2. S.D. Allen, J. Appl. Phys. $\underline{52}$, 6501 (1981).

3. R.D. Coombe et al., Appl. Phys. Lett. 37(9), 1980.

4. L.J. Rothberg et al., J. Chem. Phys. 74(4), 1981.

5. Geoffroy & Wrighton, Organometallic Photochemistry, Academic Press, N.Y. 1979, pp. 107-108.

6. J.M. Hurd et al., J. Elect. Mat. Vol. 8, No. 6, 1979.

SECTION V
DIAGNOSTICS OF CONVENTIONAL AND LASER PROCESSING

Laser Spectroscopic Investigation of Gas-Phase Processes Relevant to
Semiconductor Device Fabrication

R. F. Karlicek, Jr., V. M. Donnelly and W. D. Johnston, Jr.
Bell Laboratories, Murray Hill, New Jersey 07974

ABSTRACT

Chemical vapor deposition (CVD) and plasma etching are important gas-phase techniques used in fabricating semiconductor devices. These processes frequently involve poorly understood multicomponent gas-phase reactions which control reproducibility and product quality. Laser spectroscopic techniques have recently been developed to investigate CVD and plasma etching. These methods offer several advantages for probing complex systems. A comparison of various probing techniques will be presented, and recent results of laser spectroscopic investigations of plasma etching and CVD of silicon and III-V compounds will be reviewed.

INTRODUCTION

Gas-phase semiconductor processing techniques such as chemical vapor deposition (CVD), plasma deposition (PD), plasma etching (PE), and reactive ion etching (RIE) are widely used in fabricating microelectronic devices. These processes frequently involve poorly understood, complex gas-phase reactions which control product quality and reproducibility. In practice, it has proven possible to empirically optimize the process parameters (e.g. pressure, temperature, gas composition, etc.) to obtain acceptable results without a detailed understanding of the chemistry involved. In view of the usually large number of process variables, monitoring techniques such as optical spectroscopy can provide a fundamental understanding of the mechanisms involved and can diagnose problems when they occur.

Optical spectroscopy is ideally suited to investigating gas-phase semiconductor fabrication processes, since it is nonintrusive and can provide data in real time. Simple methods such as emission spectroscopy are used routinely in PE and PD [1],[2]. However, this technique usually provides only qualitative information about the concentration of species in plasmas, and is not possible for thermal CVD processes.

In recent years, laser spectroscopic techniques such as laser induced fluorescence (LIF) and laser Raman scattering (LRS) have been used to provide detailed mechanistic information about gas-phase reactions in surroundings ranging from the upper atmosphere [3] to piston chambers of internal combustion engines [4]. Such techniques are now also being used to study gas-phase reactions in CVD and PE, providing spacially resolved, quantitative detection of key reactive species. This paper will review this work, with emphasis on studies conducted in the authors' laboratory using lasers to probe CVD processes related to III-V semiconductor device fabrication [5].

COMPARISON OF LASER SPECTROSCOPIC TECHNIQUES

A wide variety of analytical laser spectroscopic techniques have been developed in recent years [6]. This section reviews only the salient features of LIF and LRS important for the discussion of their use as diagnostic tools for semiconductor device processing.

Laser Induced Fluorescence (LIF). LIF is an extremely useful tool for detection of gas-phase reactive species. Its advantages include high sensitivity (low detection limits) and selectivity, which is especially necessary for multi-component systems typical of semiconductor processing techniques. Its disadvantages include somewhat limited applicability (not all molecules have accessible transitions) and potential complications in its use as a quantitive technique, as will be discussed below.

The primary instrumentation requirements of LIF are contained in an apparatus used to study InP CVD (Fig. 1) [5]. Most applications require a tunable laser, although fixed frequency sources can occasionally be used. Fluorescence is collected normal to the beam axis and is imaged onto the optics of a monochromator which selects the fluorescence wavelength to be monitored and rejects scattered laser and background radiation. Rejection is especially important in plasma diagnostics, and is further improved by using a pulsed laser and gated detection electronics. Incident and transmitted laser power is monitored to correct the detected fluorescence for variations in laser intensity and for absorption in the reactor.

In LIF, a molecule is excited from an occupied electronic state (usually the ground state) to an upper state which relaxes to some lower electronic state via spontaneous emission (fluorescence). This process, sometimes called resonance fluorescence, requires the excited electronic state to be bound or only weakly predissociative and is shown schematically in Fig. 2. In some cases, laser absorption results in photodissociation of the parent molecule producing electronically excited fragments which fluoresce. This process will be referred to as laser induced photofragment emission (LIPE). The primary requirement for detection of molecules via LIF or LIPE is that a transition (at least weakly allowed) to an excited state be accessible at an available laser energy (generally 1.5 to 6.4 eV). For both LIF and LIPE, the observed fluorescence intensity is proportional to the density of molecules in the initially occupied lower state, provided laser absorption and nonradiative relaxation processes (i.e. quenching) are properly accounted for.

It is not difficult to predict a priori which molecules are good candidates for LIF, based on the wealth of published spectroscopic literature available, especially for diatomics [7]. A partial list of species relevant to CVD, PD, and PE which have either been detected or are likely candidates for LIF are shown in Table 1. Table 2 shows species which have been detected via LIPE.

The application of LIF as a quantitative tool is possible provided the detected fluorescence intensity is corrected for laser intensity variations and for quenching. For the single photon process shown in Fig. 2, and in the absence of saturation effects, fluorescence intensity varies linearly with laser intensity. If the fluorescence collection optics are focused on the center of the beam path inside the reactor and Beer's law absorption is assumed, the corrected fluorescence intensity is given by:

$$F = F_t \frac{(I_0^{in})^2}{I_t^{out} \cdot I_t^{in}} \qquad (1)$$

where F_t, I_t^{in}, and I_t^{out} are the fluorescence intensity, input, and output laser intensities at time t, and I_0^{in} is the reference beam intensity (t=0). For multiple photon excitation via a real or virtual intermediate state (see

Fig. 2), the fluorescence intensity varies superlinearly with laser intensity, and the normalization factor should be determined emperically by measuring fluorescence intensity as a function of laser power.

The excited state produced by absorption may relax via fluorescence or nonradiative collision (quenching) processes. For a simple two state quenching model [8], the fluorescence intensity is given by [5]:

$$F_{\nu_f} = C_0 \frac{k_r}{k_r + \sum_M k_{q_M} P_M} [AB] \qquad (2)$$

where F is the fluorescence intensity at frequency ν_f, [AB] is the concentration of the ground state, k_r is the radiative lifetime of the excited state, k_{q_M} is the quenching rate constant of AB by species M, and P_M is the partial pressure of species M. C_0 is a proportionality constant containing geometric, spectroscopic, and kinetic factors related to excitation and detection efficiency. For pressures encountered in most semiconductor processing techniques, quenching is important, and the constants in Eq. 2 must be measured. This can be done using pulsed excitation-time resolved fluorescence. In many instances, particularly for atmospheric CVD, quenching is dominated by collisions with molecules (atoms) present at much higher concentrations (i.e. $P_M \sim P_{total}$) and Eq. (2) can be rewritten as:

$$F_{\nu_f} = C_1 [AB^\star] \qquad (3)$$

where:

$$C_1 = \frac{k_r}{k_r + k_q P_{total}} = \text{constant}, \qquad (4)$$

so that at constant temperature and pressure, quenching effects do not preclude quantitative detection.

<u>Laser Raman Scattering</u>. In contrast to LIF and LIPE, LRS is more applicable to quantitative detection, and can be used for a much wider variety of molecules. However, the detection sensitivity of LRS is considerably less than that of LIF and LIPE.

The apparatus required for LRS is very similar to that shown in Fig. 1 for LIF. LRS systems do not require a tunable laser source, and usually employ a double monochromator to provide sufficient rejection at the laser wavelength. Since light scattering processes increase as ν^4, fixed frequency lasers operating in the UV can provide improved detection sensitivity. However, such sources can also cause fluorescence (resonance or via LIPE) which is much more intense and completely masks Raman scattering.

LRS involves inelastic scattering of photons by molecules, with the energy lost or gained by scattered photons causing changes in the rotational and/or vibrational states occupied by the molecules. All molecules possess at least one Raman-active band, but the applicability of the technique is limited by the weakness of the effect. Raman scattering cross-sections are typically three orders of magnitude less than Rayleigh (elastic scattering) cross-sections, and between five to fifteen orders of magnitude less than unquenched fluorescence. In spite of its weakness, the application of LRS in gas-phase diagnostics has been extensively studied [9]. A partial list of species relevant to semiconductor processing, detected via LRS is shown in Table 3.

Since LRS can provide information about the distribution of occupied vibrational and rotational energy levels for molecules in the region probed by the laser and collection optics, the technique has proven most useful for measuring local gas-phase temperatures. The presence of overlapping rotational side bands, however, can complicate spectra from multicomponent gas-phase systems, making simutaneous detection of several species difficult.

APPLICATION OF LASER SPECTROSCOPY TO SEMICONDUCTOR PROCESSING DIAGNOSTICS

CVD Diagnostics. One of the first applications of LIF and LRS in Si CVD diagnostics has been discussed in a series of reports by Sedgwick [10-12]. Using LRS of N_2 in a Si CVD reactor, thermal profiles in the gas were studied as a function of susceptor temperature and position in the reactor by comparing the relative intensities of the Stokes and anti-Stokes components [10]. The measured temperature profiles were then used to check the validity of simplifying assumptions usually made in modelling the hydrodynamics of gas flow in cold wall, heated susceptor CVD reactors.

Sedgwick also proposed that LRS be used to measure concentration profiles of chlorosilanes (e.g. $SiCl_4$, $SiHCl_3$, etc.) during silicon CVD. Although detection limits in the range of 10-100 ppm were measured at room temperature, experiments at high temperature revealed that intense LIF of $SiCl_2$ caused by irradiation at 488 nm, prevented detection of other reactive species via LRS. The fluorescence intensity of $SiCl_2$ was found to be about five orders of magnitude greater than the N_2 Raman cross-section. In this case, LIF was used to measure $SiCl_2$ concentration profiles from 50 μm to 1 cm above the heated Si surface [12].

Miller et al. [13] have used pure rotational LRS of N_2 to measure thermal profiles above a heated susceptor in a bell jar type CVD reactor, citing several advantages over the vibrational-rotational LRS technique used by Sedgwick. These authors also discussed the use of LIF to measure concentrations of reactive species in CVD, citing as an example LIF observed from NH ($A^3\Pi - X^3\Sigma^+$).

The increasing importance of III-V compounds in electro-optics and high speed electronics has led to the development of a series of laser spectroscopic probes for atmospheric CVD of GaAs, InP, and related ternary and quaternary compounds [5]. Using an ArF excimer laser operating at 193 nm, quantitative detection of most reactive species involved in growth was shown to be possible at conditions typically employed in CVD reactors. Detected species include InCl, GaCl, AsH_3, PH_3, P_2, As_2, and As_4 (see Tables 1 and 2).

At 193 nm, the metal chlorides undergo two photon absorption producing In^+ and Ga^+ ions which recombine with electrons to form excited In*, and Ga*, resulting in intense atomic emission. The quantitative use of this photolysis technique was verified by comparing the atomic fluorescence intensity observed after 193 nm irradiation with the intensity of LIF from InCl and GaCl excited with a tunable dye laser.

Plasma Diagnostics. PD and PE techniques are becoming increasingly important in the fabrication of microelectronic devices. PE is replacing wet chemical techniques for etching patterns in wafers, and is essential in the development of submicron features required in very large scale integration (VLSI). PD is gaining popularity in the growth of dielectrics at lower temperatures than used in conventional CVD growth. A discussion of plasma diagnostics using LIF has been presented by Miller.[14] The application of laser spectroscopic plasma diagnostics to semiconductor processing is very recent and has only been used in PE studies.

Donnelly et al. [15] have reported the use of Cl_2^+ detection using LIF to investigate the origin of anisotropic etching of Si, Al, and III-V compounds reported for Cl_2 containing plasmas [15]. Cl_2^+ is the predominant ion in a Cl_2 containing discharges and is responsible for the ion bombardment induced anisotropy. By studying the dependence of spacially resolved Cl_2^+ densities on discharge frequency and power, important information related to the frequency dependence of etch rates has been obtained.

The Cl_2^+ spectrum, recorded by monitoring LIF at 396 nm ($A^2\Pi_u$, $v'=$ 10 - $X^2\Pi_g$, $v''=1$) and scanning the laser in the vicinity of the $v'=10$ $v''=0$ transition, exhibits rotational structure which permits the calculation of gas temperature in the plasma. Measurements at the center of the plasma gave a temperature of 330 (±20)K at discharge frequencies of both 250 kHz and 13.56 MHz.

Gottscho et al. [16] have investigated CCl_4 plasmas used for Si, GaAs, InP, and Al PE using LIF dectection of the CCl radical in the discharge.[16] Using a tunable dye laser to excite $A^2\Delta$-$X^2\Pi$ and monitoring fluorescence from the excited state back to the initial state, ground state CCl densities were monitored as a function of gas composition and flow-rate, discharge power, electrode temperature, and position in the plasma. By comparing LIF intensities to plasma induced emission, it was determined that N_2 actinometry (CCl emission normalized to N_2 emission) misrepresents the CCl concentration (determined by LIF) by as much as an order of magnitude. The measured CCl concentration profiles are consistent with CCl_4 dissociation via low energy electron attachment reactions. Rotational CCl temperatures were also measured to determine the shape of thermal gradients in the plasma at different pressures and electrode temperatures.

Fluorocarbon plasmas are widely used for etching Si and SiO_2. Hargis and Kushner [17], have used a KrF excimer laser at 248 nm to excite of LIF from $CF_2(\tilde{A}^1B_1-\tilde{X}^1A_1)$. LIF from CF_2 was used to study the dependence of CF_2 production as a function of power in CF_4 and C_2F_6 containing plasmas. Higher CF_2 densities were found for C_2F_6 containing plasmas, consistent with the higher electron impact dissociation and dissociative attachment cross-sections for C_2F_6 than for CF_4.

SUMMARY

Laser diagnostic techniques are now receiving attention for use in studying semiconductor device fabrication processes. Although such techniques have received limited application thus far, they are capable of providing unique information about the gas-phase chemistry involved in PE, PD, and CVD technologies. Such information can provide improved understanding leading to refinement of these techniques.

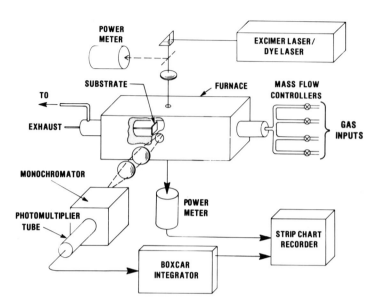

Fig. 1. Schematic apparatus used for LIF and LIPE measurements.

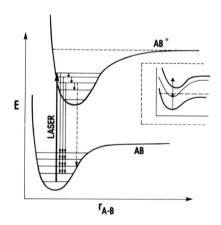

Fig. 2. LIF mechanism showing laser excitation to state AB*, vibration relaxation (small arrows), fluorescence, and quenching (dashed arrow). The inset shows two photon excitation via a real (solid curve) or virtual (dashed line) intermediate state.

TABLE I
Partial list of species of interest in CVD, PE and PD which have been detected (references from text in ( )) or may be detectable through laser-induced fluorescence (LIF).

Molecule	V_{00} (cm^{-1})	Transition	References
CF	42693	$A^2\Sigma^+ - X^2\Pi_r$	HH
CF_2	37220	$\tilde{A}^1B_1 - \tilde{X}^1A_1$	CWM (17)
$CC\ell$	35870	$A^2\Delta_r - X^2\Pi$	HH (16)
$CC\ell_2$	~17100	$\tilde{A}^1B_1 - \tilde{X}^1A_1$	TWR, RLT
O_2^+	40669	$A^2\Pi_u - X^2\Pi_g$	HH
O_2^-	25300	$A^2\Pi_u - X^2\Pi_g$	HH
SiF	22858	$A^2\Sigma^+ - X^2\Pi_r$	HH
SiF_2	44114	$\tilde{A}^1B_1 - X^1A_1$	DH
	26310	$\tilde{a}^3B_1 - X^1A_1$	RAO
$SiC\ell$	23114	$A^2\Sigma - X^2\Pi_r$	HH
$SiC\ell_2$	?	?	(12)
$C\ell_2^+$	20000	$A^2\Pi_u - X^2\Pi_g$	HH (15)
Br_2^+	21602	$A^2\Pi_u - X^2\Pi_g$	HH
NH_2	~11100	$\tilde{A}^2A_1 - \tilde{X}^2B_1$	JRR
NH	29807	$A^3\Pi_i - X^3\Sigma^-$	HH (13)
$CC\ell^+$	42350	$A^1\Pi - X^1\Sigma$	HH
OH	32684	$A^2\Sigma^+ - X^2\Pi_i$	HH
NO	43966	$A^2\Sigma^+ - X^2\Pi_r$	HH
In	-	$6^2S_{1/2} - 5^2P_{3/2}$	GSB
$GaC\ell$	29527	$A^3\Pi_0^+ - X^1\Sigma^+$	HH
$InC\ell$	27765	$A^3\Pi_0^+ - X^1\Sigma^+$	HH (5)
P_2	46941	$C^1\Sigma_u^+ - X^1\Sigma_g^+$	HH "
SiO	42641	$A^1\Pi - X^1\Sigma^+$	HH

HH = K. P. Huber and G. Herzberg, ref. 7 of text
CWM = C. W. Matthews, Can. J. Phys. 45 2355 (1967).
TWR = J. J. Tiee, F. B. Wampler, and W. W. Rice, Chem. Phys Lett. 65, 425 (1979).
RLT = R. E. Huie, N. J. T. Long, and B. A. Thrush, Chem. Phys. Lett. 51, 197 (1977).
JRR = J. W. C. Johns, D. A. Ramsay, and S. C. Ross, Can. J. Phys. 54, 1804 (1976).
DH = R. N. Dixon and M. Halle, J. Mol. Spectros. 36,192 (1970).
RAO = D. R. Rao, J. Mol. Spectros. 34, 284 (1970).
GSB = R. A. Gottscho, G. Smolinsky, and R. H. Burton, J. Appl. Phys. 53, 5908 (1982).

TABLE 2
List of species detected via laser induced photofragment emission (LIPE).

Molecule	λ_{ex}	Emitter	Ref.
NH_3	193	$NH_2(\tilde{A}^2A_1-\tilde{X}^2B_1)$	SY
PH_3	193	$PH_2(\tilde{A}^2A_1-\tilde{X}^2B_1)$	DBM
AsH_3	193	$AsH_2(\tilde{A}^2A_1-\tilde{X}^2B_1)$, As*	(5)
InCl	193, 248	In*	" , CK
GaCl	193, 248	Ga*	" , CK
$Fe(CO)_5$	248	Fe*	KNZ
$Zn(CH_3)_2$	248	Zn*	"

SY = C. L. Sam and J. T. Yardley, J. Chem. Phys. 69, 4621 (1978).

DBM = V. M. Donnelly, A. P. Baronavski, and J. R. McDonald, Chem. Phys. 43, 271 (1979).

CK = T. A. Cool and J. B. Koffend, J. Chem Phys. 74, 2287 (1981).

KNZ = Z. Karny, R. Naaman, and R. N. Zare, Chem. Phys. Lett. 59, 33 (1978).

TABLE 3
Raman Detection Limits (S/N = 3) With 248.5 nm Excitation*

Molecule	Detection Limit (mTorr)		
	Pure Gas	600 Torr He	600 Torr H_2
N_2	3	10	8
O_2	3	10	8
H_2	2	6	-
H_2O	6	20	-
CO_2	3	--	-
NH_3	1	3	-
CH_4	1	--	-
CF_4	5	--	-
SiH_4	.9	2	2
C_2F_6	5	--	-

* Data provided by P. J. Hargis, Jr., Sandia National Laboratories

REFERENCES

1. P. J. Markoux, P. D. Foo, Solid State Technology 24, 115, (1981).

2. S. Yokoyama, M. Hirose, and Y. Osaka, Japan. J. Appl. Phys. 20, 241 (1981).

3. J. Trolinger and W. W. Moore, Eds., Advances in Laser Technology for the Atomospheric Sciences, Proceedings of the Society of Photo-Optical Instrumentation Engineers, v. 125, 1977.

4. J. R. Smith in: Laser Probes for Combustion Chemistry, D. R. Crosley, Ed., (American Chemical Society, Washington, DC 1980), p. 259.

5. V. M. Donnelly, R. F. Karlicek, J. Appl. Phys. 53, 6399 (1982).

6. N. Omenetto, Ed., Analytical Laser Spectroscopy, (John Wiley and Sons, New York 1979).

7. K. P. Huber and G. Herzberg, Molecular Spectra and Molecular Structure IV, (Van Nostrand, New York 1979).

8. O. Stern and M. Volmer, Pysik. Z. 20, 183 (1919).

9. M. Lapp and C. M. Penny, Eds., Laser Raman Gas Diagnostics, (Plenum Press, New York 1979).

10. J. E. Smith, Jr., and T. O. Sedgwick, Letters in Heat and Mass Transfer 2, 329 (1975).

11. T. O. Sedgwick, J. E. Smith, Jr., R. Ghez, and M. E. Cowher, J. Cryst. Growth 31, 264 (1975).

12. J. E. Smith, Jr., and T. O. Sedgwick, Thin Solid Films 40, 1 (1977).

13. G. H. Miller, A. J. Mulac, and P. J. Hargis, Jr., NBS Special Publication #561, 1979, p. 1135.

14. T. A. Miller, Plasma Chemistry and Plasma Processing 1, 3 (1981).

15. V. M. Donnelly, D. L. Flamm, and G. Collins, J. Vac. Sci. Technol., to be published.

16. R. A. Gottscho, G. P. Davis, and R. H. Burton, J. Vac. Sci. Technol., (Proceedings of the American Vacuum Society Meeting, 11/16-19/82, Baltimore, abstract #EMTA-20), to be published.

17. P. J. Hargis, Jr. and M. J. Kushner, Appl. Phys. Lett. 40, 779 (1982).

LASER-INDUCED FLUORESCENCE DIAGNOSTICS OF $CF_4/O_2/H_2$ PLASMA ETCHING[*]

S. PANG AND S. R. J. BRUECK
Lincoln Laboratory, Massachusetts Insitute of Technology,
Lexington, Massachusetts 02173

ABSTRACT

Laser-induced fluorescence experiments have been carried out during $CF_4/O_2/H_2$ plasma etching of Si and SiO_2. Measurements of relative CF_2 radical concentrations as a function of rf power, frequency, pressure, and gas composition are reported. The results are correlated with etch rates of Si and SiO_2. The balance between CF_2 and F concentrations is shown to influence the etching process strongly.

INTRODUCTION

As semiconductor device dimensions are scaled down to the 1-μm range, dry etching fabrication processes become more important as a consequence of their ability to produce the necessary anisoptropic profiles.[1,2] Good control on etch rate, selectivity, etching profile, uniformity, and cleanliness is essential in using plasma etching in device fabrication. However, plasma etching is, in general, strongly system dependent so that etching results are sometimes not reproducible and are not easily transferred between systems. A more complete understanding of the physical and chemical mechanisms involved in plasma etching is necessary in order to further develop the technique.

In general, the controllable parameters in a plasma-etching system, e.g. rf power and frequency, gas composition and flow parameters, and total area of Si substrates exposed to the plasma (Si loading effect), are only indirectly related to the concentrations of important etchant species such as atomic fluorine. Etching results are often modified by uncontrolled variables (system cleanliness, residual impurities) and system constraints (geometry, wafer loading, and patterning). There are also questions concerning the basic surface chemistry taking place in a plasma reactor. Product species and their internal energy distributions are not fully understood even for the most widely used etching processes such as etching Si with CF_4. Similarly, the roles of ion and photon bombardment and sidewall passivation in producing the observed anisotropy and etching parameters are not resolved. A more complete understanding of the plasma-etching process is of considerable interest both with respect to basic surface chemistry and to practical applications.

A number of diagnostic techniques have been used to monitor the etching process and to gain a better understanding of etching mechanisms. Optical emission is often used for end point detection[3,4] and spectra have been

---

[*]This work was sponsored by the Department of the Air Force, in part with specific funding from the Air Force Office of Scientific Research.

analyzed for the chemical species involved in etching.[5,6] However, the emission spectrum from a plasma discharge is usually very rich and complicated, which makes the analysis difficult. In addition, only excited state species are observed and small changes in the discharge parameters can drastically alter the spectra. Further, only poor spatial resolution is attainable by emission spectroscopy. Mass spectroscopy has also been used to study the etching species.[7,8] Downstream mass spectrometric sampling can provide information on stable end products, but it is not adequate to detect reactive or unstable products. <u>In-situ</u> mass spectroscopy, on the other hand, perturbs the plasma and cannot be used on a conventional plasma-etching system. Langmuir probe measurements have also been used to monitor the plasma potential and the electron and ion densities in a plasma discharge.[9,10] However, the probe also perturbs the plasma and the probe surface is subjected to chemical reaction; the measurements are thus somewhat difficult to interpret.

Laser-induced fluorescense (LIF) is an <u>in-situ,</u> nonperturbing diagnostic technique which has the potential to probe radical species concentrations, temperatures, and internal state distributions with high spatial and temporal resolution. Typically, LIF spectra originate from a small number of excited states of a single radical species which have been populated by the incident laser source and are therefore relatively simple. A number of groups are presently using this technique to probe various plasma-etching systems.[11-13]

In this work, LIF is used to study a CF_4 plasma-etching system. CF_4 is widely used as the etching gas for Si and SiO_2. Mixing CF_4 with O_2 or H_2 provides etching selectivity between Si and SiO_2. The addition of O_2 to CF_4 discharges increases the Si etch rate much faster than the SiO_2 etch rate.[14] In contrast, H_2 addition depresses the Si etch rate relative to the SiO_2 etch rate[15] and provides the selectivity of SiO_2 over Si which is preferred when etching contact holes through SiO_2 to a poly-Si layer. Among the many reactive species in a CF_4 rf discharge, CF_2 is one of the significant radicals and has been related to plasma polymerization[16] and to selective etching of SiO_2.[17] CF_2 radicals also play an important role in controlling the concentration of more reactive species such as F radicals. We have used LIF to probe the variation of CF_2 concentration with etching parameters such as rf power, pressure, frequency, and gas composition and have examined the correlations between ground electronic state CF_2 concentration and both Si/SiO_2 etch rates and polymer film formation.

EXPERIMENT

The plasma reactor and the optical arrangement are shown schematically in Fig. 1. The reactor was a quartz chamber with 3.5"-diameter Al electrodes. A 2.5"-long Al cylinder was attached to the ground electrode to increase the area ratio between the ground and the powered electrodes. Samples to be etched were loaded onto the water-cooled powered electrode. The total gas flow rate was maintained at 10 sccm. The rf power density was variable from 0.16 to 1.45 W/cm^2 and the rf frequency could be adjusted from 4 to 14 MHz. Pressures were measured with a capacitance manometer and varied between 0.1 and 1 Torr. The gas flow was directed through an array of apertures on the periphery of the ground electrode and pumped out from a similar set of apertures on the powered electrode. The gas residence time was approximately 0.35 second at 0.1 Torr.

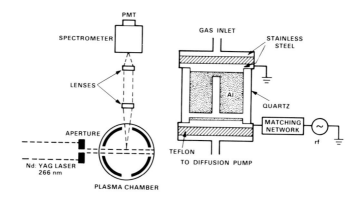

Figure 1. Schematic diagram of the plasma etching chamber and the optical arrangement used in this study.

A flashlamp-pumped, Q-switched Nd:YAG laser source with a 5-ns pulse duration operating at 10 Hz was used. The laser output was frequency quadrupled to 266 nm using KD*P crystals with an energy of approximately 1.5 mJ/pulse and was directed into the plasma-etching system through a 4" O.D. quartz vacuum jacket and slits milled in the Al cylinder. A collimated input beam geometry with a beam diameter of ~2 mm was used. The fluorescence was collected at 90° to the incident beam using BaF_2 collection optics, analyzed with a 1/4-m spectrometer, and detected with a photomultiplier. The PMT output was monitored using a fast Track/Hold amplifier and a laboratory computer system. The plasma-etching reactor could be translated relative to the optical system to monitor spatial dependencies.

RESULTS AND DISCUSSION

In a rf discharge, radicals and ions are generated when CF_4 molecules are decomposed by electron-impact-induced dissociation.[18] Some of the processes occuring in the plasma include:

$$e + CF_4 \rightarrow CF_3 + F + e$$
$$\rightarrow CF_3^+ + F + 2e$$
$$\rightarrow CF_3 + F^-$$
$$\rightarrow CF_2 + 2F + e$$
$$\rightarrow CF + 3F + e.$$

The emission spectrum (λ = 200 - 800 nm) from the plasma discharge indicates that CF_2, CF, and F are present. We use the 266-nm beam from the Nd:YAG laser to excite the CF_2 radical from a low-lying vibrational state in the ground electronic state [$\tilde{X}$ (0,1,0)] to a vibrational state in the first excited electronic state [$\tilde{A}$ (0,2,0)].[19] Fluorescence between 250 and 400 nm is observed as the CF_2 radical radiatively relaxes back to vibrational levels in the ground electronic state as shown in Fig. 2. Because of the short radiative lifetime (~60 ns) compared to the collisional deactivation time at

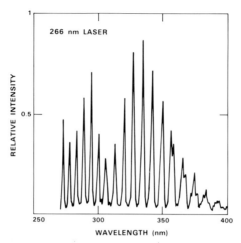

Figure 2. Laser-induced fluorescence spectra of CF_2 in CF_4 rf discharge. Rf power density - 0.64 W/cm^2, Pressure - 0.2 Torr.

low pressure (~300 ns at 0.1 Torr), the fluorescence spectrum provides information only on the initial ground electronic state CF_2 population. No collisional redistribution of the spectrum has been observed up to highest pressures used in this work.

Relative CF_2 concentrations have been measured as a function of rf power density, pressure, frequency, and gas composition. We choose to monitor the emission intensity at 330 nm, which corresponds to the $\tilde{A}$ (0,2,0) → $\tilde{X}$ (0,12,0) transition. The laser beam was directed 0.3 cm above the powered electrode; the probed volume was in the dark space of the discharge. Figure 3 shows the relative intensity of 330-nm emission as a function of rf power density. The CF_4 discharge was maintained at 0.2 Torr at 13.56 MHz with a 2" diameter Si wafer on the powered electrode. Since more CF_4 is decomposed at higher power densities, the CF_2 concentration increases with rf power density as expected. Similarly, we observe an increase of CF_2 with pressure as shown in Fig. 4. The higher the pressure at constant gas flow rate, the longer the gas residence time and the more efficient the discharge in producing radicals. As more radicals and ions are generated at higher rf power or pressure, the etch rate of Si increases. In Fig. 5, we show the dependence of the CF_2 concentration on rf frequency. The applied rf power density was 0.64 W/cm^2 and pressure was maintained at 0.2 Torr. We detected more CF_2 at 14 MHz than at 4 MHz. A similar frequency dependence of Cl_2^+ in Cl_2 discharge was observed by Donnelly et al.[13]

The effect of oxygen addition on both the CF_2 density and the Si etch rate in a CF_4 discharge is shown in Fig. 6. The plasma discharge was maintained at 0.64 W/cm^2, 0.2 Torr and 13.56 MHz, our usual etching condition. A 2"-diameter Si wafer is placed on the powered electrode. The etch rate of Si increased from 175 Å/min to 1170 Å/min with the addition of 40% O_2, while the

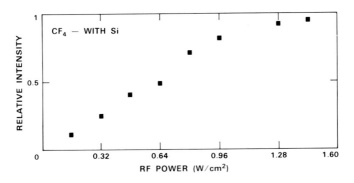

Figure 3. Relative concentration of CF_2 radicals as a function of rf power density. Pressure - 0.2 Torr, Frequency - 13.56 MHz.

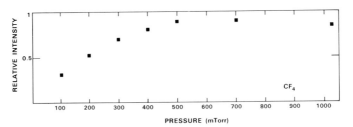

Figure 4. Relative concentration of CF_2 as a function of pressure. Rf power density - 0.64 W/cm^2, Frequency - 13.56 MHz.

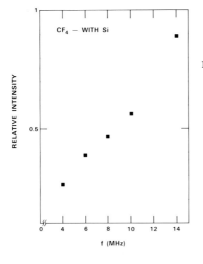

Figure 5. Relative concentration of CF_2 as a function of frequency. Rf power density - 0.64 W/cm2, Pressure, - 0.2 Torr.

CF$_2$ LIF signals decreased below the detection sensitivity for O$_2$ additions greater than 45%. These changes may be due to the reaction of O$_2$ with CF$_2$ and other fragmented species, allowing more free fluorine atoms for Si etching and for depleting the CF$_2$ concentration. The following reactions, among others, are possible:

$$CF_3 + O_2 \rightarrow COF_2 + F + O,$$
$$CF_2 + O_2 \rightarrow CO_2 + 2F,$$
$$CF_2 + O \rightarrow CO + 2F,$$
$$Si + 4F \rightarrow SiF_4.$$

Similar results are obtained for SiO$_2$ etched in a mixture of CF$_4$ and O$_2$ as shown in Fig. 7. Again, the CF$_2$ concentration decreases with O$_2$ addition, but the etch rate for SiO$_2$ does not increase as rapidly as the Si etch rate.

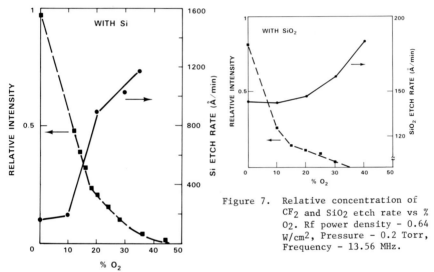

Figure 7. Relative concentration of CF$_2$ and SiO$_2$ etch rate vs % O$_2$. Rf power density - 0.64 W/cm^2, Pressure - 0.2 Torr, Frequency - 13.56 MHz.

Figure 6. Relative concentration of CF$_2$ and Si etch rate vs % O$_2$. Rf power density - 0.64 W/cm^2, Pressure - 0.2 Torr, Frequency - 13.56 MHz.

Chapman[20] has proposed that the relatively small change in SiO$_2$ etch rate compared to Si etch rate as O$_2$ is added to the CF$_4$ discharge is due to a built-in supply of liberated oxygen when SiO$_2$ is etched, and the addition of O$_2$ is superfluous. However, we do not observe a large decrease in the CF$_2$ concentration when the plasma chamber is heavily loaded with SiO$_2$ samples, indicating that oxygen liberated from SiO$_2$ etching does not change the composition of radicals in the plasma significantly. It has also been suggested that the slower etch rate in SiO$_2$ is accounted for by the strength of the Si-O bonds (~180 Kcal/mol) in SiO$_2$ compared to the Si-Si bonds (~ 80 Kcal/mol) in Si, rather than by the different reactive species involved in etching.[9] Our results are consistent with this model.

With the addition of O_2, the CF_2 radical concentration is inversely related to the Si or SiO_2 etch rates. This suggests that the concentration of atomic fluorine (the probable etching species) is in balance with the CF_2 concentration and the LIF of CF_2 may be used to monitor the etching of Si and SiO_2. Contrastingly, Millard and Kay[11] have monitored the CF_2 emission as oxygen was added to a CF_4 discharge and found the CF_2 emission to be independent of O_2 addition. They suggested that CF_2 did not react with O_2 in releasing fluorine. The apparent difference may result because the excited electronic state concentration is monitored by the emission spectrum while the ground state concentration is probed by LIF. Our results show that the CF_2 concentration decreases drastically as O_2 is added in CF_4.

Figures 8 and 9 show the result of hydrogen addition to a CF_4 discharge during Si and SiO_2 etching. In both cases, the CF_2 concentration increases and the etch rate decreases. Polymer film deposition was observed when the hydrogen percentage in the gas mixture exceeds 35%. The addition of H_2 reduced the Si etch rate faster than the SiO_2 etch rate. The highest selectivity between SiO_2 and Si was obtained near the onset of polymerization. The increase in CF_2 may be due to the reaction of hydrogen with free fluorine

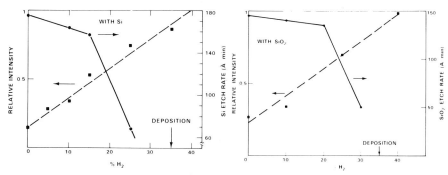

Figure 8. Relative concentration of CF_2 and Si etch rate vs % H_2.

Figure 9. Relative concentration of CF_2 and SiO_2 etch rate vs % H_2.

atoms to form HF, thereby reducing the availability of fluorine to recombine with CF_2, as follows:

$$F + H \rightarrow HF,$$
$$CF_2 + F \rightarrow CF_3.$$

Again, there is an inverse correlation between the CF_2 radical concentration and the Si or SiO_2 etch rates. The reduction in Si or SiO_2 etch rates when H_2 is added in CF_4 discharges may be due to the depletion of atomic fluorine by hydrogen and/or the formation of polymers on etched surfaces. Also, the CF_2 concentration is a good indicator of the onset of polymer deposition.

In conclusion, we have used LIF to probe the relative CF_2 concentration in a rf plasma discharge in CF_4, CF_4/O_2, and CF_4/H_2 mixtures. The CF_2 concentration increases with the rf power density, frequency, and pressure. Addition of oxygen depletes CF_2, but increases Si and SiO_2 etch rates.

Hydrogen addition to CF_4 discharges increases the CF_2 concentration, and the etch rates for Si and SiO_2 decrease; as CF_2 concentration is further increased, etching of Si or SiO_2 stops, and polymer deposition occurs. By replacing the fixed frequency laser source with a tunable source obtained by frequency doubling the output of a tunable dye laser, these measurements may be extended to monitoring CF_2 vibrational and rotational temperatures. Additional LIF measurements probing Si product species such as SiF, SiF_2 and SiF_4 are also possible. These additional measurements should add significantly to our understanding of etching Si in CF_4 plasma discharges.

ACKNOWLEDGMENT

The authors wish to thank T. O. Herndon for providing the design of the plasma system and for helpful discussions and L. J. Belanger for expert technical assistance.

REFERENCES

1. J. W. Coburn, Plasma Chemistry and Plasma Processing 2, 1 (1982).
2. D. L. Flamm and V. M. Donnelly, Plasma Chemistry and Plasma Processing, 1, 315 (1981).
3. E. O. Degenkolb and J. E. Griffiths, Appl. Spectrosc. 31, 40 (1977).
4. K. Hirobe and T. Tsuchimoto, J. Electrochem. Soc. 127, 234 (1980).
5. W. R. Harshbarger, R. A. Porter, T. A. Miller, and P. Norton, Appl. Spectrosc. 31, 201 (1977).
6. J. E. Greene, J. Vac. Sci. Technol. 15, 1718 (1978).
7. G. Smolinsky and M. J. Vasile, Int. J. Mass. Spectrom. Ion Phys. 16, 137 (1975).
8. D. L. Smith and R. H. Bruce, J. Electrochem. Soc. 129, 2045 (1982).
9. J. A. Thornton, J. Vac. Sci. Technol. 15, 188 (1978).
10. C. H. Steinbruchel, presented at the Electrochem. Soc. Meeting in Detroit, recent news paper 361 (1982).
11. P. J. Hargis, Jr. and M. J. Kushner, Appl. Phys. Lett. 40, 779 (1982).
12. R. A. Gottscho, G. Smolinsky, and R. H. Burton, J. Appl. Phys. 53, 5908 (1982).
13. V. M. Donnelly, D. L. Flamm, and G. Collins, J. Vac. Sci. Technol. 21, 817 (1982).
14. C. J. Mogab, A. C. Adams, and D. L. Flamm, J. Appl. Phys. 49, 3796 (1978).
15. L. M. Ephrath, J. Electrochem. Soc. 124, 2846 (1977).
16. M. M. Millard and E. Kay, J. Electrochem. Soc. 129, 160 (1982).
17. D. L. Flamm, Solid State Tech. 22, 109 (April, 1979).
18. H. F. Winters, J. W. Coburn, and E. Kay, J. Appl. Phys. 48, 4973 (1977).
19. D. S. King, P. K. Schenck, and J. C. Stephenson, J. Mol. Spectrosc. 78, 1 (1979).
20. B. N. Chapman, Glow Discharge Process, Wiley, New York, 1980.

SPECTROSCOPY AND PHOTOREACTIONS OF ORGANOMETALLIC MOLECULES ON SURFACES

C. J. CHEN, AND R. M. OSGOOD, JR.
Columbia Radiation Laboratory and Department of Electrical Engineering,
Columbia University, New York, NY 10027

ABSTRACT

A study of the UV photochemistry of organometallic molecules in the vapor and adsorbed phases is discussed. The gas-phase spectra is interpreted on the basis of molecular orbital theory and experimental data. The absorption spectra of the surface adlayers are determined by computer subtraction of the gas-phase spectra and an intepetation is provided. The influence of metal-substrate microstructure on UV photochemical reactions of metal alkyls is briefly discussed.

INTRODUCTION

Since the development of laser photochemical direct writing [1], there has been an increasing interest in the understanding of the UV photodissociation mechanism of organometallic molecules. While gas-phase ultraviolet absorption spectra can provide significant information on the dissociation process, the existing spectroscopic data are not complete and an analysis of the excited states has not been made [2-5]. Although one observation of the chemisorbed monolayer of DMCd (dimethyl cadmium) has been reported [6,7], the spectrum of the physisorbed molecular layer has not been measured. The difficulty of measuring the spectrum of the physisorbed layer stems from the fact that at high temperatures the physisorbed layers always coexist with a relatively dense ambient gas . As a consequence, the spectrum of the adlayer is obscured by that of the gas.
In this paper, we report on a study of the UV spectroscopy of adsorbed metal-alkyl molecules. The spectra, which include both the chemisorbed and physisorbed layers, are interpreted by comparison with our recent measurements of gas-phase metal alkyl molecules as well as by an analysis based on molecular-orbital considerations. In addition, a recent experiment to study the photodissociation of these same adsorbed molecules on metal features is described.

EXPERIMENTAL

A sketch of the apparatus is shown in Fig. 1. A nitrogen-purged, 0.3-m scanning monochromator with a 1200-groove-per-millimeter grating and a deuterium lamp provides a spectrally-tunable UV probe with 0.6 Å resolution. The power supplies for the anode and the filament of the deuterium lamp are both highly stabilized to provide a constant light intensity. A PDP-11 microcomputer controls the scanning of the monochromator, collects and stores the readings of the photomultiplier, and then performs scheduled computation.
The absorption cell is made of 316 stainless steel with both ends precisely ground. Ten to thirty suprasil (fused silica) discs can be fit in the cell, separated with C-shaped spacers of 25-μm thickness. The cell is enclosed in a copper thermal enclosure with thermal insulation. The temperature of the cell is regulated to within $\pm$ 0.2°C by a dry-ice bath and an electronic thermal controller.

The gas-handling system, with a diffusion pump, is made of stainless steel. It was baked to 200° C in vacuum before use. The cell is directly connected with the gas-handling system . The pressure is read with a digital capacitance manometer to 0.01 torr.

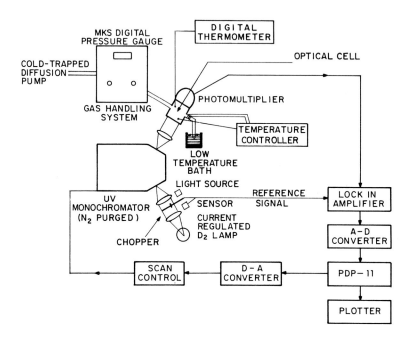

Fig. 1 Experimental apparatus.

RESULTS AND DISCUSSION

a) GAS SPECTRA

The gas spectra of DMZn, DMCd and DMHg are shown in Fig. 2. In general, the overall structure is similar; each consists of a weak absorption knee and a strong peak with almost equally spaced bands. However, for DMCd, another weak absorption peak in the short wavelength region is apparent. We will not discuss the detailed assignment of the electronic states here; instead, only our general conclusions will be summarized (Fig.3). The weak absorption feature at the long wavelength end results from a vibronically allowed quadrapole transition to a totally dissociative potential surface. The transition leads to the immediate formation of a metal atom in the ground state and two methyl radicals. The strong absorption feature, whose cross section is typical for an allowed dipole transition, produces a methyl radical and an

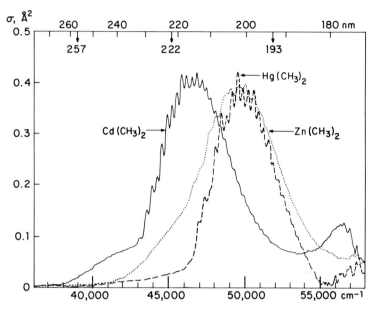

Fig. 2 UV absorption spectra of dimethyl zinc, dimethyl cadmium and diemthyl mercury.

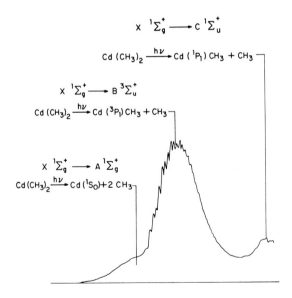

Fig. 3 The photofragmentation mechanism of organometallics.

excited metal monomethyl which dissociates after radiative emission to the
ground state. A third feature is just observable on the blue side of the
strong absorption band. In this VUV band the photon energy exceeds the sum of
the dissociation energy of the molecule into an excited metal atom and two
methyl radicals.

b) SPECTRA OF THE CHEMISORBED MONOLAYER

In the case of DMCd a chemisorbed monolayer forms first on the substrate.
Since this layer cannot be removed by pumping, the measurement is simple,
requiring no subtraction of the gas spectra (Fig. 4). Note that there is no
chemisorbed layer for the related compound DMHg. This is consistent with the
fact that, unlike DMCd, DMHg is air and moisture stable. We believe that the
DMCd reacts with the OH radical on the silica surface and produces cadmium
monomethyl with its cadmium atom firmly bonded on the surface.

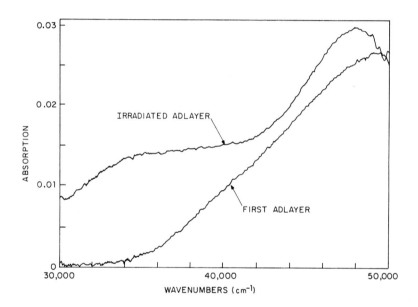

Fig. 4 The absorption spectrum of the chemisorbed $Cd(CH_3)_2$.

If the monolayer is irradiated with an 193-nm laser beam, the spectrum
changes radically, thus indicating that the monolayer is activated or dissociated by ultraviolet light. Exposure to air also changes the spectrum
strongly. Note that at 257 nm, the absorption strength of the chemisorbed
layer is about 7.8 times greater than for an equivalent quantity of molecules
in the gas phase.

c) SPECTRA OF THE PHYSISORBED LAYER

The spectra of the physisorbed DMCd layers at 0° C is shown in Fig. 5. Twenty surfaces were used to obtain this spectra in a cell, with a free path of 0.405 mm. Under these conditions the absorbtion due to the gas is only about 30% of the total absorbtion signal. Thus, even the unprocessed cell spectra are radically different from the gas spectra. The gas portion of the spectra is then subtracted accurately by an on-line computer. Several features of the absorption spectra of the physisorbed layers are notable. First, the strong absorbtion peak is slightly redshifted and its vibrational structure is almost completely washed out. Note, however, that there still appears to be some residual vibronic structure. Second, there is a strong pressure and temperature dependence to the adsorbtion depth of the adlayer. Third, there is a long wavelength tail extending directly to visible wavelengths. The wavelength dependence of this tail is very flat and the pressure dependence of it is radically different from that of the main peak. At low pressures the dependence of this tail is nonlinear; in contrast, the linear dependence of the absorption in the main peak is consistent with the measurements of the DMCd isotherm.

The interpretation of the physisorbed layer spectra is as follows. Most of the molecules in the physisorbed layer are in a liquid-like environment, in which the dense molecular environment can broaden spectral features due to shift in the intromolecular potential of the upper and lower energy states.

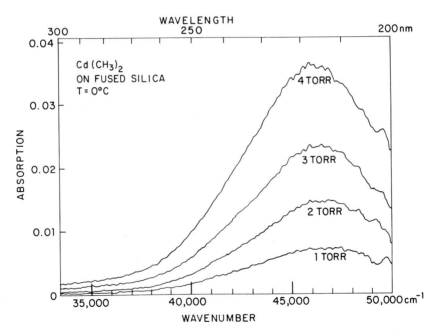

Fig. 5 The absorption spectra of the physisorbed $Cd(CH_3)_2$ at 0° C.

The long-wavelength tail is due to the Rayleigh scattering by the
nonuniformity thickness of the adsorbed layer. This nonuniformity increases
near the condensation point. Note that the high surface density and the
slight spectral redshift of the adsorbed-layers may play an important role in
photochemically producing the first metal-atom clusters on the surface.

LOCAL-FIELD-ENHANCEMENT OF SURFACE PHOTOCHEMISTRY

We have recently studied the photochemistry of adsorbed organometallic
layers on metal particles. These studies are important in clarifying the
early stages of film growth from small metal nuclei.

It is well known that, the free electrons in metal microstructures can
exhibit a plasma resonance at a particular wavelength determined by the
dielectric function and the geometry of the metal structure [9]. An
interesting fact is that for cadmium spheres with diameter about 10 - 50 nm
a strong plasma resonance exists near 257 nm. At plasma resonance, the
electric field intensity on and near the cadmium spheres will be considerably
greater than that of the incident field; and, consequently, the rate of
photochemical reactions on and near the spheres should be correspondingly
greater.

This effect was observed directly in an experiment described as follows.
Small cadmium spheres of diameter 10-30 nm were made on a very thin
(d $\sim$ 100 Å) carbon film supported on a 3-mm diameter copper grid. The film
was then enclosed in an optical cell with quartz windows filled with 1 torr of
DMCd and 1000 torr of argon gas. The film was then irradiated with a slightly
defocused 257-nm laser beam of approximately 1 mW/cm^2 intensity. After a one
minute exposure, a thin deposition of cadmium was observed. The transmission-
electron-microscope photographs of the cadmium deposition at resolution $\sim$10Å
revealed two interesting features (Fig. 6); viz, the small spheres grew into

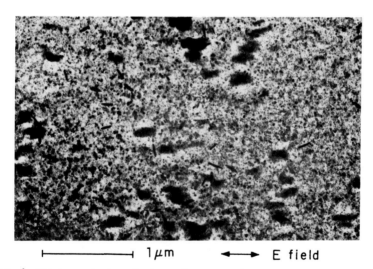

Fig. 6 The transmission-electron-microscope photograph of photodeposited
cadmium on a carbon film covered with cadmium spheres, which were
prepared separately.

prolate spheriods of dimension ∼ 0.1 μm with the major axis parallel to the electric field of the incident light, and around each spheriod there was an interference pattern with a thick elliptical core of dimension 0.1 μm x 0.2 um and a very thin elliptical ring of dimension 0.25 μm x 0.4 μm. This latter observation is consistent with the theoretical model of the interference pattern of the reradiated retarded field of a resonanting dipole with the incident field. A more detailed account of this experiment is to be published elsewhere [10].

CONCLUSION

In this paper, we have discussed the effects of solid surfaces on the photochemistry and spectroscopy of adsorbed metal-alkyl molecules. Several of the results including the spectral redshift and the enhanced reaction rate on small metal features are important in understanding both the rate and the spatial localization in photodeposition.

We would like to acknowledge significant contribution to this work by Heinz Gilgen and Abraham Szöke.

REFERENCES

1. D.J. Ehrlich, R.M. Osgood, Jr., and T.F. Deutsch, IEEE Journal of Quantum Electronics, 16 1233 (1980).

2. G. Herzberg, Molecular Spectra and Molecular Structure III. Electronic Spectra and Electronic Structure of Polyatomic Molecules, D. Van Nostrand, (1966).

3. H.W. Thompson and W. Linnett, Proc. Roy. Soc. A156 108 (1936).

4. C. Jonah, P. Chandra and R. Bersohn, J. Chem. Phys., 55 1903 (1971).

5. M.E. Kellman, P. Pechukas and R. Bersohn, Chem. Phys. Letters, 83 304 (1981).

6. D.J. Ehrlich and R.M. Osgood, Jr., Chem. Phys. Lett., 79 381 (1981).

7. Y. Rytz-Froidevaux, R.P. Salathe', H.H. Gilgen and H.P. Weber, Appl. Phys. A27 133 (1982).

8. See, for example, D.M. Young and A.D. Crowell, Physical Adsorption of Gases, Butterworths, (1962).

9. See, for example, J. Gersten and A. Nitzan, J. Chem. Phys., 75 1139 (1981).

10. For a preliminary account see paper Phys. 96, C.J. Chen and R.M. Osgood, Jr., 184th Annual American Chemical Society Meeting, Kansas City, MO.

THE SPECTROSCOPY AND PHOTOLYSIS OF METALLO-ORGANIC PRECURSORS TO III-V COMPOUNDS

MARTIN R AYLETT AND JOHN HAIGH
British Telecom Research Laboratories, Martlesham Heath, Suffolk, UK.

ABSTRACT

This paper describes the deposition by light-stimulated breakdown of gallium and indium on borosilicate glass, gallium arsenide and indium phosphide substrates, from precursors whose ultraviolet (uv) spectra have recently been reported. Some preliminary work on the deposition of indium phosphide is also reported, using an indium-phosphorus complex whose uv spectrum is also given.

INTRODUCTION

Deposition of metals by light-stimulated breakdown of metallo-organic vapours is attracting increasing attention [1,2] Its potential capabilities include localised selected-area deposition ("writing") and implantation without the need for a deposition mask. Developments of the technique towards epitaxial deposition of III-V compounds would make available new, unique, capabilities. These might include:- a) the growth of alloy compositions with lateral compositional variation (which would allow, in optoelectronic devices for example, the production of lasers with different emission wavelengths on the same chip) and b) a new lower-temperature deposition technique, possibly when combined with metallo-organic chemical vapour deposition (MOCVD). An approach in the latter direction has been initiated by Frolov [3].

We have recently presented [4] the ultraviolet (uv) vapour-phase spectra of the compounds $GaMe_3$, $GaEt_3$, $AlEt_3$, $InMe_3$, $InEt_3$, and InC_5H_5. The spectra show reasonably intense bands at 190 - 250 nm wavelength, indicating that optical power may be coupled into the molecules at wavelengths within the silica transmission range. This makes it possible to consider photolytic breakdown of these species - that is, direct absorption of a photon by the molecule leading to dissociation - as an approach to III-V compound deposition. However it must be stressed, as has been pointed out recently [5,6] that light-stimulated decomposition may occur by routes other than photolysis, not all of which may admit of the advantages discussed above. If we consider firstly deposition on semiconducting substrates, then since these are strongly absorbing in the uv/visible region the light flux incident on the substrate will create large numbers of phonons, electrons and holes. The presence of these must increase the possibility of a catalysed pyrolysis reaction occurring on the surface of the substrate. Secondly in the 190 - 300 nm band the photon energy exceeds the work function of the semiconductor, so that if the ambient pressure is low there is the possibility of electrons being ejected and interacting with the vapour [6]. This again will modify the course of the reaction.

Ultraviolet laser sources have been extensively used in the light-stimulated deposition of metals because of the technological emphasis on highly spatially confined deposition. It is worth pointing out the value of broad-band sources where there is no immediate need for spatial confinement of the light flux. Their main advantage is that it is easier to ensure efficient photolytic coupling of energy into a range of molecules of unknown absorption spectra from a broad-band source than from a narrow-band fixed frequency source. This is particularly important for the alkyl compounds of metals of groups II-IV of the

Periodic Table, because although some of them have ultraviolet spectra which are purely continuous, others have sharp lines superimposed on the continua [7]. If a narrow-band source is being used, small frequency shifts in the source or spectral shifts due to, for example, pressure changes, may give rise to unwanted variations in the power coupling because of the presence of such fine-structure in the spectrum.

The present paper discusses the light-stimulated decomposition of some of the compounds listed above, as a step towards III-V synthesis, and also of the volatile complex $Me_3In.PMe_3$.

EXPERIMENTAL

The method of obtaining the uv spectra of the vapours has been recently described [4].

The apparatus for light-stimulated decomposition is shown in Figure 1. It is made entirely in silica and borosilicate glass except for two stainless steel and Viton couplings at the substrate pedestal mount and at the mass spectrometer outlet, and for PTFE taps. The apparatus is pumped to about 10^{-2} torr by a rotary pump with a liquid nitrogen trap.

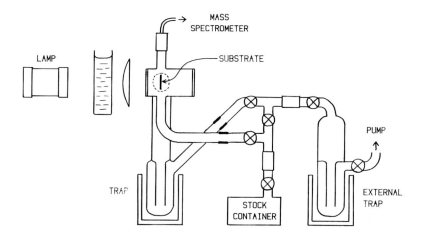

Fig. 1. Schematic diagram of the decomposition apparatus.

The lamp is a Varian VIX 300 UV high-pressure xenon arc, giving at the focus about 20 watts cm^{-2} uv flux over an area of 0.25 - 0.5 cm^2. The infrared content is reduced by a 1 cm path-length water filter.

Gallium trimethyl and indium trimethyl were electronic grade samples supplied by, respectively, Labolac SA and Alfa Ventron. Indium cyclopentadienyl and indium trimethyl - phosphorus trimethyl complex were supplied by the Chemistry Department, Queen Mary College, London University. The metallo-organic compounds were sublimed or distilled into the trap from stock containers. The stock container was then removed, the pumping direction reversed, and the vapour slowly pumped from the warmed trap via the deposition chamber to the external trap. This two-stage pumping process allowed some degree of control over the flow rate of the vapour, and also permitted the removal of any volatile decomposition products (alkanes, cyclopentadiene, etc) which might otherwise accumulate in the stock container, or be produced by trace hydrolysis in the apparatus. The mass spectrometer (SX300, VG Gas Analysis Ltd) gave a measure of the point of onset of decomposition, by the appearance of hydrocarbon fragments. It also allowed the assessment of reproducibility of the decomposition rate.

Deposits were obtained on borosilicate (Pyrex) glass, and on gallium arsenide (100) and indium phosphide (100) single crystal surfaces. They were analysed by SEM EDAX and by Auger spectroscopy.

DISCUSSION

a) Indium trimethyl

Figure 2a shows that deposition of indium from $InMe_3$ on Pyrex yields droplets. Auger analysis indicates these to be pure indium. The appearance of the deposit indicates that the temperature has exceeded the melting point (156°C) at some stage. At this temperature pyrolysis of the vapour can take place [8], so that it is likely that such pyrolysis will play a part in the build-up of the deposit. The deposit on gallium arsenide is more uniform, with only occasional large droplets (Fig. 2b).

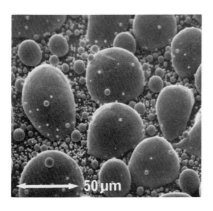 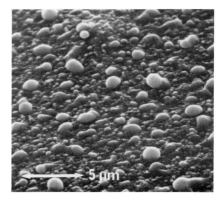

Fig. 2. Deposition of indium from $InMe_3$ vapour.
    a) on Pyrex glass   b) on gallium arsenide

b) Indium cyclopentadienyl (InCp)

This compound was examined because it contains only one indium-to-carbon bond, the structure being analogous to ferrocene [9]. It seems possible therefore that photodissociation to indium may be produced by a single photon absorption, whereas in the case of the trialkyls such an absorption, by breaking only one bond [10], will leave a radical which must decompose further to liberate the metal.

The decomposition of the compound in the presence of a Pyrex substrate gave a deposit which over part of its area consisted of droplets of pure indium. However Auger analysis indicated that the deposit was heterogeneous, and some areas consisted essentially of carbon. The difference in this behaviour from that found for the trimethyl lies in the propensity for further photolysis or pyrolysis of the organic component of the InCp decomposition products. The following reaction scheme, although hypothetical, illustrates this point:-

$$InC_5H_5 \rightarrow In + C_5H_5 \cdot$$

followed by

$$2\ C_5H_5 \cdot \rightarrow \text{(structure)}\ (C_{10}H_{10})$$

The product $C_{10}H_{10}$, dihydrofulvalene, is a conjugated diene and will absorb very strongly in the uv, undergoing photochemical condensation reactions as a result [11]. Other reaction routes from $C_5H_5 \cdot$ may be postulated as alternatives, but also lead to strongly absorbing dienes. Thus further photochemical action will take place in all cases, leading ultimately to a carbon-rich solid which presumably will develop where the beam intensity is highest. Hence in order to be able to use this, or related, potentially attractive indium precursors it will be necessary to investigate carefully the photochemistry of the organic decomposition products, possibly with a view to choosing a wavelength which is inactive to the latter.

c) Gallium trimethyl

Deposition of gallium trimethyl on gallium arsenide yields droplets which Auger analysis shows to be gallium with some carbon.

d) Indium trimethyl - phosphorus trimethyl complex

$Me_3In.PEt_3$ has been pyrolysed by workers in our laboratory and elsewhere to yield indium phosphide [12,13], although it has not yet been found possible to obtain a stoichiometric product without adding phosphine to the gas stream. The related complex $Me_3In.PMe_3$ has a uv spectrum (fig 3) which shows a very strong absorption at 200 nm. The light-stimulated breakdown, when carried out with an indium phosphide substrate, gave a deposit which was mostly indium, but in places consisted of whisker growths of indium phosphide (Fig. 4) which carried droplets of indium at their tips. This indicated that deposition of indium phosphide occurred by a vapour-liquid-solid mechanism, suggestive cf a deficient supply of phosphorus. Similar structures were observed when a gallium arsenide substrate was used. It remains to be seen whether this deficiency was simply due to loss of the volatile phosphorus component following breakdown of the complex by heat.

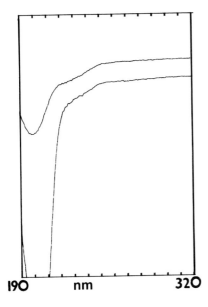

Fig 3.
UV spectrum of $Me_3In.PMe_3$.
Transmittance plotted vertically on arbitrary scale at two pressures.

Absorbance greater than 100 000 neper cm^{-1} litre mol^{-1}.

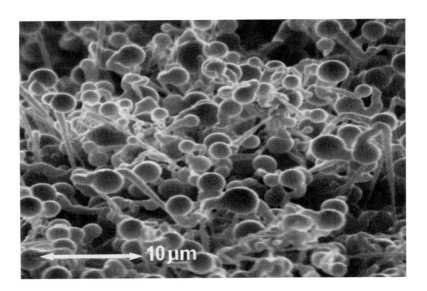

Fig 4. Crystalline growth of InP from decomposition of $Me_3In.PMe_3$.

CONCLUSIONS

These results show, encouragingly, that uv/visible light may be used to bring about the deposition of gallium and indium metals. A number of compounds of these metals which absorb uv light have been shown to be decomposed by it. It is still unclear whether the reaction is wholly or even partly photolytic. Indium cyclopentadienyl, which is attractive on photochemical grounds as a precursor, gives films containing carbon because of photochemical or pyrolytic reactions undergone by its organic decomposition products. It may be possible to overcome this problem. Indium alkyl - phosphorus alkyl complexes are indicated to be useful precursors to InP, but as with MOCVD reaction there is loss of phosphorus. However lowering the temperature may reduce this loss.

ACKNOWLEDGEMENTS

We thank Professor M M Faktor and Dr H Chudzynska, London University, for the synthesis of some of the compounds, and Mr C G Tuppen for Auger analyses. Acknowledgement is made to the Director of Research, British Telecom, for permission to publish this work.

REFERENCES

1. D. J. Ehrlich, R. M. Osgood and T. F. Deutsch, IEEE Journal of Quantum Electronics QE-16, 1233 (1980).

2. S. D. Allen, J. Appl. Phys. 52, 6501 (1981).

3. I. A. Frolov, B. L. Druz', P. B. Boldyrevskii and E. B. Sokolov, Izv. Akad. Nauk SSSR Neorg. Mat. 13, 906, (1977).

4. J. Haigh, Journal of Materials Science, to be published.

5. Y. Rytz-Froidevaux, R. P. Salathé, H. H. Gilgen and H. P. Weber, Applied Physics A, 27, 133 (1982).

6. P. A. George and J. L. Beauchamp, Thin Solid Films, 67, L25 (1980).

7. H. W. Thompson and J. W. Linnett, Proc. Roy. Soc. 156A, 108, (1936).

8. M. G. Jacko and S. J. W. Price, Can. J. Chem. 42, 1198 (1964).

9. S. Shibata, L. S. Bartell and R. M. Gavin, J. Chem. Phys. 41, 717 (1964).

10. Z. Karny, R. Naaman and R. N. Zare, Chem. Phys. Letters 59, 33 (1978).

11. For illustrations of the photochemistry of dienes see: Aspects of Organic Photochemistry, W. M. Horspool (Academic Press, London 1976).

12. H. Renz, J. Weidlein, K. W. Benz and M. H. Pilkuhn, Electronics Letters 16, 228 (1980).

13. R. W. Moss and J. S. Evans, Journal of Crystal Growth 55, 129 (1981).

SECTION VI
PHOTODEPOSITION OF SEMICONDUCTORS

SEMICONDUCTOR THIN FILMS GROWN BY LASER PHOTOLYSIS

J.G. EDEN, J.E. GREENE, J.F. OSMUNDSEN, D. LUBBEN, C.C. ABELE, S. GORBATKIN AND H.D. DESAI
University of Illinois, Urbana, IL 61801

ABSTRACT

Thin ($\leq$ 1.2 μm) Ge and Si films have been grown with rates up to 3.6 μm/hr by laser-induced chemical vapor deposition (LCVD) on a variety of substrates. Germanium films grown on amorphous SiO_2 (quartz) by photodissociating GeH_4 in He at 248 nm (KrF laser) exhibit grain sizes of 0.3 - 0.5 μm that increase only slightly up to the pryolytic threshold for GeH_4 (280°C). On (100) NaCl, however, Ge films grown at a substrate temperature of 120°C are expitaxial. The activation energy for the LCVD growth of Ge films (from GeH_4) on SiO_2 is measured to be 85 ± 20 meV which suggests that germanium is arriving at the substrate in atomic form. The wavelength and intensity dependence of the initial film growth rate supports the conclusion that this process is photolytic and is initiated by the absorption of a single photon.

INTRODUCTION

Several groups have recently demonstrated the growth of Ge, Si, SiO_2 and Si_3N_4 films on a variety of substrates by photodissociating GeH_4, $Ge(CH_3)_4$ or SiH_4 alone or in the presence of N_2O or NH_3 [1-4]. These experiments have generally utilized excimer lasers since the photon energies available (3.5 $\leq$ hν $\leq$ 6.4 eV) enable most chemical bonds to be broken with a single photon. Hanabusa et al [2] have reported the growth of Si films by photo-dissociating SiH_4 in the infrared with a CO_2 laser but this process requires collisions (i.e., high pressure) in order to effect film growth. The attractiveness of growing semiconductor films by photolytic, laser induced chemical vapor deposition (LCVD) is due to: 1) minimal heating of the substrate which allows for lower temperature processing than that afforded by conventional CVD and 2) the independently adjustable wavelength and intensity of the laser which permit control over the nature and rate of the photo-induced gas reaction. The only drawback of photolytic LCVD is that the bond to be broken within the semiconductor-bearing polyatomic molecule fixes the maximum allowable wavelength of the laser.

In an earlier paper [3], it was shown that polycrystalline Ge films could be grown at room temperature on amorphous SiO_2 (quartz) by photodissociating GeH_4 (He carrier gas) with an ArF (193 nm, hν = 6.4 eV) or KrF (248 nm, hν = 5.0 eV) laser which establishes a wavelength threshold $hν_{MIN} \sim$ 4.0 eV for the process, which is consistent with the known energy of the GeH_3-H bond (3.3-3.8 eV). The low temperature of the substrate in these initial studies, however, restricted the grain sizes to $\sim$ 0.3-0.5 μm and the film conductivity was low due to intergranular voids.

EXPERIMENTAL PROCEDURE

In this paper, the LCVD growth of Ge films on amorphous SiO_2, (100) NaCl and $1\bar{1}02$ sapphire at substrate temperatures up to ~ 500K is reported. Figure 1 is a schematic diagram of the experimental apparatus used to grow the films and to spectroscopically examine the gas phase excited species produced by the excimer laser. The rectangular (2.9 cm x 0.5 cm) output beam from a KrF laser (20 Hz, 10-40 mJ/pulse) is focussed into the reactor by a 20 cm focal length cylindrical lens. In order to compress the long dimension of the pump beam, the lens is mounted with its axis perpendicular to the optical axis of the propagating laser beam. With this arrangement, the substrate area illuminated by the pump is typically 0.5 x 0.5 cm^2 when the lens focus is positioned 2 cm beyond the substrate.

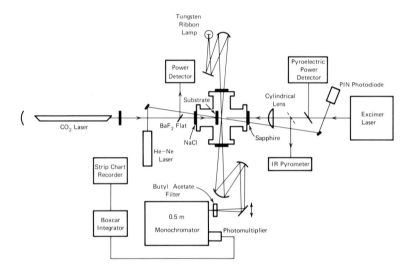

Fig. 1. Partial schematic diagram of the experimental apparatus used to grow Ge and Si films by photolytic LCVD. This arrangement allows the study of the spatially and spectrally-resolved emission that is generated by the laser-excited GeH_4 gas.

Substrate temperatures up to ~ 300°C are obtained while still maintaining spatial selectivity by irradiating the substrate with a CO_2 laser (maximum of 11 W TEM_{00}). An IR pyrometer monitors the substrate temperature (which requires a sapphire entrance window) and the results were verified by measuring the CO_2 laser power necessary to melt tin, indium or zinc pellets (melting points of 232, 155 and 420°C, respectively) on the substrate. A pyroelectric detector monitors the average power of both lasers and the thickness of the growing Ge or Si films is measured in transmission using a low power He-Ne laser [3].

The reactor is evacuated by a liquid-N_2 trapped diffusion pump and the system has a base vacuum of < 10^{-7} Torr. For most of the experiments to be described later, the reactor was statically filled with a 5% GeH_4/He gas mixture.

Spontaneous emission, from electronically excited atomic and molecular species near the substrate that are produced by the laser, is collected at 90° with a telescope composed of 7 cm dia. mirrors and is imaged onto the entrance slits of a 0.5 m Jarrell-Ash monochromator. By translating the final (planar) mirror of the telescope in the manner shown, spatially-resolved scans (in the direction normal to the substrate) of the fluorescence emanating from the gas phase near the surface are obtained. To reject stray pump laser (248 nm) radiation scattered into the detection system, a butyl acetate filter [7] is situated in front of the monochromator.

RESULTS AND DISCUSSIONS

The results of measurements of the initial Ge film growth rate R_0 versus SiO_2 substrate temperature T_s are shown in Fig. 2. Note that these experiments were conducted well below the pyrolytic threshold of GeH_4 (~280°C). In contrast to the weak temperature dependence of R_0, the film incubation time drops rapidly, reaching ~ 60s for $T_s \simeq$ 400K. An Arrhenius plot of $\ln R_0$ as a function of $(kT_s)^{-1}$ is presented in Fig. 3 for the growth of Ge on amorphous SiO_2. The measured activation energy of 85 ± 20 meV is considerably smaller than those typical of dissociative absorption and suggests that germanium is transported to the substrate in atomic form and not as GeH. This is also much less than the activation energy for pyrolysis of GeH_4 (1-2 eV). This supports the conclusion that the production of Ge is occurring near the substrate but in the gas phase.

Although not indicated in Fig. 1, Ge films have also been grown by passing the excimer beam parallel to and ~ 1 mm away from the substrate surface. This further substantiates the photolytic nature of the growth process since the substrate is not heated by the excimer laser at all. Also, in this configuration, film growth rates were observed to be one-to-two orders of magnitude lower than those obtained with normal incidence.

A segment (330-440 nm) of the spectrum that is observed when ~ 1.7 Torr of GeH_4 (in 32 Torr He) is photolyzed at 248 nm is illustrated in Fig. 4. The $^2\Delta \rightarrow ^2\Pi$ band of GeH is clearly present as are several atomic Ge lines, most of which terminate on the $^1D_2$ metastable state. Although not shown here, all of the neutral Ge resonance transitions between λ = 250 nm and 300 nm were also observed.

For the spatially-resolved measurements, the $5^1P_1 \rightarrow 4^1D_2$ line of Ge at 303.9 nm was chosen for initial studies and a representative scan is shown in Fig. 5 where the substrate is located at x = 0.

For the gas pressure and laser intensities studied here, a luminous region extending ~ 1 cm from the substrate was observed. Figure 5 illustrates the asymmetry of this emission about x = 0.5 cm which appears to arise from: 1) the interaction of laser-produced excited species with the surface or 2) diffusion. By adjusting the substrate temperature and gas pressure, this luminous region can be moved away from the substrate. As this happens, the emission profile becomes symmetric as would be expected.

The tungsten ribbon lamp and spherical mirrors illustrated at the top of Fig. 1 were used to measure the spatial resolution of the detection system. The inset of Fig. 5 shows a scan of the tungsten ribbon lamp after it had been imaged (1:1) to a point in front of the substrate. The FWHM of this scan is 2 mm which is precisely the physical width of the lamp's filament. An advantage of this system is that it does not require mechanical apertures to define the region viewed by the detection system.

Clearly, the photodissociation of GeH_4 produces a variety of atomic and

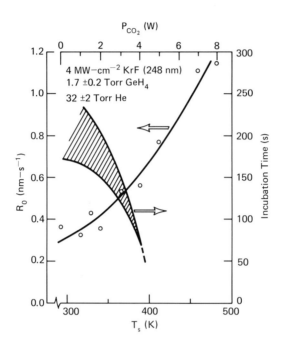

Fig. 2 Dependence of the intial Ge film growth R_0 on the substrate temperature T_s when GeH_4 is photodissociated at 248 nm. The rapid decline of the incubation time with T_s is also shown.

molecular species some of which demand the absorption of more than one KrF photon. The 5^1P_1 state of neutral Ge, for example, lies ~ 5 eV above ground. To investigate this further, the KrF intensity dependence of several neutral Ge and GeH lines was determined and the results are presented in Fig. 6. For $2 \le I_{KrF} \le 4$ MW - cm^{-2}, the transition intensity varied as $I_{KrF}^{1.4 \pm 0.1 K_{KrF}}$ for each line investigated. Since the KrF threshold intensity for the growth of Ge on SiO_2 is ~ 1 MW - cm^{-2}, it is unlikely that the intensity dependence depicted in Fig. 6 is due to saturation effects. Still, the reasons for the dependence are presently unclear and additional measurements in this area are being made in an effort to unravel the gas phase photochemistry with the goal of correlating excited state densities and kinetic behavior with the quality of the resulting Ge film.

Ge films grown on amorphous SiO_2 at room temperature are polycrystalline with average grain sizes of 0.3-0.5 μm, but, as mentioned earlier, intergranular voids cause the films to be highly resistive. As the substrate temperature is increased, the grains enlarge only slightly (0.5-0.7 μm at 250°C) until pyrolytic threshold is reached (280°C) at which point the grain

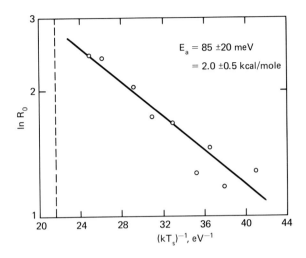

Fig. 3. Variation of R_0 with T_s^{-1} showing that R varies as $\exp(-E_a/kT)$ where E_a = 0.085 eV.

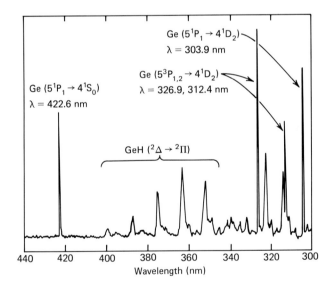

Fig. 4. A portion of the emission spectrum observed when GeH_4 is photolyzed at 248 nm (KrF laser).

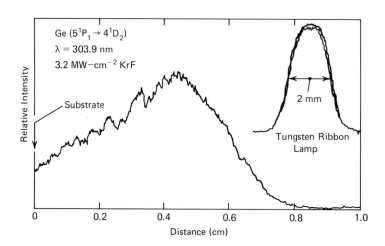

Fig. 5. Spatially-resolved emission profile that is observed from electronically excited Ge at 304 nm. The resolution of the detection system is less than 0.2 mm. The inset shows a scan of the tungsten ribbon that has been imaged (1:1) to a point ~ 1 cm from the substrate.

size rapidly increases to ~ 10 μm. X-ray diffractometry and transmission electron microscopy show a slight (111) orientation to the grains.

Films were also grown on (100) NaCℓ for substrate temperatures up to 150°C. In this case X-ray diffraction shows only the (400) peak and the films are highly conducting. TEM and electron channeling studies are underway to further characterize these films.

In summary, crystalline Ge films have been grown on quartz and (100) NaCℓ by photodissociating GeH_4 over a heated substrate with an excimer laser. Polycrystalline Si films have also been grown on quartz. From the film growth rate and spectroscopic measurements made to date, two major conclusions can be drawn:

1) The wavelength and intensity dependence of R_o indicate that the film growth process is photolytic and is initiated by the gas phase absorption of a single KrF photon. The subsequent absorption of one or more photons is required to produce the Ge and GeH excited states that are observed.

2) The substrate temperature dependence of R_o yields an activation energy $E_a < 0.1$ eV which suggests that germanium is arriving at the surface in atomic form.

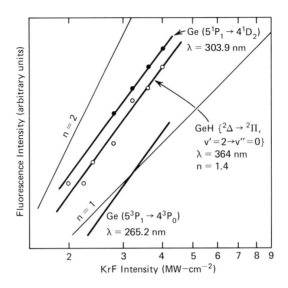

Fig. 6. The dependence of various Ge and GeH emission line intensities on the KrF pump intensity. The threshold for photodissociative growth of Ge (from GeH_4) on amorphous SiO_2 is ~ 1 MW-cm^{-2}.

ACKNOWLEDGMENTS

The authors wish to thank P.J. Hargis, Jr. and J.T. Verdeyen for many interesting discussions and suggestions and Y. Moroz, R. Witt and J. Keller for excellent technical assistance. Also, the support of this work by the Air Force Office of Scientific Research (H. Schlossberg) under contract 79-0138 and the Office of Naval Research under contract N00014-81-K-0568 is gratefully acknowledged.

REFERENCES

1. D.J. Ehrlich, R.M. Osgood, Jr. and T.F. Deutsch, IEEE J. Quant. Electron. QE-16, 1233 (1980).

2. M. Hanabusa, A. Namiki and K. Yoshihara, Appl. Phys. Lett. 35, 627 (1979).

3. R.W. Andreatta, C.C. Abele, J.F. Osmundsen, J.G. Eden, D. Lubben and J.E. Greene, Appl. Phys. Lett. 40, 183 (1982).

4. P.K. Boyer, G.A. Roche, W.H. Ritchie and G.J. Collins, Appl. Phys. Lett. 40, 716 (1982).

5. Bond Dissociation Energies in Simple Molecules, B. deB. Darwent, ed., NSRDS-NBS 31, National Bureau of Standards, Washington, DC, (1970), p. 31.

6. K.C. Kim, D.W. Setser and C.M. Bogan, J. Chem. Phys. 60, 1837 (1974).

7. P.J. Hargis, Jr., Appl. Opt. 20, 149 (1981); P.J. Hargis, Jr., and M.J. Kushner, Appl. Phys. Lett. 40, 779 (1982).

LASER STIMULATED GROWTH OF EPITAXIAL GaAs

WALTER ROTH, HERBERT KRÄUTLE, ANNEMARIE KRINGS AND HEINZ BENEKING
Institute of Semiconductor Electronics, Sommerfeldstraße, D-5100 Aachen,FRG

ABSTRACT

Stimulated growth of single crystalline GaAs has been obtained by irradiation of (100) oriented GaAs substrates inside an MOCVD reactor with a pulsed Nd-YAG laser.
Process temperatures have been varied between $540^{\circ}C$ and $360^{\circ}C$. In the non-irradiated areas, below $480^{\circ}C$ substrate temperature the growth rate decreases rapidly, whereas in the irradiated part of the substrate epitaxial layers could be grown in the whole temperature range investigated. Below $450^{\circ}C$, the growth is reaction limited.

INTRODUCTION

Laser induced decomposition of metal-organic compounds has been successfully demonstrated for various materials. Using UV lasers the molecules can be decomposed with low power light sources. This process depends sensitively on laser wavelength because of its photochemical nature. Submicrometer resolution in metal patterns has been achieved /1/.
A technique using thermal effects of a laser beam is the so called "Graphoepitaxy", a crystallisation of amorphous films which are deposited on structured non lattice matched, nonsinglecrystalline substrates. This process was first carried out by laser heating /2/. However, recent publications report on the advantages of other power sources like strip heater arrangements /3/.
In this paper we describe a method, which uses a laser stimulated MOCVD-process with Trimethylgallium (TMG) and Arsine for epitaxial growth on (100) GaAs. The temperature range of a GaAs-MOCVD-process extends from 500 to 700 $^{\circ}C$ with a preferred growth temperature at about 650 $^{\circ}C$. The lower temperature limit is given by the decomposition rate of the Arsine molecules, which decreases rapidly below 500 $^{\circ}C$. However, when special arrangements are used, process temperatures down to 450 $^{\circ}C$ can be realized /4/. In our process the laser beam stimulates the cracking and growth reactions, leading to single crystalline layers at extremely low temperatures.

EXPERIMENTAL PART

The experimental arrangement shown in fig. 1 shows the MOCVD-reactor, which has been especially designed for laser irradiation of the sample during growth. The L-shaped quartz reactor allows irradiation with a horizontal beam maintaining a natural flow of the heated gases, because a convection induced vertical flow is achieved in the direction of the exaust. The process temperature is controlled by two thermocouples sticking inside the narrow quartz tubes, which hold the graphite susceptor. The samples are situated on the front side of the susceptor with an angle of 7° to the vertical axis. This arrangement keeps the wafer in position without special clamping and allows an effective irradiation of the wafer surface with the laser beam. Simultaneously the graphite susceptor can be heated from the rear with a spot heater as reported earlier /5/. The gases enter the reactor through the mixing head on the left. The laser entrance window is continously flushed with pure hydrogen, which prevents deposition of Ga and As. The laser used is a frequency doubled Nd-YAG laser (λ= 530 nm) with 3 ns pulse width and a maximum pulse energy of 200 mJ. Maximum pulse repetition frequency is 10 Hz.

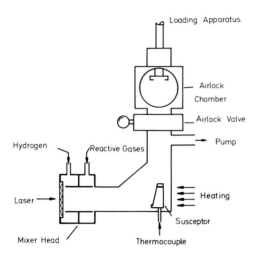

Fig. 1: MOCVD reactor designed for laser stimulated growth

Standard process parameters in our experiments were a pressure of 950 mbar, a hydrogen flow rate of 4000 sccm/min, TMG flow-0.3 sccm/min, AsH_3 flow-12sccm/min. The substrates were loaded through the airlock system into the evacuated reactor, and flushed with H_2 for 10 min. Then the temperature was raised linearly to the process temperature, after that the arsine flow was raised. The whole system was allowed to stabilize for 10 min, TMG flow and laser were simultaneously switched on. Growth was maintained for one hour. After the TMG and the laser were turned off, arsine flow was lowered to zero within two minutes and temperature was linearly reduced to room temperature (5 min). The surface of the samples was controlled by an SEM and a phase contrast optical microscope. Layer thickness was measured with an optical microscope, after the sample had been stained.

RESULTS

Fig. 2 shows the growth rate of GaAs deposited within and outside the laser irradiated area as a function of substrate temperature. In the range of 540 °C to 480 °C no strong difference in growth rate can be seen between the irradiated and nonirradiated part. However, the morphology is very different. Whereas the irradiated area is a bright single crystalline layer, the unirradiated part shows increasing roughness and polycrystalline growth with decreasing process temperature. However, for lower flow speeds in other reactors monocrystalline growth has been realized in this temperature range /4/. Below 480 °C, growth rate in the non irradiated areas drops rapidly, and is below the measuring sensitivity at 450 °C, whereas in the laser stimulated region only a slight decrease occurs. At 450 °C a laser stimulated growth rate of about 3μm/h is obtained.

Fig. 3 shows the influence of laser power on morphology at 450 °C. Without laser illumination, only few whiskers are grown, which is typical for arsenic limited growth. At an energy density of the laser pulse of about 70 mJ/cm^2 a very rough polycrystalline layer is formed. The optimum energy density is 120 mJ/cm^2, which allows to grow a smooth monocrystalline layer. Power ratings above 150 mJ/cm^2 caused severe destruction of the wafer. Layers grown at 450°C,

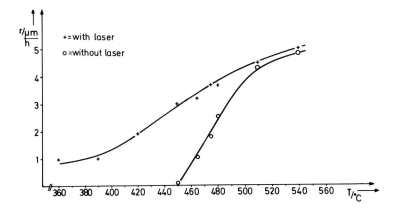

Fig. 2: Growth rate of GaAs versus temperature

120 mJ/cm^2 laser power, and 10 Hz pulse repetition frequency, were p-type with $p = 3 \cdot 10^{17} cm^{-3}$. Photoluminescence-measurements show strong carbon-luminescence, which would explain the high p-doing of the layers.

Fig. 4 shows the influence of the total pressure on stimulated growth rate using the same flow rates as in fig. 2. No significant influence on growth rate can be seen at 450°C. The slight decrease of growth rate with decreasing pressure is within our measuring accuracy. Moreover, variations of the TMG or AsH$_3$ concentration by a factor of two result only in 10% variation in growth rate at 450 °C, whereas at 650 °C the growth rate depends linearly on TMG partial pressure. These results indicate that the stimulated growth is controlled by surface reactions and not by diffusion.

Regarding the given temperatures it should be pointed out that the surface of the wafer might be even cooler (~10°C) because of the location of the thermocouples inside the susceptor.

GROWTH MODEL

In the pulse irradiated area growth takes place in two steps, characterized by strongly different duration and temperature. During the laser irradiation of 3 ns the surface temperature raises to about 1000 °C and thus the energy needed for crystal formation is provided. Temperature falls below 500 °C within less than 1 µs. In this time interval the reaction of the gas molecules, their surface movement and epitaxial growth takes place. However, this time is far too short to supply the amount of reactive material from the gas phase to the surface, to explain the measured growth rate.

This indicates that during the long periods between the pulses, where surface temperature is too low for growth, the reactive gas molecules must be accumulated at the surface. The adsorption including desorption can be described with Eq. 1 /6/.

$$\frac{dN_a}{dt} = (N-N_a) \cdot k_a - N_a \cdot k_d \tag{1}$$

where N_a is the number of adsorbed molecules, N the number of sites available

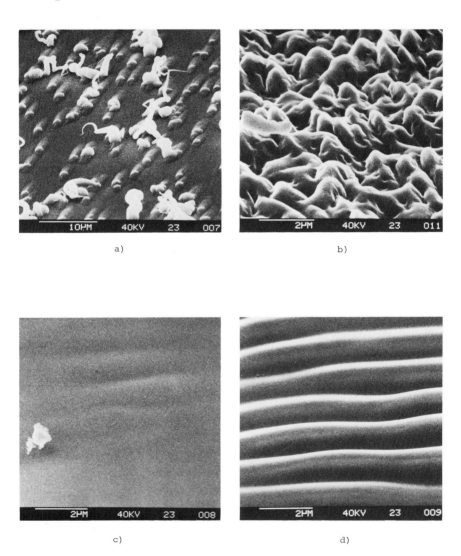

Fig. 3: Morphology of GaAs surfaces grown at 450 °C for different laser powers. a) no laser, b) 70 mJ/cm², c) 120 mJ/cm², d) 150 mJ/cm²

for adsorption, k_a an adsorption constant and k_d an desorption constant. The number of adsorbed molecules is:

$$N_a(t) = N_\infty (1-\exp(\frac{-t}{\tau}))\qquad(2)$$

where $N_\infty = \frac{k_a}{k_a+k_d} N$ is the saturation value and $\tau = 1/(k_a+k_d)$ is the time constant of the adsorption process. If a constant percentage of the adsorbed molecules form a crystalline layer at every laser pulse, the thickness of these layers versus time interval between two pulses should be described by eq. (2).

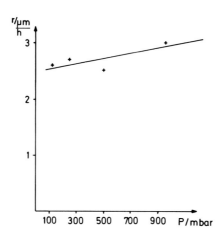

Fig. 4: Growth rate under laser stimulation at 450 °C versus pressure

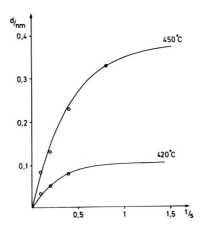

Fig. 5: Deposited layer thickness per shot versus time between pulses. The thick drawn graphs are theoretical fits.

Therefore we made growth experiments with different pulse repetition frequencies. Fig. 5 shows the measured values of layer thickness per shot versus time. The thick drawn lines are calculated fits, using time constants of 0.42 s for 450 °C and 0.28 s for 420 °C. The saturation values are 0.38 nm and 0.105 nm for 450 °C and 420 °C respectively. The decreasing saturation layer thicknesses with decreasing temperature show that the process cannot be simply explained by physical adsorption. For physical adsorption the Langmuir and BET theories show constant or at least increasing thicknesses of equilibrium adsorbed layers with decreasing temperature /6/. Therefore other mechanisms must be involved. We assume that at 450°C catalytic effects of the GaAs surface cause a partial reaction of the molecules leading to the adsorption of thicker layers at higher temperatures.

CONCLUSIONS

We have shown that the GaAs MOCVD process can be stimulated by laser radiation. In the irradiated areas monocrystalline layers were grown at a rate of 3 μm/hour which is 50 % of the rate at 640 °C whereas growth had ceased in the unirradiated areas. For laser stimulated growth we propose the following model: At low temperatures reactive molecules (AsH_3-and TMG-derivatives) adsorb at the GaAs surface, including partial reaction with increasing temperature, and react within ns of heat treatment completely to GaAs and grow epitaxially on the substrate.

ACKNOWLEDGEMENTS

The authors would like to thank Lili Vescan for fruitful discussions. The work was supported by the Ministerium für Wissenschaft, Nordrhein-Westfalen.

LITERATURE

1. R.M. Osgood jr. talk given at Microelectronics-Structures and Complexity, Lex Deux Alpes, 14.-20.03.1982.
2. M. W. Geis, D. C. Flanders and H. I. Smith, Appl. Phys. Lett. 35, 71 (1979).
3. M. W. Geis, H. I. Smith, B. Y. Tsaur, J. C. C. Fan, D. J. Silversmith and R. W. Mountain, submitted to J. Electr. Chem. Soc.
4. H. Kräutle, H. Roehle, A. Escobosa and H. Beneking, accepted for publication in J. Electron. Mat.
5. H. Beneking, A. Escobosa, H. Kräutle, J. Electron. Mat., 10, 473-480 (1981).
6. Y. Brunauer, L. E. Copeland and D. L. Kantro, The Solid Gas Interface, Marcel Dekker Inc., New York, 77 (1967).

LASER INDUCED CHEMICAL VAPOR DEPOSITION OF HYDROGENATED AMORPHOUS SILICON

RENZO BILENCHI, IVA GIANINONI AND MIRELLA MUSCI
CISE S.p.A., P.O.Box 12081, 20100 Milano, Italy

ROBERTO MURRI
Istituto di Fisica, Università di Bari, 70100 Bari, Italy

ABSTRACT

Some results on hydrogenated amorphous silicon growth by CO_2 laser photodissociation of silane are reported. A 100 W CW CO_2 laser was used as the excitation source. A horizontal configuration was adopted, where the laser beam is sent parallel to the substrate surface inside a flux reactor, and its energy is used to excite and dissociate the silane molecules flowing near the solid surface. The laser has no direct heating effect on the substrate, which is independently heated by an oven.
The photoproduced radicals by interacting with the surface grow a film at a rate strongly depending on silane pressure, substrate temperature and laser intensity. This experimental configuration allows depositions on large areas, owing to the large number of reactant molecules involved in the photochemical process. Moreover, material can be produced with a continuously variable hydrogen content, since the substrate temperature required for obtaining depositions can be as low as room temperature and adjusted independently of the other process parameters.
The film properties are similar to those of the glow discharge deposited material. The film amorphousness and the hydrogen presence either in monohydride and dihydride groups are evidenced by x-ray patterns and ir spectra. Results on the electrical and optical properties are also reported.

INTRODUCTION

In recent years it has been extensively demonstrated that the technique of excitation and dissociation of gas phase molecules by resonant absorption of both coherent and incoherent e.m. radiation provides an efficient and useful method to produce chemical surface reactions. In particular, metal and semiconductor depositions have been performed by UV laser photolysis, mainly with the aim of obtaining surface patterns and controlled surface microstructures.
The purpose of our work, instead, is to achieve large-area silicon depositions at low substrate temperatures by using CW CO_2 lasers. Areas up to 25 cm^2 have been deposited by means of a source supplying 100 W of output power. However, the process can be easily scaled up since at present multikilowatt CO_2 sources are commercially available.
The reactant gas is SiH_4 that exhibits a large resonant absorption for some high gain CO_2 laser lines[1][2]; the deposited material is amorphous silicon, with hydrogen content depending on some process parameters.
It is of general importance, in the technology of semiconductor devices, to set up low-temperature processing techniques. In the particular case of hydrogenated amorphous silicon (a-Si:H) production, conventional CVD thermal processes are ruled out, since to obtain hydrogen incorporation it is essential to operate

at temperatures lower than 500°C. Hydrogenated amorphous silicon has turned out to be a promising material for applications to electronic and optoelectronic devices. Current techniques for preparing a-Si:H are glow discharge and reactive sputtering; however there is a need for new deposition methods to improve the material properties, whose dependence on the growth kinetics is critical though not yet clearly established.

We have previously verified that silane is efficiently dissociated in the homogeneous phase by CW CO_2 laser radiation [3] (the maximum dissociation efficiency occuring for the P(20) emission line at 10.59 µm), and that silicon depositions at low substrate temperatures can be obtained when the beam is either normal or parallel to the substrate surface [4]. The main advantage of the parallel configuration, which we are using at present, is that it permits deposits on large areas, since a great number of molecules can be involved in the dissociation process. In addition, there are no limits in the choice of the substrate material that can be either absorbent or trasparent to the laser radiation without affecting the substrate temperature and, consequently, the properties of the deposited material.

EXPERIMENTAL TECHNIQUES

Fig.1 shows the flux reactor used for a-Si:H photodepositions. It consists of a 600-mm-long quartz tube housing a hollow graphite cylinder, with a 14 mm internal diameter and 200 mm long, heated by an oven. SiH_4 was directly injected

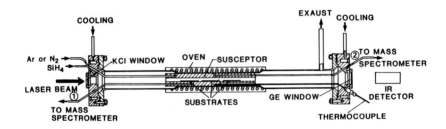

Fig. 1. Flux reactor used in the photodeposition arrangement.

into the reaction region, while the carrier gas inlet was set near the front window to prevent SiH_4 back diffusion and therefore laser energy absorption before the useful reaction zone. Glass, sapphire or crystalline silicon substrates were set in a suitable groove at the bottom of the graphite susceptor. The substrate temperature was measured by means of a termocouple plunged in the susceptor. Extraction probes 1 and 2 allowed the gaseous species to be analyzed by means of a quadrupole mass spectrometer. A thermopile monitored the laser absorption during the deposition process. The laser was operated without grating at about 100 W of output power with 6 mm beam diameter. In this arrangement the laser energy was used to excite and dissociate the silane molecules flowing near the solid surface and had no direct heating effect on the substrate. By varying the flow rate of the carrier gas it was possible to adjust the residence time of the reactant molecules independently of the partial SiH_4 pressure, thus optimizing the dissociation efficiency. The choice of the carrier gas was determined by its thermal conductivity. In fact, only gases with low thermal conductivity, such as N_2 or Ar, prevent the rapid transfer of the absorbed energy to the whole gas volume and so enable the laser radiation to be efficiently exploited in a limited region near the substrate surface. Several substrates of various kinds of materials could be simultaneously processed. The overall area deposited in one run was limited in the longitudinal direction by the length of the graphite susceptor (the power attenuation length being 600 mm in typical operating conditions) and the diffusion of the produced radicals. As a matter of fact we obtained deposited strips 12 mm wide with a total length up to 200 mm. The mass spectrometer was a Balzers 511; it was used to monitor the process during deposition and to find the best operating conditions by comparing the amount of silane dissociation with the laser either on or off and for different flow rates, partial pressures, substrate temperatures and laser intensities. The film thickness was evaluated by interferometric measurements and verified with an alpha-step profiler.

RESULTS

As the laser was introduced into the reactor, the onset of silane dissociation was marked by the mass spectrometer as a sudden rise in the molecular hydrogen signal and a simultaneous drop in each SiH_n^+ (n=0 to 4) signal. Peaks of $Si_2H_n^+$ (n=1 to 6) also appeared indicating disilane formation in the gaseous phase, due to the high density of free radicals in the laser beam volume. At the same time, depositions were obtained on the substrates set about 1 mm under the laser beam. Dissociation was evident even at room temperature, but the deposition rate was low and the deposited films, looking yellowish because of the high hydrogen content, had a poor adherence. At $T \geqslant 200^oC$ the deposition rates became significant and the produced films were scratch-resistant and adherent, as pointed out by the scotch-tape test.

The most important process parameters affecting the gaseous dissociation and the deposition rate were silane pressure, substrate temperature and laser intensity. The reaction efficiency is critically dependent also on the choice of the carrier gas. H_2 and He were ruled out because of their high thermal conductivity, whereas Ar provided the highest deposition rates. The film thickness was measured in different axial positions along the reactor and for various partial pressures of silane, versus the substrate temperature. Fig.2 shows the deposition rate, 20 mm apart from the silane injector, versus substrate temperature, for two different mixtures of silane and argon. The deposition rate, incident laser intensities being equal, is critically dependent on the partial silane pressure, owing to the larger radiation absorption. At $T=250^oC$ the absorption was 20% higher for curve (a) than for curve (b). In the pressure conditions of curve (a) the amount of absorbed laser radiation was constant over the whole temperature range, while the homogeneous phase dissociation was increasing with temperature probably because of the lower dissociation energy of the heated molecules. The maximum deposition rate was limited by the onset of powder nucleation in the gaseous phase. When the pressure is well below the gas-phase nucleation threshold, as in the case of curve (b), the deposition rate increases with T_s up to 425^oC even if at this temperature thermal decomposition begins and the gaseous mixture becomes more transparent to the laser radiation. The absorbed laser energy was 64% at $T_s=250^oC$ and 59% at 425^oC. In any case, the deposition rate has the same trend versus T_s as the silane dissociation efficiency, thus evidencing the dominant role of the homogeneous decomposition reaction: the dissociation occurs in the gaseous phase and the produced radicals diffuse to the substrate growing a film; when the concentration of free radicals becomes too large, condensation may occur producing polisilane powders. The proportionality between deposition rate and dissociation efficiency is evidenced by their dependence on the laser intensity, shown in Fig.3. The dissociation efficiency was evaluated in relative units by comparing the ratio between the molecular hydrogen signal and the residual undissociated silane with the laser either on or off; the substrate temperature was kept constant at 330^oC. The non linear power dependence of silane dissociation should be expected because of the absorption of many ir photons necessary for dissociating one molecule.

The deposition rates are high in comparison with those obtained with the current methods (typically 100 Å/min in glow discharge) and could be enhanced if more radiation intensity is supplied.

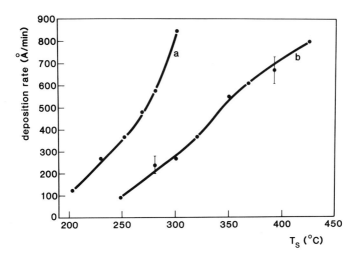

Fig. 2. Deposition rate versus substrate temperature: (a) total pressure (SiH$_4$+Ar) 5 torr, silane pressure 2.41 torr, flow rate 3 sccm; (b) total pressure 3.8 torr, silane pressure 1.7 torr, flow rate 2.2 sccm. In both cases the laser intensity was 180 W/cm^2.

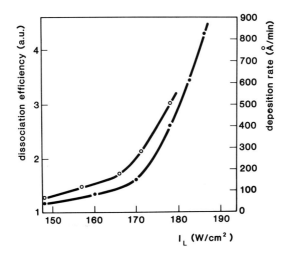

Fig. 3. Deposition rate (●) and dissociation efficiency (○) versus laser intensity: pressures and flow rate as in Fig.2, curve (b); T_S=330°C.

MATERIAL ANALYSES

Investigations were performed on morphology, composition and electrical and optical properties of the deposited material.

X-ray diffraction analyses confirm the amorphousness of the material. Fig.4 shows (111) Bragg reflection patterns referred to a 3-μm-thick film grown on a sapphire substrate at a temperature of 340°C, before and after thermal annealing. The very large broadening of the peak [5] (8° full width at half intensity) proves the amorphousness of the as-grown sample; the 2° shift towards the smaller angles, with respect to the (111) crystalline reflection, is a feature already noticed [6] in thin a-Si:H films obtained by glow discharge. Thermal annealings of the sample induce a progressive crystallization, as shown by the narrowing of the peak and by the rise of the weaker (220) and (311) reflections at higher Bragg angles.

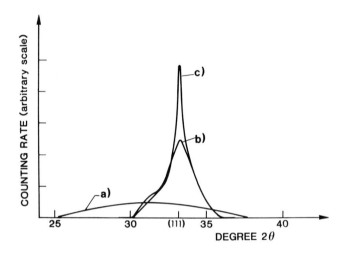

Fig. 4. (111) Bragg reflection patterns of a 3-μm-thick film deposited on a sapphire substrate at T_s=340°C: (a) before thermal annealing; (b) and (c) after 5-h annealings at T=550°C and T=650°C, respectively. The x-ray diffractometer was operated with a Co tube.

The hydrogen content and its bond distribution were evaluated by vibrational absorption. Curve (a) in Fig.5 reports the relative transmittance in the range 2500-400 cm^{-1} of a 1-μm-thick film grown on a single-crystal silicon wafer at T_s=320°C. In agreement with the spectra [7] of a-Si:H deposited by glow discharge at low temperatures (about 25°C) and high pressures (about 1 torr), our film presents abundance of dihydride groups (SiH$_2$) identified by stretching mode ω_1=2100 cm^{-1} and bending mode ω_3=890 cm^{-1}. Monohydride groups (SiH) are less evident and are identified by the stretching mode ω_2=2000 cm^{-1}. The large peak near 640 cm^{-1} is attributed to ω_4 and ω_5 wagging modes of SiH and SiH$_2$ groups, respectively. Curves (b) and (c) in Fig.5 show the vibrational spectra of the same sample after two successive 30-min annealings at 350°C and 450°C, respectively, and indicate that the SiH bond is stronger, as generally verified in a-Si:H.

Spectrophotometric measurements in the range 500-900 nm, carried out by a Cary 219 spectrophotometer, gave the absorption coefficient values and the absorption edge shapes of our samples. The optical absorption in the gap region

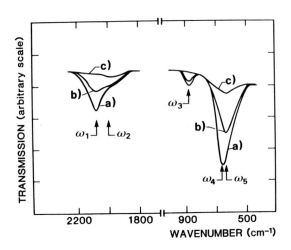

Fig. 5. Infrared spectra of a sample deposited on a single-crystal silicon substrate at $T_s=320°C$: (a) as-grown material; (b) and (c) after 30-min annealings at $T=350°C$ and $T=450°C$, respectively.

turned out to depend on specific growth parameters, particularly on the substrate temperature and the consequent hydrogen content. Absorption coefficient α at 2 eV increases about one order of magnitude by increasing the substrate temperature T_s from 220°C to 350°C. The α value evaluated at 620 nm was $5.5 \cdot 10^3$ cm^{-1} for a sample grown at $T_s=247°C$ and $3.57 \cdot 10^4$ cm^{-1} for a sample grown at $T_s=330°C$. By using the absorption coefficient data we determined the optical gap E_o, defined as the intercept at the $(\alpha h \nu)^{1/2}$ versus $h\nu$ curve in the high absorption region [8]. For a-Si:H deposited at $T_s=247°C$ E_o was found to be equal to 2 eV and to 1.56 eV for a sample deposited at $T_s=330°C$.

Electrical measurements of conductivity and photoconductivity equally presented a remarkable dependence on the substrate temperature. The dark conductivity, measured at room temperature using the Van der Pauw method, was generally rather low. Typical values $2 \cdot 10^{-8} \leqslant \sigma_{RT} \leqslant 5 \cdot 10^{-6}$ Ω^{-1} cm^{-1} for the substrate temperature range 220-350°C were obtained. The increase in the dark conductivity with the substrate temperature was also noticed in the material obtained with conventional methods. The behaviour of the dark conductivity as a function of the temperature in the range 90-700°K was also investigated in order to obtain information on the gap state distributions. From the variation in σ versus 1/kT it was possible to deduce the occurrence of three different transport mechanisms, in agreement with results already obtained [9], and to locate the states inside the gap. For instance, for a sample grown at $T_s=250°C$, the presence of localized states at 0.46 eV above the Fermi level was evidenced. The photoconductivity spectra were measured by using a monochromatic chopped light (10^{13}-10^{14} photons cm^{-2}) emitted by a Xenon lamp. The photoresponse at λ=550 nm and for the substrate temperature range 220-350°C had values $10^{-7} \leqslant i_{ph} \leqslant 10^{-3}$, where i_{ph} represents the number of charge carriers flowing round the circuit for each photon entering the sample.

The values obtained for the most important material properties are consistent with the results of the glow discharge technique used by one of us in previous works [9]. However, further work is required to systematically evaluate the dependence on the process parameters of the various material properties, since indications were obtained that they are affected by deposition rate and laser intensity as well as by substrate temperature.

As a conclusion, a CW CO_2 laser was used to deposit a-Si:H at low substrate temperatures with high growth rates (up to 900 Å/min). In the adopted horizontal configuration the homogeneous reaction is dominant: the radicals photoproduced in a localized region just above the substrate diffuse to the solid surface growing a film. A large number of silane molecules are involved in the photo-chemical excitation, thus providing an overall deposition area up to 25 cm^2. The process could be easily scaled up for larger area depositions by using a more powerful laser that supplies comparable intensity on a wider beam section. Further work is in progress with this aim using a 1 kW laser having a uniform intensity distribution on a 25x10 mm rectangular beam section. This particular source would also help in improving the deposition uniformity in the transverse direction, which at present is limited by the gaussian intensity distribution. The analyses on the deposited material properties show that they are very similar to those of the plasma-deposited amorphous silicon and that such a material could be successfully used in a-Si:H electronic devices.

ACKNOWLEDGEMENTS

The authors wish to thank Prof. E. Mantica of Politecnico of Milan for providing the ir spectroscopy and Dr. A. Ferrario for valuable discussions. The technical assistance of Mr. F. Crociani is also greatfully acknowledged.

REFERENCES

1. T. F. Deutsch, J. Chem. Phys. 70, 1187 (1979).

2. N. V. Karlov, N. A. Karpov, Yu. N. Petrov and O. M. Stel'makh, Sov. Phys. JETP 37, 1012 (1973).

3. R. Bilenchi and M. Musci, Proc. European Conference on Optical Systems and Applications, Utrecht (1980).

4. R. Bilenchi and M. Musci, Proc. Eighth International Conference on CVD, Paris (1981).

5. M. H. Brodsky, R. S. Title, K. Weiser and G. D. Pettit, Phys. Rev. B1, 2632 (1970).

6. C. Messana, B. A. De Angelis, G. Conte and C. Gramaccioni, J. Phys. D: Appl. Phys. 14, L91 (1981).

7. C. C. Tsai and D. Fritzsche, Solar Energy Materials 1, 29 (1979); M. H. Brodsky, M. Cardona and J. J. Cuomo, Phys. Rev. B16, 3556 (1977).

8. J. Tauc in: Amorphous and Liquid Semiconductors, J. Tauc ed. (Plenum, New York 1974) Chap. 4.

9. V. Augelli, R. Murri and L. Schiavulli, Thin Solid Films, 90, 153 (1982).

This work was partially supported by the Progetto Finalizzato Chimica Fine e Secondaria of the Italian National Council of Research, Rome, CNR/CISE Contract no.81.01735.95.

DIRECT WRITING USING LASER CHEMICAL VAPOR DEPOSITION

S. D. ALLEN, A. B. TRIGUBO, AND R. Y. JAN
Center for Laser Studies, University of Southern California, University Park
DRB 17, Los Angeles, California 90089-1112 USA

ABSTRACT

Metal, dielectric and semiconductor films have been deposited by laser chemical vapor deposition (LCVD) using both pulsed and cw laser sources on a variety of substrates. For LCVD on substrates such as quartz, the deposition was monitored optically in both transmission and reflection using a collinear visible laser and the depositing CO_2 laser. Deposition initiation and rate were correlated with irradiation conditions, the laser generated surface temperature, and the changing optical properties of the filmμsubstrate during deposition. Single crystallites of W greater than 100 μm tall were deposited using a Kr laser on Si substrates.

INTRODUCTION

Laser chemical vapor deposition (LCVD) is one of several recently developed laser deposition techniques [1]. The goals of these new methods are predominantly twofold: 1) maskless pattern generation by direct laser writing and 2) deposition of materials with novel properties such as controlled structure and grain size, increased adherence, modified electrical properties, and enhanced deposition at low temperatures. These effects can be achieved by localizing the heated area in the thermal processes and by absorbing the laser energy directly into the reactive species in the photochemical processes.

LCVD is an adaptation of conventional CVD using a laser heat source. The laser is focused through a transparent window and the transparent gaseous reactants onto an absorbing substrate, creating a localized hot spot at which the deposition reaction takes place. Although the process is thermal, it can be employed for deposition on heat sensitive structures because the heating is localized. The very rapid deposition rates (>100 μm/sec) achievable with LCVD, in combination with fast laser heating rates (~ 10^{10} °C/sec) should allow the deposition of very small area (≤1 μm diameter) coatings with a minimum heat affected zone in the substrate. Modification of structural and electrical properties can be achieved by control of the laser heated surface temperature, growth rate, dopants, and post growth annealing. Metal [2,3], semiconductor [4], and dielectric [3,4] films have been deposited by LCVD on a variety of substrates using both pulsed and cw lasers in this laboratory. In this paper we will discuss the LCVD of metal films on quartz and Si substrates using CO_2 and Kr lasers.

For the deposition of a reflecting (i.e., metal) film on a highly absorbing substrate using a constant intensity optical heat source, it would be expected that the film would be optically self-limited to a thickness on the order of the optical absorption depth or several hundred Å. As the film is deposited the absorbed laser intensity decreases and therefore the substrate temperature and the deposition rate decrease. A comparison of the optical constants of most metals and quartz at 10.6 μm shows that the absorptivity changes by approximately an order of magnitude once several hundred Å of metal are deposited and the surface temperature should decrease accordingly. The LCVD process, in this case, can be characterized by an initial surface temperature rise to near the deposition temperature, a decrease in the surface temperature as the film is deposited, and, finally, attainment of an equilibrium temperature which may or may not be above the minimum deposition temperature. The effective deposition rate, defined as the deposit thickness divided by the irradiation time, is thus a complicated function of not only the irradiation conditions and the reaction kinetics but also the optical constants of both the substrate and the LCVD film.

EXPERIMENTAL

LCVD Ni, Fe, W/SiO$_2$

For the LCVD of W from $WF_6 + H_2$ on quartz substrates using a CO_2 laser, the expected optical self-limiting does occur, with the deposited film thickness under most conditions independent of the irradiation time with a maximum film thickness is 2500 - 5000 Å depending on irradiation conditions and reactant concentration. At the other extreme, the LCVD rate for Ni from Ni(CO)$_4$ is linear with irradiation time up to a film thickness of several thousand Å for a range of incident intensities. LCVD Fe from Fe(CO)$_5$ is an intermediate case with the film thickness, 1, proportional to the irradiation time, $\tau^{0.8}$, for an incident power of 2.2 W and to $\tau^{0.5}$ for an incident power of 5.5 W [3].

In order to understand this behavior, optical monitoring of the LCVD film deposition was undertaken with the apparatus shown in Fig. 1. The laser is an electrically pulsed, line tunable cw CO_2 with maximum output power of 40 W.

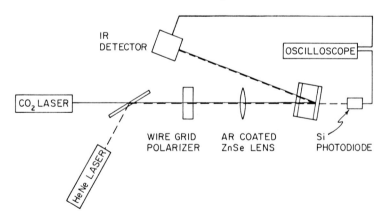

Fig. 1. Schematic diagram of the LCVD apparatus.

Attenuation of the beam is provided by current control and a wire grid polarizer. A removable power meter and/or fluorescent viewing plates are used to check power stability and beam quality. A He-Ne beam is folded into the optical path of the CO_2 laser with a ZnSe Brewster angle beam splitter to allow visible optical monitoring of the LCVD metal film thickness on quartz substrates. Both beams are focused through a NaCl window onto the substrate with a 10 inch focal length 10.6 μm AR coated ZnSe lens. The CO_2 beam profile at the substrate was measured by pinhole scans and is approximately gaussian with a D_{1/e^2} = 600 μm. The beam diameter of the He-Ne laser at the focus is much smaller. The temporal intensity profile of the CO_2 pulses of 1 ms or longer is essentially a step function with some initial overshoot as measured using a HgCdTe detector. The transmitted He-Ne beam and the reflected CO_2 beam are detected with a Si photodiode and either a HgCdTe or Ge:Au detector respectively. Signals from both detectors are recorded on an oscilloscope.

Representative transmission and reflection curves are given in Figure 2 for the W from WF_6 (P = 45 T) + H_2 (P = 400 T) system for different laser intensities and an irradiation time of nominally 100 ms. The upper curve is the He-Ne intensity and the lower curve the reflected CO_2 intensity as measured by the Ge:Au detector. At the lower incident power (4.7 W, Fig. 2a) a delay time of approximately 67 msec is observed before significant deposition takes place as evidenced by a steep decrease in the He-Ne transmission and an increase in the CO_2 reflectance. (The initial decay in the He-Ne transmission is due to substrate heating and subsequent defocusing of the He-Ne beam and is reversible.) A comparison of the delay times for several different incident intensities showed that the data could be fit by a very simple model assuming no deposition until a "threshold temperature" was reached and one dimensional heat flow in the laser heated substrate. Under these conditions, the surface temperature is proportional to the incident intensity and the square root of the irradiation time if we further assume that the optical and thermal

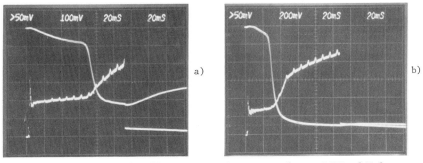

Fig. 2. Transmission and reflection vs. time curves for cw LCVD of W from WF_6 + H_2. The upper and lower curves are the transmitted He-Ne and reflected CO_2 intensities respectively. Laser power: a) 4.7W; b) 7.0W.

properties of the quartz substrate are constant. As shown in Table 1, the product of the incident power and the square root of the delay time before deposition begins is a constant, indicating that there is some validity to the simple model.

Calculations of the on-axis surface temperature generated by a gaussian laser source [5,6] do not yield reasonable results under the previous

TABLE 1
Relative and calculated surface temperature for different irradiation conditions (W from $WF_6 + H_2$)

P (W)	τ (msec)	$P\tau^{\frac{1}{2}} \alpha\ T_s$ (W msec$^{\frac{1}{2}}$)	T_s (calc) (°C)
4.7	55.8	35.1	810
7.0	22.5	33.2	880
10.0	10.9	33.0	950
15.0	4.9	33.2	990

assumptions, however. For quartz it is necessary to take into account the temperature dependence of the thermal properties such as heat capacity and thermal diffusivity. The formalism developed for the calculation of the laser heated surface temperature for Si [7,8] cannot be used for quartz because of the large differences in the thermal properties of the two materials. Iterative calculations using the measured thermal properties of fused quartz [9] yield the temperature vs. irradiation time curves given in Figure 3 for incident intensities corresponding to the experimental conditions of Table 1. The on-axis surface temperatures calculated for the irradiation times at which deposition begins are also given in Table 1. The calculated temperatures are not constant, but the range of values is small and falls well within the optimum temperatures used in conventional CVD for this system [10].

In terms of the model of LCVD discussed previously in which the process could be described by an initial heating period, deposition initiation, surface temperature decrease for deposition of a metal on an absorbing substrate, and attainment of an equilibrium surface temperature, the difference in effective deposition rate measured for Ni, Fe, and W is predominantly due to the large differences in the threshold deposition temperatures for the reactions. The Ni from $Ni(CO)_4$ deposition occurs at a very low temperature (~100°C, Ref. [10]) and for the irradiation conditions chosen for LCVD Ni, the equilibrium surface temperature is greater than this deposition temperature. A deposition rate which is constant with increasing irradiation time would therefore be expected once the LCVD film thickness exceeded several hundred Å. For W from $WF_6 + H_2$, the deposition temperature is almost an order of magnitude larger [10] and the equilibrium temperature calculated using the W optical constants is less than the deposition temperature and severe optical self-limiting occurs. The deposition temperature for Fe from $Fe(CO)_5$ is an intermediate case and the observed optical self-limiting is less severe than for LCVD W.

The LCVD Ni, Fe, and W deposits were hard, shiny, and metallic. Adherence was good for the Ni and Fe coatings up to a thickness of approximately 1 μm. LCVD W coatings greater than about 3000 Å thick also showed some indication of peeling. Resistivity measurements of Ni and W films 500 - 1500 Å thick in both sheet and line geometries yielded values of 3-10 times the bulk

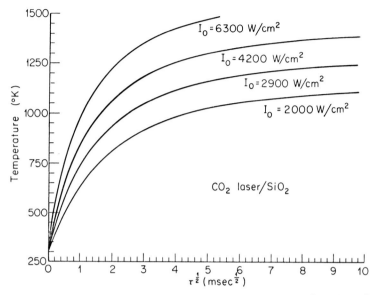

Fig. 3. Calculated surface temperature for fused quartz as a function of irradiation time for several incident laser intensities.

resistivities of the pure metal. These values of the resistivity are quite good for thin films deposited under unoptimized conditions. The lines were drawn by translating the substrate relative to the laser beam. The LCVD Ni and Fe films examined by scanning electron microscopy (SEM) revealed no surface microstructure to less than the resolution of the instrument (100 Å). LCVD W films varied from essentially featureless to a surface nodular structure (diameter approximately 2000 Å) to small crystallites (approximately 4000 Å) depending on irradiation conditions.

LCVD W/Si

An apparatus similar to Figure 1 but without the He-Ne optical monitoring was used to deposit W from WF_6 (200 T) + H_2 (400 T) on Si substrates using a Kr laser. The blue-green (468 - 530 nm) lines of the Kr laser are strongly absorbed by the Si and most gaseous reactants are transparent in the visible, satisfying the LCVD requirements. The laser is focused with a 6.5 cm focal length lens onto the substrate yielding a beam diameter of approximately 20 μm at the focus. The intensity profile deviates considerably from TEM_{00}, having a large TEM_{01*} component. Lines and spots were deposited at scan speeds of 0.2 - 2.0 mm/sec at laser powers of 3 - 4 W. For the slower speeds and higher incident powers, melting of the substrate was observed. Because the absorptivities of the Si and the W are similar in this wavelength region, it was possible to deposit thicker lines than could be achieved on fused quartz substrates. Multiple irradiations could also be used to build up deposit thickness. Unfortunately, these thicker lines (1 = several microns) peeled when the substrate was stressed during removal from the mount.

A curious growth pattern was observed for some spot depositions. Single crystal W spikes (Figure 4) could be deposited with dimensions on the order of 40 - 50 μm wide and 50 - 120 μm tall. These are similar in geometry to the polycrystalline C and Si rods deposited by LCVD by Bauerle et. al., [11,12], but the appearance of one or at most a few large crystals has not previously

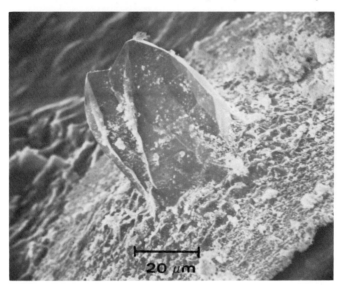

Fig. 4. SEM of LCVD W deposited on a Si substrate using a Kr laser.

been observed. The growth rates measured for these crystallites approach a mm/sec. Such structures have not been observed for LCVD W on SiO_2 using the CO_2 laser for similar reactant concentrations. It appears that the difference in growth habit is related to the large difference in the laser heated areas in the two cases. Examination of a LCVD W spot on Si (Figure 5) where single crystal growth did not take place reveals the familiar "volcano" shape observed in LCVD with the CO_2/SiO_2 system [2]. In the center of the volcano are small crystallites which are miniature versions of the large single crystal of Figure 4. Because the Kr laser irradiates an area on the order of 10 μm as opposed to the hundreds of microns irradiated by the CO_2 laser, it is possible for one or several of these crystallites to dominate the growth. LCVD W spikes have been deposited with 1 - 4 crystallites apparent in the SEM photographs.

CONCLUSIONS

Metal films with good physical properties have been depsoited by LCVD on fused quartz and Si substrates at scan speeds of cm/sec and deposition rates approaching mm/sec. Using UV laser sources it is possible to achieve deposit geometries on the order of 1 - 2 μm with good prospects for further reduction of dimensions [13,14]. LCVD is thus an excellent candidate process for direct writing of metal patterns for microelectronics and other applications. LCVD film growth initiation and deposition rate for the CO_2/SiO_2 system have

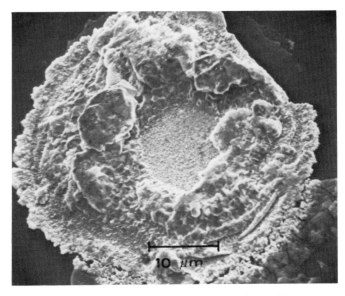

Fig. 5. SEM of LCVD W deposited on a Si substrate using a Kr laser.

been monitored optically and the deposition initiation can be explained qualitatively using a simple threshold temperature model and laser heated surface temperature calculations which include temperature dependent thermal properties of the quartz substrate. LCVD of single crystal rods greater than 100 μm tall of W on Si substrates has been observed.

ACKNOWLEDGMENTS

This work was supported in part by a grant from AFOSR under the technical administration of H. Schlossberg.

REFERENCES

1. See, for example, other papers in these proceedings.

2. S. D. Allen, J. Appl. Phys. 52, 6501 (1981).

3. S. D. Allen and A. B. Trigubo, J. Appl. Phys., to be published (2/83).

4. S. D. Allen, A. B. Trigubo, and M. L. Teisinger, J. Vac. Sci. Tech. 20, 469 (1982).

5. W. W. Duley, CO_2 Lasers: Effects and Applications (Academic Press, New York, 1976).

6. J. F. Ready, Effects of High-Power Laser Radiation (Academic Press, New York, 1971).

7. Y. I. Nissim, A. Lietoila, R. B. Gold, and J. F. Gibbons, J. Appl. Phys. 51, 274 (1980).

8. J. E. Moody and R. H. Hendel, J. Appl. Phys. 53, 4364 (1982).

9. A. Goldsmith, T. E. Waterman, and H. J. Hirschhorn, Handbook of Thermophysical Properties of Solid Materials (Macmillan, New York, 1961).

10. C. F. Powell, J. H. Oxley, and J. M. Blocher, Jr., Vapor Deposition (Wiley, New York, 1966).

11. G. Leyendecker, D. Bauerle, P. Geittner and H. Lydtin, Appl. Phys. Lett. 39, 921 (1981).

12. D. Bauerle, P. Irsigler, G. Leyendecker, H. Noll, and D. Wagner, Appl. Phys. Lett. 40, 819 (1982).

13. G. Tisone and A. W. Johnson, private communication.

14. D. Ehrlich, R. M. Osgood, Jr., and T. F. Deutsch, Amer. Vac. Soc. Meeting, Nov. 1981.

IR LASER-INDUCED DEPOSITION OF SILICON THIN FILMS

T. R. GATTUSO, M. MEUNIER, D. ADLER and J. S. HAGGERTY,
Massachusetts Institute of Technology, Cambridge, MA 02139

ABSTRACT

The deposition of a-Si:H by means of CO_2 laser-induced pyrolysis of silane gas is described. Deposition rates were found to increase with increasing silane flow rate, reactor pressure, laser power and substrate temperature. Spin density decreased and both optical gap, and hydrogen content increased with decreasing substrate temperature. Electrical conductivities are reported.

I. INTRODUCTION

There has been a growing interest in a class of thin film amorphous semiconductors deposited in the presence of hydrogen [1] because their electronic properties make them potential candidates for photovoltaic [2] and other device applications. In particular, hydrogen saturates dangling bonds and relieves strains in hydrogenated amorphous silicon (a-Si:H), resulting in a much lower defect density and consequently in the ability to control the Fermi level by substitutional doping. This material is usually produced by the glow-discharge decomposition of silane [3] or by reactive sputtering in argon/hydrogen mixtures [4]. Chemical vapor deposition (CVD) also has been used to prepare amorphous films [5], but they contain insufficient H_2 (≤ 1 at. %) to achieve good electronic properties because of the necessarily high substrate temperatures (T_s ~ 600°C). In the laser CVD process, high deposition rates can be achieved at low substrate temperatures, leading to films containing adequate hydrogen.

In this process, the reactant gases are heated directly by absorbing light emitted from an IR laser, consequently the reaction zone can be precisely controlled. The laser beam does not provide a surface that dominates various heterogeneous nucleation and reaction effects so this process is distinct from those that induce localized pyrolysis reactions [6-8] by laser-heated substrates. Bilenchi et al. [9] recently reported depositing amorphous silicon onto substrates by a technique very similar to the one described in this paper. Other reported laser CVD work has employed ultraviolet wavelengths capable of inducing photochemical decomposition [10].

II. LASER-INDUCED PYROLYSIS OF SILANE

A. Optical Absorption

The optical absorption coefficients (α) of the reactant gases determine the fraction of the incident laser power absorbed by the gas. The effective absorption coefficient is a function of the difference between the positions of the emission lines and adsorption lines and their respective linewidths. The silane absorption line nearest the principle CO_2 laser emission line (CO_2 P(20) = 944.195cm^{-1}) is at 944.213cm^{-1} [11]. Natural and Doppler broadening are not sufficient to cause coupling [12].

At system pressures above a few torr, collisions between like or unlike gas molecules cause the absorption line widths to broaden. Lorentz broadening results from transitions that occur between the two potential energy curves of the colliding molecules [13]. For many gases, this broadening has been found to be proportional to the pressure [12]. We have found good agreement between calculated and measured P(20) absorptivities of SiH_4 for pressures up to 0.9 atm [14]. Pressure broadening results in very efficient energy transfer.

Figure 1 shows the optical absorptivities we measured as a function of SiH_4 partial pressure for various H_2/SiH_4 ratios [15]. Hydrogen, which is transparent, has a dramatic effect on silane absorptivity. At a silane partial pressure of 1 Torr the absorptivity increases by over two orders of magnitude as the $H_2:SiH_4$ ratio is increased from 0 to 9. The maximum in the data for $H_2/SiH_4 = 1.3$ is not a real pressure broadening maximum and suggests the onset of some sort of saturation [16].

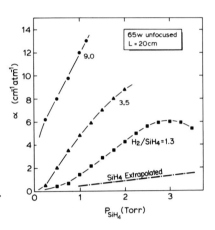

Fig. 1. The absorption coefficient of SiH_4 as a function of silane partial pressure and the hydrogen to silane ratio for the P(20) CO_2 laser line.

B. Silane Pyrolysis

The overall chemical reaction of interest in this research is:

$$SiH_4(g) \rightarrow Si(s) + 2H_2(g) . \qquad (1)$$

Photons from the CO_2 laser light do not interact with silane to form silicon according to Equation (1) in a single absorption event because photon energies an order of magnitude higher are required to break chemical bonds. When an infrared photon is absorbed, the absorbing molecule makes a transition to an excited vibrational level. Collisions distribute the absorbed energy and return the absorbing molecule to the ground state where it is again able to absorb another photon. The overall effect is an increase in temperature. Deutsch [16] found no evidence for multiphoton, collisionless processes in silane at CO_2 P(20) fluences up to 150 J/cm^2. CO_2 laser pyrolysis of silane is essentially a thermal process in which the entire mixture is heated if one species in a mixture of gases absorbs.

The definition of the mechanisms for thermal decomposition of silane is the subject of much research. Deutsch [16] observed molecular hydrogen lines in the luminescence of silane excited by high energy CO_2 laser pulses. Mass spectroscopic analyses gave no evidence of Si_2H_6, and it was concluded that the dominant initial dissociation step is the formation of $SiH_2 + H_2$. Bilenchi et al. [9] concluded from mass spectroscopic evidence that dissociation occurs in the gas phase in CO_2 laser-induced pyrolysis of silane. They observed SiH_2, SiH_3 and molecular hydrogen in the product vapor. They also observed only weak dependence of deposition rate on substrate temperature. Scott et al. [17] concluded that $SiH_2(g)$ is the precursor for silicon deposited from silane for a process employing a cooled substrate in a hot-walled reactor in agreement with predictions by Sladek [18] based on his general model for homogeneous CVD. Scott et al. [17] hypothesize that rapid surface reactions were responsible for the reduction in the H:Si ratio in deposited films. Other researchers have made different observations. This chemistry is complex and laser excitation introduces possibilities for atypical reaction paths.

III. DEPOSITION EXPERIMENTS AND RESULTS

A. Deposition System

The apparatus that was used is shown in Figure 2. Substrates are mounted on a temperature controlled stage in a hermetic reaction cell; substrate temperature is monitored by means of a thermocouple in contact with the stage. Although substrate heating is not necessary for deposition to occur, the substrate temperature is expected to have a significant effect on the properties of the resultant films and is expected to be an important variable in process optimization. Generally, substrate temperatures have been in the 200 to 400°C range for these experiments.

A Coherent Radiation Everlase 150 untuned CO_2 laser or an Advanced Kinetics MIRL 50 grating-tuned CO_2 laser were used in a cw mode. The axis of the laser beam is made to pass through the cell, parallel to the substrate plane at a distance of approximately one beam diameter. The unfocused beam diameters are 6 mm; a lens with a focal length of 12.7 cm was used in the experiments involving a focussed beam. A thermopile was used to monitor the laser power transmitted through the cell. Incident laser intensities have been in the 100 to 1000 watts/cm^2 range.

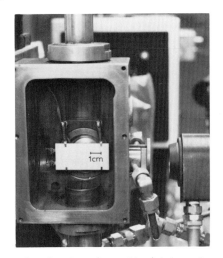

Fig. 2. Reaction cell with heated substrate stage.

Pure silane (4 to 10 Torr), has been used in most of the experiments. SiH_4/He and SiH_4/H_2 mixtures have been used in a few experiments. Films have been deposited with both vertical and horizontal substrate orientations, and under both constant volume (static cell) and constant pressure (flowing gas) conditions. In the flowing gas experiments silane is admitted through a 1 mm ID cylindrical nozzle below the substrate stage. The gas passes through the laser beam and out the top of the cell through a filter and throttling valve assembly that maintains a constant pressure. A variety of substrate materials including borosilicate glass, aluminum, aluminum oxide, single crystal silicon and borosilicate glass coated with platinum, molybdenum or indium-tin oxide has been used. Deposition rates were measured by an interferometric technique employing reflected He-Ne laser light.

B. Deposition Rates

Figure 3 shows plots of thickness and deposition rate as functions of time constructed from the positions of the maxima and minima of a typical reflectance versus time record. An index of refraction of 4.6 was used in the thickness calculations in agreement with values from the literature [19] and film thicknesses measured by profilometry [20]. The general shapes in Figure 3 are typical; growth rates increase with time until reaching a constant, steady state rate. The long time required to reach steady state is surprizing.

The maximum deposition rate achieved by this process is somewhat higher than 160 Å/min. This is comparable to deposition rates for a-Si in normal CVD [21] for which maximum deposition rates are limited by the onset of crystallinity as the substrate temperature is increased. Under high deposition rate conditions, the amount of retained hydrogen decreases as T_s is increased, resulting in degradation of elecrical properties. In the laser CVD process high deposition rates can be achieved at low T_s, thus eliminating the need for post-deposition hydrogenation.

The deposition rate in the flowing gas experiments was found to depend quite strongly on the silane flow rate, as shown in Figure 4. Under normal constant pressure conditions only about 1% of the silane is consumed in a single pass through the cell, so this effect is not associated with depletion of the available reactant or with thermodynamic driving forces. The result may reflect the transport of reactants to the reaction zone because the steep temperature gradients characteristic of laser heating oppose diffusion of gas molecules into the beam [22]. Alternatively, it may reflect a change in absorption of laser energy and/or a change in gas thermal conductivity. Although not fully explained, it means that flow rates must be controlled very precisely.

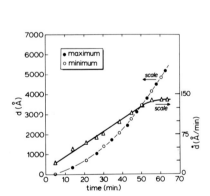

Fig. 3. Thickness and deposition rate versus time for P_{SiH_4} = 6 Torr, T_s = 300°C and 70W of laser power.

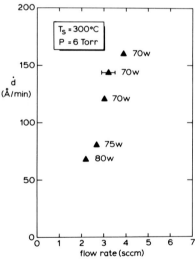

Fig. 4. Steady state deposition rate versus silane flow rate for constant substrate temperature, cell pressure and (nominally) laser power.

Deposition rates in the laser CVD process increase with increasing substrate temperature, laser power and silane pressure. The maximum deposition rate is limited by the onset of powder production. It is expected that the range for film production can be extended by using mixtures of silane and either H_2 or HCl to suppress the onset of homogeneous reactions.

C. Film Characteristics

Films produced under the conditions described above have been determined to be amorphous by electron diffraction. This was expected based on the low substrate temperatures used. With clean substrates film adhesion was found to be very good. Occasionally a deposit would peel and curl, indicating a state of tensile stress in the film. In almost all of these cases the origin of the peeling could be traced to contamination (generally particles) on the substrate surface. Peeling of films back from substrate edges also was observed.

One of the most important properties for device applications is the concentration of unpaired spins [23] which can be evaluated by electron spin resonance (ESR). Unpaired spins always arise from defect configurations which, if sufficiently concentrated, pin the Fermi level and preclude fabrication of good devices. Ordinarily, the incorporation of hydrogen in the film decreases the defect concentration sufficiently to unpin the Fermi level and allow substitutional doping. Figure 5 shows the spin concentration N_s as a function of substrate temperature T_s for a-Si:H films deposited by laser CVD. The g value is ~ 2.0055 in agreement with that obtained in undoped glow-discharge films [3]. The magnitude of N_s in the laser CVD films is about a factor of 100 lower than in conventional CVD films [5,24] and

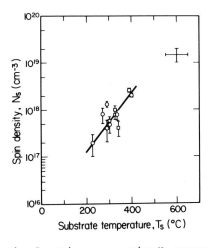
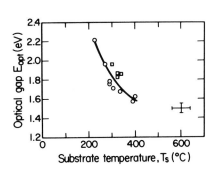

Fig. 5. Spin concentration N_s versus substrate temperature T_s for films made with (o) Laser Power = 40W, SiH_4 = 8.8 Torr; (□) Laser Power = 60W, SiH_4 = 7.0 Torr; (+) Normal CVD [5,24].

Fig. 6. Optical gap E_{opt} (eV) versus substrate temperature T_s (°C) for films produced at laser powers of 40W (o) and 60W (□) and normal CVD (+) [27].

about a factor of 10 higher than in the best glow-discharge films [3]. N_s appears to be independent of the laser power, but it decreases with decreasing T_s, due to increased H which saturates dangling bonds. Conventional CVD films ($T_s \approx 600°C$) contain < 0.5 at. % H_2 [5], in contrast with ≈ 4 at. % determined by the effusion technique for one of our films deposited at $T_s \approx 400°C$.

The measurement of optical absorption α versus photon energy $h\nu$ provides information about the "optical" gap E_{opt} defined by the expression [25,26], $(\alpha h\nu)^{1/2} = (h\nu - E_{opt})$. Figure 6 shows E_{opt} as a function of T_s for films produced at laser powers of 40 and 60 watts (6 mm diameter beam). Values of E_{opt} between 1.5 and 2.0 eV are in agreement with those of glow-discharge films [3]. The decrease of E_{opt} with increasing T_s is most likely due to the decreasing H concentration in the films. We should expect that the admixture of the stronger Si-H bonds (~ 3.4 eV) to the Si matrix (the Si-Si bond energy is ≈ 2.4 eV) tends to increase E_{opt}. It is less clear why E_{opt} depends on the laser power.

Figure 7 represents an Arrhenius plot of the conductivity, σ, as a function of temperature for two films made at $T_s = 400°C$ and $305°C$, using a planar configuration with a distance of 5×10^{-2} cm between two aluminum contacts. Activation energies of $E_0 \sim 0.27$ eV ($T_s = 400°C$) and $E_0 \sim 0.44$ eV ($T_s = 305°C$) were deduced from the high-temperature regions and most likely represent the energy difference between the Fermi level and the nearest mobility edge. The increase of E_0 with decreasing T_s is probably due to the effects of hydrogen which both increases the gap and tends to unpin the Fermi level. The curvature of the Arrhenius plot at lower temperatures can be explained by the onset of electronic transport by hopping between localized states near the Fermi level, both between the nearest neighbors and more distant sites (variable-range hopping) [28].

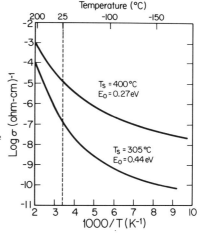

Fig. 7. Log of conductivity versus 1/T for films made with laser power = 40W, SiH_4 pressure = 8.8 Torr, (A) $T_s = 400°C$, (B) $T_s = 305°C$. Activation energies E_0 are deduced from the high temperature region.

IV. SUMMARY

Hydrogenated, amorphous silicon films have been deposited by CO_2 laser induced pyrolysis of SiH_4 gas. The films reflect the qualities anticipated on the basis of perceived process attributes; low substrate temperatures result in hydrogen levels usually achieved with glow-discharge processes in films having the structural quality of those produced by CVD. The combination of these effects is reflected in measured spin densities, optical absorptivities, optical gaps and conductivities. These individual properties can be varied through process variables while maintaining high growth rates.

V. ACKNOWLEDGEMENTS

The financial support of the 3M Corporation and the extensive contributions of Mr. John Flint are gratefully acknowledged.

VI. REFERENCES

1. J. C. Knights and G. Lucovsky, CRC Critical Reviews in Solid State and Materials Science, 9, 211-83 (1980).

2. D. E. Carlson, Sol. En. Mat., 3, 503-18 (1980); Y. Hamokawa, J. de Physique, C4, 1131-42 (1981).

3. H. Fritzche, Sol. En. Mat., 3, 447-501 (1980).

4. W. Paul and D. Anderson, Sol. En. Mat., 5, 229-316 (1981).

5. M. Hirose, J. de Physique, C4, 705-14 (1981).

6. C. P. Christensen and K. M. Lakin, Appl. Phys. Lett., 32, 254-5 (1978).

7. V. Baranauskas, C. I. Z. Mammana, R. E. Klinger and J. E. Greene, Appl. Phys. Lett., 36, 930-2 (1980).

8. S. D. Allen, J. Appl. Phys., 52, 6501-5 (1981).

9. R. Bilenchi and M. Musci, Proc. 8th Int. Conf. in Chemical Vapor Depositon Electrochemical Society, 275-83 (1981). R. Bilenchi, I. Gianinoni and M. Musci, J. Appl. Phys., 33, 6479 (1982).

10. T. F. Deutsch, D. J. Ehrlich and R. M. Osgood, Jr., Appl. Phys. Lett., 35, 175-7 (1979).

11. J. W. C. Johns and W. A. Kreiner, J. Mol. Spec., 60, 400-11 (1976).

12. A. C. G. Mitchell and M. W. Zemansky, Resonance Radiation and Excited Atoms, Cambridge University Press, Cambridge (1961).

13. H. Okabe, Photochemistry of Small Molecules, Wiley, New York (1978).

14. R. A. Marra and J. S. Haggerty, Ceramic Engineering and Science Proceedings, 3, 1-2, (1981).

15. T. R. Gattuso, M. Meunier, and J. S. Haggerty, "Laser Induced Deposition of Thin Films, MIT-EL82-022, May 1982.

16. T. F. Deutsch, J. Chem. Phys., 70, 1187-92 (1979).

17. B. A. Scott, R. M. Plecenik and E. E. Simonyi, Appl. Phys. Lett., 39, 73-5 (1981).

18. K. H. Sladek, J. Electrochem. Soc.: Sol. St. Sci., 118, 654-7 (1971).

19. D. C. Booth, D. D. Allred and B. O. Seraphin, Sol. En. Mat., 2, (1979).

20. J. T. Hilman, B. S. Thesis, M.I.T., June 1982.

21. J. Bloem and L. J. Giling, Current Topics in Materials Science, ed. E. Kaldis, 1, 147-342 (1978).

22. S. K. Friedlander, Smoke, Dust and Haze, Wiley, New York (1977).

23. D. Adler, J. de Physique, C4, 14 (1981).

24. Hasegawa, S., et al., Phil. Mag. B, 43, 149-56 (1981).

25. Tauc., J., Optical Properties of Solids, ed. F. Abeles, North-Holland, Amsterdam (1970) pp. 227-313.

26. Cody, C. D., et al., Solar Cells, 2, 227-43 (1980).

27. Janai, M., and Karlsson, B., Sol. En. Mat., 1, 387-95 (1979).

28. Mott, N. F., and Davis, E. A., Electronic Processes in Non-Crystalline Materials, 2nd Ed., Clarendon Press (1979).

SECTION VII
PHOTOCHEMICAL DOPING

PULSED UV EXCIMER LASER DOPING OF SEMICONDUCTORS*

T. F. DEUTSCH
Lincoln Laboratory, Massachusetts Institute of Technology,
Lexington, Massachusetts 02173

ABSTRACT

UV excimer lasers have been used to dope semiconductors by a one-step process in which the laser serves both to release dopant atoms from a parent molecule and to melt the surface, allowing incorporation of dopant atoms by liquid state diffusion. The technique has been used to dope Si, GaAs, and InP. Shallow junctions formed by the technique have been fabricated into efficient Si and GaAs solar cells.

INTRODUCTION

The use of lasers in the doping of semiconductors has been studied extensively. Pulsed lasers have been used to anneal damage caused by ion-implantation of dopants. More recently, laser-induced diffusion of dopant films [1-6] and laser-induced recrystallization of doped amorphous films to form epitaxial junctions [7] has been explored. These techniques use the pulsed laser to produce melting of a surface layer which, in the case of laser annealing, can regrow epitaxially from an undamaged substrate or which, in the case of laser-induced diffusion, allows liquid-state diffusion of dopant atoms. The pulsed laser delivers heat only to a thin surface layer, avoiding undesired diffusion in other parts of the substrate or unwanted reactions between, for example, the aluminum metallization on a Si wafer and the substrate.

Photochemical techniques for semiconductor processing have been under intensive investigation at M.I.T. Lincoln Laboratory and elsewhere [8]. This paper discusses the use of pulsed UV excimer lasers to dope semiconductors by a one-step process in which the laser serves both to release dopant atoms from an appropriate parent molecule and to melt a thin layer on the semiconductor surface, allowing incorporation of dopant atoms by liquid state diffusion. Figure 1 shows a schematic diagram of the process.

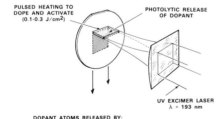

Fig. 1. Schematic diagram of pulsed excimer laser doping of semiconductors.

---

*This work was sponsored by the Department of the Air Force, in part under a specific program sponsored by the Air Force Office of Scientific Research, by the Defense Advanced Research Projects Agency, and by the Army Research Office.

UV excimer lasers offer some unique advantages for semiconductor processing. They can produce high average powers; commercial lasers with 193 nm powers in excess of 10 W are available. They can be operated at different UV wavelengths by changing gases and they can be scaled to produce yet higher output powers. The 193 nm output of the ArF laser, corresponding to a photon energy of 6.4 eV, is capable of photodissociating most molecules of interest as dopant carriers. Because the excimer laser is a pulsed source, it cannot be tightly focused on a substrate to produce highly localized doping; a 1 mJ pulse focused on a 100 μm square region corresponds to an energy density of 10 J/cm^2, above the damage threshold for many materials. Hence pulsed laser doping is best suited for large-area processing, such as the production of junctions for solar cells.

EXPERIMENTAL

A pulsed UV excimer laser was used to irradiate various semiconductor samples. The excimer laser was operated with either ArF or XeF, producing 7-ns-long pulses at 193 nm or 351 nm respectively. The laser beam was brought to a line focus near the surface of the sample by a 5 cm-focal-length quartz cylinder lens. The beam size at the sample surface, measured between half-power points, was 0.27 mm wide by 10 mm long. The laser was generally operated at 2-4 Hz, with typical fluences at the substrate of 0.1-1 J/cm^2.

The samples were enclosed in a 1-cm-long stainless-steel cell which was translated normal to the beam axis. Scan rates of 0.25-8 mm/min were examined; at 2 Hz a typical scan rate of 1 mm/min corresponds to ~ 32 pulses per focal area.

A variety of doping gases including BCl_3, PCl_3, H_2S, $Cd(CH_3)_2$ and $Al(CH_3)_3$ were used. Gas pressures were chosen to give 193 nm absorptions of 10-50% in a 1-cm path. As discussed in more detail below, at 351 nm these gases were not absorbing and gas pressures up to 700 Torr were used.

RESULTS

Si

The electrical properties of UV excimer laser doped Si have been examined and the technique used to produce junctions which were then fabricated into solar cells. B, P, and Al doping were examined [9-11]. Figure 2 shows the profile of B concentration vs depth obtained by secondary-ion mass spectroscopy (SIMS) for an n-type (100) Si wafer (2-5 Ω-cm) doped using ArF radiation. The SIMS signal is dominated by instrumental background below ~ 10^{17} cm^{-3}. The estimated junction depth, obtained by extrapolating the linear portion of the B depth profile to the substrate doping level of 2 x 10^{15} cm^{-3}, is about 0.35 μm. The sheet resistance of the B-doped layer was about 50 Ω/☐.

Boron doping of Si using BCl_3 gas was examined at two different laser wavelengths using both single crystal and polycrystalline material. The single crystal Si samples had either (100) or (111) orientation and resistivities of 300-500 Ω-cm. The amorphous Si films, which were used in investigations of the doping of noncrystalline Si, were produced by chemical vapor deposition (CVD) at 625°C on Si substrates covered with a 2000 Å thick layer of thermal oxide. Some of the CVD Si samples were subsequently annealed at 900°C for 30 minutes to provide polycrystalline samples. Prior to irradiation all sample surfaces were cleaned with organic solvents and etched in buffered HF. The CVD Si samples were irradiated using both 193-nm ArF laser radiation and 351 nm XeF laser radiation. At 193 nm the absorption coefficient of BCl_3 was measured to be 0.0019 cm^{-1} Torr^{-1}, giving ~ 10% absorption for 50 Torr BCl_3 in a 1 cm cell. At 351 nm, BCl_3 had no measurable absorption even at pressures of 700 Torr in a 1 cm cell. The sheet resistance of irradiated strips was measured using a four point probe. In addition, some irradiated samples were fabricated into specimens suitable for van der Pauw measurements of sheet resistance and mobility.

Figure 3 shows the sheet resistance of 5000-Å-thick CVD Si films on SiO_2 versus fluence at the substrate for both ArF and XeF laser irradiation. The curves are quite similar, with the lowest sheet resistances obtained with ArF-laser radiation, $\sim 60\ \Omega/\square$, about 1/3 of those obtained with the XeF laser. Figure 3 also shows sheet resistance versus fluence for B doping of single-crystal, 500 Ω-cm, n-Si using ArF radiation; at fluences above 0.4 J/cm^2 the results are almost identical to those obtained for CVD Si.

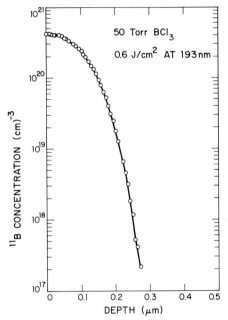

Fig. 2. ^{11}B concentration vs depth for Si sample doped using 50-Torr BCl_3 and a 193 nm fluence of 0.6 J/cm^2 at the sample.

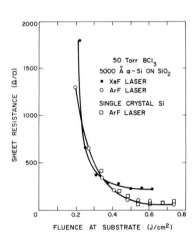

Fig. 3. Sheet resistance of single crystal and CVD Si as a function of ArF or XeF laser fluence at the substrate. The sample scan rate is 1 mm/min, the laser pulse rate 2 Hz, and the gas pressure 50 Torr BCl_3.

The steep rise of the curves at fluences below ~ 0.2 J/cm^2 is probably due to the threshold for melting of the Si film. In the case of P doping using PCl_3, similar sheet resistance versus fluence curves were obtained for single crystal substrates. When we attempted to P dope CVD Si films under the same conditions, high sheet resistances, typically 500-1000 $\Omega/\square$, were obtained and we could not obtain a reliable sheet resistance versus fluence curve. The reasons for this difference are not known.

Table I summarizes the results of van der Pauw measurements made on single-crystal, amorphous, and polycrystalline Si that was B doped using the ArF laser. Doping profiles of B doped Si produced under similar conditions, e.g., Fig. 2, show total B doses of 2-3 x 10^{15}/cm^2, in good agreement with the carrier densities obtained here, and doping depths of a few thousand angstroms. Hence all the B atoms introduced by the UV doping process are electrically activated. Somewhat higher mobilities were obtained with single crystal or polycrystalline (annealed CVD) Si than with amorphous CVD Si. The shallow doping depths imply carrier densities in the 10^{20} cm^{-3} range and the low mobility observed in single-crystal Si is due to this high doping density.

TABLE I
Electrical Properties of UV Laser Doped Si. Conditions: 0.7 J/cm^2 at 193 nm, 50 Torr BCl$_3$, 1 mm/min scan at 2 Hz. Approximately 35 pulses per focal area.

	Sheet resistance ($\Omega/\square$)	Surface carrier density (cm^{-2})	300 K mobility (cm^2/V-s)
single crystal Si	46	3.3 x 10^{15}	41
5000 Å CVD Si (amorphous)	68	3.7 x 10^{15}	24
5000 Å CVD Si annealed for 30 min at 900°C (polycrystalline)	61	2.2 x 10^{15}	47

In earlier, closely related, experiments involving Cd doping of InP, gas phase photodissociation was found to be essential for producing good ohmic contacts [12]. In order to clarify the doping mechanism operative with 351 nm XeF radiation, which does not produce gas phase photodissociation, the sheet resistance of single crystal Si was measured as a function of BCl$_3$ pressure for fixed XeF laser fluence and sample scan speed. In previous studies of laser photodeposition adsorbed films had been shown to play an important role [13]. The role of adsorbed surface layers of BCl$_3$ in the doping process was investigated by irradiating a sample in an evacuated cell (P ~ 2 x 10^{-5} Torr). The cell was then filled with 100 Torr BCl$_3$, re-evacuated, and another portion of the sample irradiated. Figure 4 shows the results of the measurements; exposure of the sample to BCl$_3$ prior to irradiation leads to a sheet resistance of 650 $\Omega/\square$ while adding BCl$_3$ gas to a pressure of 500 Torr reduces the sheet resistance by a factor of ~ 6. In order to verify the existence of an adsorbed BCl$_3$ layer an adsorption isotherm was measured using a quartz crystal oscillator. From a plot of adsorbed mass versus BCl$_3$ pressure one finds that an adsorbed layer does indeed remain after the cell is evacuated. Similar adlayer doping effects were observed with PCl$_3$ on Si. However, it should be pointed out that not all doping gases form adlayers that contribute to doping. For example, no such doping effect has been seen in the doping of GaAs using H$_2$S discussed below.

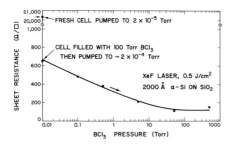

Fig. 4. Sheet resistance of CVD-Si as a function of BCl$_3$ pressure for a 351 nm fluence of 0.5 J/cm^2. The scan rate is 1 mm/min and the laser pulse rate is 2 Hz.

The data of Fig. 4 provide evidence that molecular dissociation at the Si surface is an important source of B atoms, since the 351 nm radiation is not adsorbed in the gas phase. Molecules adsorbed on the Si surface can be dissociated by pyrolysis, or possibly by photolysis. The latter process can occur if the absorption spectrum of an adlayer on the heated substrate is sufficiently red-shifted to cause some absorption at 351 nm. Since similar doping effects have been seen by other workers using much longer wavelengths (0.73 μm) [14]; we believe pyrolysis is the more likely mechanism.

The observed doping effects are qualitatively consistent with the efficient incorporation of B atoms from the adlayer. The 650 $\Omega/\square$ sheet resistance observed for the sample irradiated after exposure to BCl_3 corresponds to a carrier density of $2-4 \times 10^{14}/cm^2$, the uncertainty arising from the possible range of mobilities, while the calculated surface density for a monolayer of BCl_3 is 2×10^{14} molecules/cm^2.

The pressure dependence of the sheet resistance, shown in Fig. 4, is also in qualitative agreement with the BCl_3 adsorption isotherm which shows that the thickness of the adlayer increases rapidly up to a pressure of 50-100 Torr, and then grows less rapidly. Adlayer formation can occur between pulses, allowing each pulse to incorporate atoms from a freshly formed molecular adlayer. If pyrolysis of molecules striking the hot surface was the dominant dopant supply process a stronger pressure dependence of the sheet resistance than that shown in Fig. 4 would be expected, since the number of molecules striking a surface depends linearly on pressure.

The dependence of sheet resistance on UV dose (fluence x pulses/area) was investigated by irradiating single crystal Si samples with ArF radiation at a fixed fluence and gas pressure, but at different scan rates. The results for both P and B doping, expressed in terms of sheet resistance versus number of ArF laser pulses per focal area, are displayed on Fig. 5. The number of pulses per focal area is taken as the number of pulses delivered in the time in which the sample translates one beam width (~ 0.3 mm). The curves show a (dose)$^{-n}$ dependence, where n is ~ 0.6. With the assumption the carrier mobility is substantially constant for the various doses, the sheet resistance curves show the dependence of the reciprocal of carrier concentration on UV dose.

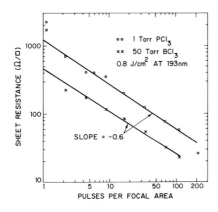

Fig. 5. Sheet resistance of single crystal Si as a function of the number of pulses per focal area for B and P doping. The 193 nm fluence was 0.8 J/cm^2, the BCl_3 pressure was 50 Torr and the PCl_3 pressure was 1 Torr.

The doping process involves two simultaneous steps, release of dopant atoms at the surface of the semiconductor and incorporation of those atoms by diffusion. Either of these steps can be rate limiting, depending on the particular conditions. From the depths of doping observed, typically several thousand angstroms, we infer that diffusion occurs with diffusion constants typical of molten silicon. If diffusion limits the doping depth attained during each pulse time, τ_p, the total doping dose is proportional to the diffusion length in the molten Si, L. In this case

$$L \approx (2 \, D \, N \, \tau_p)^{1/2} \qquad (1)$$

where D is a time averaged diffusion constant and N is the number of pulses. Thus the doping density varies as $N^{0.5}$. The 0.6 exponent obtained from Fig. 5 is qualitatively consistent with diffusion-limited conditions.

The laser doping technique was applied to the formation of junctions that could be fabricated into solar cells. ArF radiation was used to B dope n-type wafers which were then fabricated into solar cells up to 0.5 x 1 cm^2 in area [10]. The best 0.5 cm^2 cell had an open-circuit voltage V_{oc} of 0.56 V, a short-circuit current density J_{sc} of 25.5 mA/cm^2 and a fill factor of 0.72, resulting in a measured efficiency of 10.3% without correcting for the contact finger area. An antireflection coating would be expected to significantly increase the efficiency.

GaAs

Doping GaAs is more difficult than doping Si and the laser and electron beam processing techniques that have been so extensively applied to Si have not been equally successful in GaAs [15,16]. There has, for example, been only one report of successful GaAs solar cell formation using beam processing [17]. The high vapor pressure of As near the melting point can lead to material loss. An encapsulating layer or cap can be used to prevent such loss; however, the encapsulant can diffuse into the GaAs and can introduce stress into the surface of the material. Furthermore, beam heating can introduce slip planes and other defects which degrade the electrical properties of the GaAs [16]. Thus pulsed laser annealing of ion-implanted GaAs requires a compromise between the conflicting requirements of a laser energy high enough to anneal out damage and activate dopants yet low enough to avoid the introduction of electrically active defects. The laser-induced diffusion technique has been used to dope GaAs with Mg, but the resulting diodes were not useful solar cells [18].

The UV excimer laser technique has been used to dope GaAs and to produce p-n junctions [19]. S doping of GaAs using H_2S, a common doping gas used in systems for growing GaAs by chemical vapor deposition (CVD), was examined at two different laser wavelengths, one of which was not absorbed by the H_2S. This allowed us to compare the doping obtained when photolysis was operative with that obtained when only pyrolysis could occur. At the 193 nm wavelength of the ArF laser the absorption coefficient of H_2S was measured to be 0.2 cm^{-1} Torr^{-1}, giving 60% absorption for our typical operating conditions of 5 Torr H_2S in a 1-cm-long cell. At the 351 nm wavelength of the XeF excimer laser H_2S had no measurable absorption even at pressures of 700 Torr in a 1-cm-long cell and linear gas phase photolysis does not occur. Better solar cells were obtained using the ArF laser and we concentrate on results obtained with that wavelength.

The doping concentration profiles of ArF irradiated samples were obtained using secondary ion mass spectrometry (SIMS). Fig. 6 shows the profile obtained from an ArF irradiated sample; the irradiation conditions for this sample, which was produced at an early stage of the experiments, differ somewhat from the optimum solar cell conditions established later. For these conditions the junction depth, obtained by extrapolating the linear portion of the ^{32}S concentration versus depth curve to a solar cell substrate doping level of $\sim 10^{17}$ cm^{-3}, would be ~ 0.15 μm. The S concentration at the surface, $\sim 8 \times 10^{18}$ cm^{-3}, combined with the 0.15 μm depth of the doped region, gives a surface dopant concentration of 10^{14} cm^{-2}, within the range of values obtained from the van der Pauw measurements discussed below.

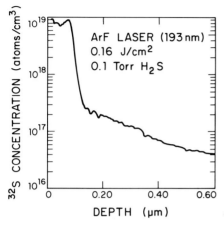

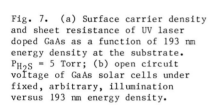

Fig. 6. Concentration of S versus depth for GaAs sample doped using 0.16 J/cm² of 193 nm radiation and 0.1 Torr H_2S. The instrumental background level is ~ 3 x 10^{16} atoms/cm³.

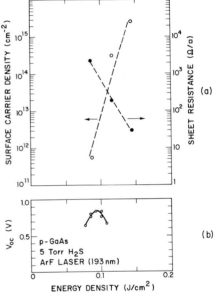

Fig. 7. (a) Surface carrier density and sheet resistance of UV laser doped GaAs as a function of 193 nm energy density at the substrate. P_{H_2S} = 5 Torr; (b) open circuit voltage of GaAs solar cells under fixed, arbitrary, illumination versus 193 nm energy density.

Figure 7a shows the variation of the electrical properties of laser-doped GaAs, obtained from van der Pauw measurements, with ArF laser energy density, while Fig. 7b shows the dependence of the open circuit voltage, V_{oc}, of small test cells on laser energy density at the sample surface. The latter curve shows that there is only a relatively narrow range of energy densities over which optimum solar cell performance can be obtained; this range is about ± 10% from the optimum. This contrasts with our previous experiments using laser-doping to make Si solar cells; in this case the incident energy density could be varied by about ± 25% around a nominally optimum value without significant variation in V_{oc}. Only limited studies of the effect of H_2S pressure on solar cell V_{oc} were made, since pressure variations change the gas transmission at 193 nm and hence the energy reaching the substrate. The pressure used here, 5 Torr, was approximately optimum for maximizing solar cell V_{oc}.

Figure 7a gives some indication of the reason for the more critical nature of GaAs junction formation. The electrical properties of the doped material, namely the sheet resistance and the surface carrier density, change by decades for variations of less than 50% in the laser beam energy density; although only 3 samples were examined the trend is clear. The surface mobility, as obtained from the van der Pauw measurements, decreased from 4500 to 80 cm^2/V-s as the energy density was increased over the same range covered by Fig. 7a. Thus, increasing the doping concentration is accompanied by a more rapid decrease in electron mobility than that which would be expected on the basis of the known variation of mobility with carrier concentration and may well reflect the effect of laser-induced, electrically active, defects. The narrow range for maximum V_{oc} probably results from the strong dependence of both doping density and mobility on laser energy density.

In order to evaluate the importance of gas phase photolysis in the doping process, similar solar cell and electrical measurements were made on GaAs samples that had been processed using 351 nm XeF laser radiation, which is not absorbed by H_2S. We were still able to make solar cells, although the open circuit voltage obtained under optimum conditions was ~ 20% less than that obtained using ArF radiation. The optimum laser energy density with XeF, 0.3 J/cm^2, was about three times that for ArF radiation and the energy density was less critical; a ± 25% variation had little effect on V_{oc}. The higher optimum energy density found for XeF is due in part to the fact that the optical absorption length in GaAs at 351 nm is about twice that at 193 nm. The allowable range of H_2S pressure was greater; V_{oc} was essentially constant for gas pressures ranging from 5 to 500 Torr. The dependence of the electrical properties of GaAs doped using XeF radiation on laser energy density was qualitatively similar to the behavior of the ArF laser irradiated samples shown in Fig. 7a. Likewise, the ^{32}S profile obtained for the XeF irradiation conditions, 0.23 J/cm^2 and 500 Torr H_2S, that produced maximum V_{oc} was essentially the same as that in Fig. 6, indicating that the junction depth is ~ 0.15 μm.

GaAs solar cells were formed by S doping a p/p$^+$ substrate, producing a n$^+$/p/p$^+$ shallow homojunction structure. The epilayer and substrate were doped with Zn to concentrations of about 1×10^{17} and 5×10^{18} cm^{-3} respectively. The best 3 x 3 mm square cell fabricated from ArF irradiated material was antireflection (AR) coated with an 800 Å thick, electron beam evaporated, Ta_2O_5 film having a refractive index of 2.0. The open circuit voltage, V_{oc}, was 0.775 V, the short circuit current density, J_{sc}, was 22.3 mA/cm^2 (not corrected for contact finger area), and the fill factor was 0.62, resulting in a measured AM1 efficiency of 10.8%. This efficiency compares quite favorably with the value of 12% obtained for ion-implanted, cw Nd:YAG laser annealed, GaAs solar cells of somewhat smaller area [17]. Values of J_{sc} before and after AR coating, together with our analytic model of GaAs solar cells [20], were used to deduce a junction depth of about 1000 Å, consistent with the SIMS results.

Although more extensive measurements of the electrical properties of laser chemically doped GaAs are needed to fully characterize the doping process, several conclusions can be drawn from the above data. In contrast to the behavior of laser doped Si, where the incident energy can be varied by a factor of two with only small changes in sheet resistance, the electrical properties of laser doped GaAs can vary by decades for such a change in laser energy. The behavior shown in Fig. 7a suggests a process with an activating energy is occurring; similar variations in electrical properties with annealing temperature have been observed in recent experiments on strip heater annealing of GaAs [21]. While the formation of p-n junctions which function as efficient solar cells requires close control over laser parameters, the low sheet resistances obtained compare favorably to those produced using other beam processing techniques and suggest that ohmic contact formation is a possible application for the technique.

InP

The doping of InP is made difficult by the same decomposition considerations that apply to GaAs. ArF laser radiation has been used to produce ohmic contacts to p-InP using Zn or Cd released by the photolysis of $Zn(CH_3)_2$ or $Cd(CH_3)_2$ [12]. In contrast to junction formation, ohmic contact formation is relatively uncritical and resistance-area products of 1.9×10^{-4} Ω cm^2 were obtained. This value is essentially comparable to the 3×10^{-4} Ω-cm^2 obtained using conventional thermal alloying and the $(0.5-2) \times 10^{-4}$ Ω cm^2 obtained using laser annealing of Zn^+ implants.

CONCLUSIONS

The use of pulsed UV excimer lasers to dope semiconductors has been demonstrated. Both photolytic and pyrolytic mechansims can serve to release dopant atoms, with the photolytic mechanism being somewhat more efficient. The pyrolytic process has the significant advantage that it does not require a match between the laser wavelength and an absorption band of the parent gas molecule. The adlayers formed by some gases can serve as a source of doping atoms. Such layers may be useful as finite surface sources of dopant atoms for applications requiring doping at levels below the limit imposed by the solid solubility.

The doping of Si is possible over a relatively large energy window; by contrast doping of GaAs and InP requires close control of the laser energy. Efficient Si solar cells have been made from junctions formed by laser doping and the process is compatible with continuous doping of Si ribbons that are being developed for low-cost Si solar cells.

ACKNOWLEDGMENTS

D. J. Silversmith, D. J. Ehrlich, R. M. Osgood, Jr., J. C. C. Fan, G. W. Turner, R. L. Chapman, R. P. Gale, D. D. Rathman, R. W. Mountain, and Z. L. Liau contributed actively to various phases of this work.

We thank J. W. Burke for experimental work throughout these experiments, M. J. Button for the van der Pauw measurements, G. W. Iseler for the InP samples, M. K. Connors, F. M. Davis, G. H. Foley, and R. F. Murphy for technical assistance.

REFERENCES

1. R. T. Young, R. F. Wood, J. Narayan, C. W. White, and W. H. Christie, IEEE Trans. Electron Devices ED-27, 807 (1980).

2. J. Narayan, R. T. Young, R. F. Wood, and W. H. Christie, Appl. Phys. Lett. 33, 338 (1978).

3. J. C. Muller, E. Fogarassy, D. Salles, R. Stuck, and P. M. Siffert, IEEE Trans. Electron Devices EDL-27, 815 (1980).

4. E. Forgassy, R. Stuck, J. J. Grob, and P. Siffert, J. Appl. Phys. 52, 1076 (1981);

5. K. Affolter, W. Luthy, and M. von Allmen, Appl. Phys. Lett. 33, 185 (1978).

6. S. Wu, Solid State Technol. 25, 71 (June, 1982).

7. R. T. Young, J. Narayan, and R. F. Wood, Appl. Phys. Lett. 35, 447 (1979).

8. D. J. Ehrlich, T. F. Deutsch, R. M. Osgood, Jr., and D. J. Silversmith, Proceedings Fourteenth Conference on Solid State Devices, (Jpn. J. Appl. Phys., Tokyo, 1982), p. 335.

9. T. F. Deutsch, J. C. C. Fan, G. W. Turner, R. L. Chapman, D. J. Ehrlich, and R. M. Osgood, Jr., Appl. Phys. Lett. 38, 144 (1981).

10. J. C. C. Fan, T. F. Deutsch, G. W. Turner, D. J. Ehrlich, R. L. Chapman, and R. M. Osgood, Jr., Proceedings of Fifteenth IEEE Photovoltaics Specialists Conference, (Institute of Electrical and Electronics Engineers, New York, 1981), p. 432.

11. T. F. Deutsch, D. J. Ehrlich, D. D. Rathman, D. J. Silversmith, and R. M. Osgood, Jr., Appl. Phys. Lett. 39, 825 (1981).

12. T. F. Deutsch, D. J. Ehrlich, R. M. Osgood, Jr., and Z. L. Liau, Appl. Phys. Lett. 36, 847 (1980).

13. D. J. Ehrlich and R. M. Osgood, Jr., Chem. Phys. Lett. 79, 381 (1981).

14. G. B. Turner, D. Tarrant, G. Pollack, R. Pressley, and R. Press, Appl. Phys. Lett. 39, 967 (1981).

15. C. L. Anderson, H. L. Dunlap, L. D. Hess, G. L. Olson, and K. V. Vaidyanathan in Laser and Electron Beam Processing of Materials, edited by C. W. White and P. S. Peercy (Academic Press, New York, 1980), p. 334.

16. J. C. C. Fan, R. L. Chapman, J. P. Donnelly, G. W. Turner, and C. O. Bozler in Laser and Electron-Beam Solid Interactions and Materials Processing, edited by J. F. Gibbons, L. D. Hess, and T. W. Sigmon (North-Holland, New York, 1981), p. 261.

17. J. C. C. Fan, R. L. Chapman, J. P. Donnelly, G. W. Turner, and C. O. Bozler, Appl. Phys. Lett. 34, 780 (1979).

18. R. T. Young, J. Narayan, R. D. Westbrook, and R. F. Wood in Laser Solid Interactions and Laser Processing-1978, edited by S. D. Ferris, II, J. Leamy, and J. M. Poate, AIP Conf. Proc. 50, (American Institute of Physics, New York, 1979), p. 579.

19. T. F. Deutsch, J. C. C. Fan, D. J. Ehrlich, G. W. Turner, R. L. Chapman, and R. P. Gale, Appl. Phys. Lett. 40, 722 (1982).

20. J. C. C. Fan, C. O. Bozler, and B. J. Palm, Appl. Phys. Lett. 35, 875 (1979).

21. R. L. Chapman, J. C. C. Fan, J. P. Donnelly, and B. Y. Tsaur, Appl. Phys. Lett. 40, 805 (1982).

SUBMICROMETER-LINEWIDTH LASER DOPING*

J. Y. TSAO AND D. J. EHRLICH
Lincoln Laboratory, Massachusetts Institute of Technology
Lexington, Massachusetts 02173

ABSTRACT

Dopant patterns of 250-nm linewidth have been written in silicon by localized heating with a cw laser beam, and then transferred into positive and negative surface-relief patterns by preferential etching. The tightly focused beam both generates free dopant atoms and simultaneously promotes solid-state diffusion into the substrate. Because of the nonlinear dependence of diffusion rates on temperature, the linewidths of the patterns are substantially narrower than those of both the temperature and the laser-beam profiles on the surface. In addition, an enhancement is observed in diffusion rates under the strong thermal gradients associated with highly localized heating.

INTRODUCTION

The use of laser and electron beams to confine thermal processes to shallow semiconductor surface layers is now well established. Confining such processes to very small lateral dimensions, however, has not received as much attention. In this paper we describe an application of highly localized heating in which laser-driven solid-state diffusion of dopants produces high-spatial-resolution dopant patterns in Si. The process first generates free dopant atoms by thermal decomposition of an encapsulating vapor, then diffuses these atoms into the bulk Si under a sharply defined temperature gradient. The linewidths obtained are substantially narrower than the diffraction-limited intensity modulation at the laser beam focus. In addition, the results suggest that localized heating can produce enhanced impurity diffusion rates. We have also used this process, in combination with preferential etching, to write submicrometer-linewidth surface-relief patterns on Si substrates. A previous report of the process has been published in Ref. 1.

EXPERIMENTAL

The B and P dopants used in this study were derived from vapor-phase (10-200 Torr) $B(CH_3)_3$, BCl_3 and PCl_3, by local pyrolysis using a 514.5-nm argon-ion laser beam. The majority of these experiments used pyrolytically deposited B. For the first experiments, a 0.1-0.6 W, 514.5 nm TEM_{00} beam was focused at ~ f/3 through a multielement lens. Si substrates were translated in the laser focus at rates of 0.9-440 μm/s by computer-controlled stepping motors. Optimal focusing was determined by autocollimation and could be maintained over scans of length > 1 cm. For the most recent experiments, the laser beam was focused through an inverted microscope column equipped with an f/1 reflective microscope objective. In-process viewing was possible with a vidicon.

---

*This work was supported by the Defense Advanced Research Projects Agency, the Department of the Air Force, in part under a specific program sponsored by the Air Force Office of Scientific Research, and by the Army Research Office.

The Si substrates, with (111) and (100) surface orientations, were cleaned with organic solvents, stripped of native oxide in buffered HF, then transferred into a 0.5-cm-path-length reaction chamber which was pumped and then filled with the appropriate vapor. The substrates were irradiated at power levels 10-20% below the melting threshold. Under all the dopant atmospheres, melting can be readily determined on Si surfaces by the onset of a rapid etching reaction [2]. After doping the wafer surfaces appear specular; no evidence of the laser track, i.e., surface roughening or reflow, is seen under Nomarski microscopy. The boron-doped regions were delineated by differential etching either in a $KOH:H_2O$:isopropanol [3] or in a tetramethylammonium hydroxide (TMAH) [4] solution. The samples were then examined by Nomarski optical and scanning electron microscopy (SEM); some secondary-ion mass spectroscopy (SIMS) measurements were also made.

RESULTS

Figure 1 shows an SEM photograph of B-doped lines laser-patterned in a (100) substrate after preferential etching for 25 s in TMAH. The relief profile has a linewidth of 250 nm, considerably narrower than the 1-2 μm spot size of the focused beam. The oscillation in the scan is due to vibration of the stepping-motor-driven translation stages.

At laser powers high enough to cause Si melting a central groove is etched. At these power levels the preferential etches reveal heavy boron doping in the wings of the scanned beam thermal gradient. Figure 2 shows an SEM photograph of a (100) substrate which has been melted under a $B(CH_3)_3$ atmosphere, and then etched for 5 minutes in TMAH. Despite the removal of ~ 3 μm of undoped substrate material, some of the central etched grooves remain. Also evident in Fig. 2 is the faceting along (111) planes of the positive relief. This is due to the anisotropic etching rate of TMAH: (100) surfaces are etched ~ 20x faster than (111) surfaces [4]. In contrast, as shown in the optical micrograph in Fig. 3, the TMAH etching of a laser doped (111) surface delineates the doped regions with a squarer relief profile. The terracing of the background surface is due to the instability of the (111) surface to an etch that preferentially etches non-(111) surfaces.

A SIMS analysis was also made of the depth profiles of large-area B-doped samples. Figure 4 shows profiles for the (111) wafer orientation using 19-μm/s and 440-μm/s scan speeds, a nominal 2 μm focal spot, and 0.4-μm steps between raster scans. Absolute depths and densities were determined by cross calibration with an implanted standard. Both profiles show shallow distributions with B-concentrations peaking in the high 10^{20} cm^{-3} range, although the sharply falling near-surface concentration spike on profile (b) may be a measurement artifact. The B detection limit is below 10^{15} cm^{-3}. As discussed below, the profiles indicate a complicated accelerated diffusion behavior, particularly in the low-concentration tails of the diffused distributions.

MECHANISM FOR LATERAL CONFINEMENT

The mechanism for the laser doping can be described as two sequential processes. First, the parent molecules must adsorb and then thermally crack on the surface, and second, the surface-adsorbed dopant atoms must diffuse into the solid. For the pressures (1-200 Torr) and local temperatures (1000-1400°C) used in these experiments, the first process can be considered extremely rapid compared to the second. For example, in the laser-thermal deposition of Si from its halides under similar experimental conditions, the Si atom flux produced in the surface reaction is greater than 10^5 atoms/(lattice site sec) [5]. Even in the most extreme case, however, in which the dopant atom concentration drops to zero from its solid solubility in a few lattice spacings, the solid-state diffusion flux is less than $< 10^3$ atoms/(lattice site sec). Therefore, solid-state diffusion is the rate-limiting step, and the step which will determine the

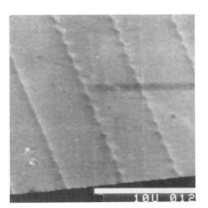

Fig. 1. Scanning electron micrograph (SEM) of (100)-oriented substrate laser-doped with boron from $B(CH_3)_3$ after 25 s of etching in TMAH solution.

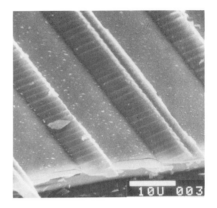

Fig. 2. SEM micrograph of (100)-oriented substrate after laser irradiation above the melting threshold in a $B(CH_3)_3$ ambient, and then a 5 min etch in TMAH solution.

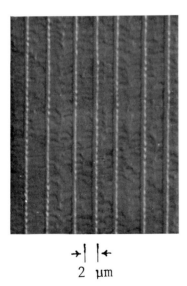

Fig. 3. Photomicrograph of (111)-oriented substrate laser doped with boron from $B(CH_3)_3$ after etching in TMAH solution.

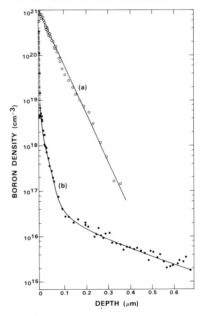

Fig. 4. Boron depth profiles determined by SIMS analysis of a raster-scanned 2000 Ω-cm Si (111) sample. Scan speeds are (a) 19 µm/s and (b) 440 µm/s.

spatial profile of the overall laser doping process. This is not the case for similar experiments using a partially photochemical technique to locally diffuse materials into InP [6] and Al [7].

The very high lateral confinement observed in laser chemical doping is therefore due to the localized thermal profiles, and the consequent strong spatial variation in dopant diffusivities, associated with the tightly focused irradiation. The expected degree of confinement can be estimated by calculating the temperature distribution and its consequences on thermally activated solid-state diffusion. The beam energy is deposited in a shallow surface layer. This results in a strongly peaked lateral temperature profile close to the surface. To illustrate this, Fig. 5 shows the result of a calculation of the surface temperature profile, $T(x)$, in unmelted Si using the simplest form of the treatment due to Lax [8]; the temperature-dependent thermal conductivity of Si which causes a slight further peaking of the profile is neglected.

Figure 5 also shows the lateral variation of the Si diffusion coefficient calculated from $D(x) \sim \exp[-E_a/kT(x)]$, where E_a is the activation energy for boron diffusion (3.69 eV), and a peak temperature of $T(0) = 1350°C$ was assumed. As shown in the figure, the nonlinear dependence of D on temperature causes the lateral variation in D to be substantially narrower than that in T. A third curve shows the variation of the low-concentration diffusion length, proportional to $\sqrt{D(x)}$, for a constant B concentration on the surface. The absolute B concentrations will scale with the surface concentration and dwell time. For moderate doping densities this last profile is the predicted dopant concentration variation in a thin layer near the surface. Note that the 1/e width of the doped line is a factor of 5 narrower than that of $T(x)$, and that the factor is even larger at lower points in the profiles. The predicted width is in good agreement with the low-doping-density results obtained in the experiment. At high densities (> 10^{19} cm^{-3}), solubility saturation effects cause a flattening of the profiles. Note, however, that very strong lateral edge definition is still predicted.

ACCELERATED DIFFUSION

Similarly, we can predict the depth profile of the dopant distribution using an effective laser dwell time, t, as calculated from Ref. 9, and the ordinary concentration- and stress-independent diffusivity, D. For shallow surface layers, the temperature, and therefore the diffusivity, varies only slowly with depth. This leads to the well-known complementary-error-function depth distribution. For four overlapping passes at the two scan speeds used in Figs. 4(a) and (b) the predicted diffusion lengths, $2\sqrt{Dt}$, are ~ 300 and 70 Å, respectively. As shown in Fig. 6, however, the observed profiles are broader and cannot be accounted for by the spot size and temperature uncertainties of the experiment. Note that the threshold melting is accompanied by pronounced etching and can be reasonably ruled out. In particular, the shape of the observed dopant profile is skewed towards depths exceeding several thousand angstroms, where the dopant concentration greatly exceeds the error-function extrapolations from the near-surface concentrations. Interestingly, these same depths also correspond to approximately an optical-absorption length, the region of the strongest vertical thermal gradient.

Several possible causes of accelerated diffusion have been considered. In addition to diffusion driven by a dopant concentration gradient, diffusion can be driven by thermal, stress, and electrical potential gradients [10]. To place these additional diffusion fluxes in perspective, the ordinary concentration-gradient-driven flux can be estimated from the data in Fig. 4(a) to be ~ $2 \cdot 10^{12}$ cm^{-2} s^{-1} at a depth of ~ 260 nm.

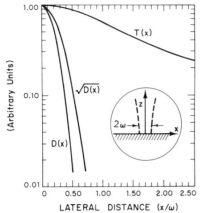

Fig. 5. Normalized lateral distribution for surface temperature T(x) and the corresponding spatial variation of the boron diffusion <u>coef</u>ficient D(x) and diffusion length ∝ [$\sqrt{D(x)}$], for the conditions of the experiment. Since the beam spot size 2ω is ~ 1-2 μm, submicrometer diffused linewidths are predicted.

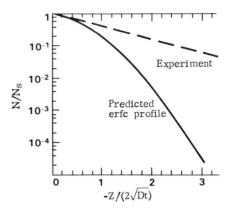

Fig. 6. Experimental (dashed line) and predicted (solid line) depth profiles normalized to surface concentration for the data of curve (a) in Fig. 5. The prediction is for the conventional concentration-gradient-driven diffusion flux without additional terms pertinent to small-geometry laser diffusions.

The best documented of the additional fluxes is due to electromigration, which arises because electrically activated dopant atoms are charged. Then, even in the absence of externally imposed electric fields, the space-charge field $\nabla\psi$ created by the dopant concentration gradient ∇N can drive diffusion [11]. This can be modeled as

$$J_{\nabla\psi} = \frac{-eN D \nabla\psi}{kT} = \frac{-D}{\sqrt{1+4n_i^2/N^2}} \nabla N , \qquad (1)$$

where n_i is the intrinsic carrier density at the temperature of the diffusion. Because this diffusion flux is more important at higher dopant concentrations, it has the effect of squaring up the dopant profile in the shallower, high-concentration surface layer, while leaving the dopant profile in the deeper, low-concentration layers unaffected. This is exactly opposite, however, to what we observe, viz., enhanced diffusion deeper in the solid.

A second possibility, thermomigration, arises because diffusion is a thermally activated process, and can be characterized [10] by a flux given by

$$J_{\nabla T} = -DN S_T \nabla T , \qquad (2)$$

where the Soret coefficient is $S_T = Q^*/RT^2$, and Q^* is the "heat of transport" for impurity motion. In fact, some evidence has already been presented that such diffusion can be important in determining the dopant profile in laser-<u>melted</u> Si [12]. In this case, where the laser heats but does not melt the lattice, a simple thermal model predicts that the maximum temperature gradient in the depth direction is on the order of 10^7 K/cm. For substitutional impurities in Si, the heat of transport is probably very similar to the ~ 3 eV activation energy for vacancy formation [13]. By using the parameters $D = 10^{-11}$ cm^2/s,

$N = 10^{18}$ cm^{-3}, and $T = 1300$ K, this Soret flux can be estimated to be $\sim 3.5 \times 10^{12}$ cm^{-2} s^{-1}. This is comparable to the ordinary concentration-gradient-driven flux, and shows that such normally small effects may be important in small-geometry laser-solid interactions. However, this flux is in the wrong direction to account for these observations, since substitutional impurities will tend to migrate toward regions that are hotter and hence have larger vacancy concentrations. This would tend to drive the impurity back towards the surface. For interstitial impurities in Si, as boron is believed to be under some conditions [14], the Soret flux is more difficult to estimate, though it is expected to also drive the impurities back towards the surface.

In addition to Soret diffusion, temperature gradients can lead to stress gradients $\nabla\sigma$, which in turn can interact with the excess volume V* associated with the impurity atoms and cause a net stress-gradient-driven diffusion flux [10]

$$J_{\nabla\sigma} = \frac{DN}{RT} V^* \nabla\sigma \quad . \tag{3}$$

A simple thermal-stress model, in which a small hot zone of Si expands thermally but is constrained by the surrounding colder lattice, gives as an upper bound estimate for the stress gradient $d\sigma/dr|_{max} \sim 10^{14}$ dyn/cm^3. If we estimate V* for substitutional B in Si to be approximately -30% of the volume of a lattice site, then the diffusion flux due to such a stress gradient is $J_{\nabla\sigma} \sim 10^{11}$ cm^{-2} s^{-1}. We note that this extra flux has the correct sign to be consistent with our observations, since B is smaller than Si, and would tend to migrate towards the interior regions of higher stress. However, it is probably too small to account for our observations. For interstitial B, the flux is more difficult to estimate; in any case, however, it has the wrong sign, since V* will be positive for interstitials.

We conclude that these additional fluxes alone cannot account for the substantial enhanced diffusion we observe, although in small geometries they may be comparable with the ordinary concentration-gradient-driven flux. It is very likely, therefore, that the diffusivity itself, which determines the magnitude of all of the diffusion fluxes, has been enhanced by the unusual conditions of the experiment. Such an enhancement could have several causes. First, previous studies have shown that substantial enhancements in diffusivity can occur by the injection of Si self-interstitials generated during surface oxidation [14,15]. Rapid thermal cycling with a scanned laser spot in a halide atmosphere may have similar effects, though such surface-generated defects would not be expected to enhance the diffusivity more away from than at, the surface. Second, mobile defects may be caused by the large thermal stresses ($\sim 10^{10}$ dyn/cm^2) that peak in the interior of the solid; such defects would be expected to enhance the diffusivity away from the surface, as observed. In particular, since such stresses are comparable to the yield stress of Si [16], it is not unlikely that these defects involve the generation and motion of dislocations [17].

CONCLUSION

In conclusion, we have described a technique for direct local doping of Si. The process has potential use as a simple, mask-free means to define surface relief with a resolution beyond that of optical lithography, and also as a means to fabricate shallow-diffused device structures. The localization achieved is consistent with the predicted thermal gradient in the beam focus. Recent experiments have indicated that lines as narrow as 1000 Å may be possible. Still better resolution may be possible with the use of a high brightness, moderate-energy electron beam [18]. In addition, new factors appear to contribute to accelerated absolute diffusion rates for a scanned beam relative to uniform heating conditions. These rates may be due to the large stresses which are developed under the sharp temperature gradients.

ACKNOWLEDGMENTS

We would like to thank J. Sedlacek and D. J. Sullivan for their important technical contributions, P. Nitishin for numerous scanning electron micrographs, and H. Zeiger, D. C. Shaver, and C. H. Tsao for helpful discussions.

REFERENCES

1. D. J. Ehrlich and J. Y. Tsao, Appl. Phys. Lett. 41, 297 (1982).

2. D. J. Ehrlich, R. M. Osgood, Jr. and T. F. Deutsch, Appl. Phys. Lett. 38, 1018 (1981).

3. G. L. Kuhn and C. J. Rhee, J. Electrochem. Soc. 120, 1563 (1973).

4. M. Asano, T. Cho and H. Muraoka, Electrochem. Soc. Extended Abstracts 76-2 911 (1976).

5. D. J. Ehrlich, R. M. Osgood, Jr. and T. F. Deutsch, Appl. Phys. Lett. 39, 957 (1981).

6. D. J. Ehrlich, R. M. Osgood,Jr. and T. F. Deutsch, Appl. Phys. Lett. 36, 916 (1980).

7. D. J. Ehrlich, R. M. Osgood, Jr. and T. F. Deutsch, Appl. Phys. Lett. 38, 399 (1980).

8. M. Lax, J. Appl. Phys. 48, 3919 (1977); and M. Lax, in Laser-Solid Interactions and Laser Processing, edited by S. D. Ferris, H. J. Leamy and J. M. Poate (Amer. Inst. of Phys., New York, 1979).

9. Y. I. Nissim, A. Lietoila, R. B. Gold and J. F. Gibbons, J. Appl. Phys. 51, 274 (1980).

10. P. G. Shewmon, Diffusion in Solids (McGraw Hill, New York, 1963); see also D. Shaw, Ed., Atomic Diffusion in Semiconductors (Plenum Press, London, 1973).

11. K. Lehovec and A. Slobodsky, Solid-State Electron. 3, 45 (1961).

12. L. F. Dona Dalle Rose and A. Miotella, in Laser and Electron-Beam Interactions with Solids, edited by B. R. Appleton and G. K. Celler (North-Holland, Amsterdam, 1982), pp. 425-430.

13. J. A. Van Vechten, Phys. Rev. B 10, 1482 (1974).

14. S. M. Hu, J. Appl. Phys. 45, 1567 (1974).

15. A. M. Lin, R. W. Dutton, and D. A. Antoniadis, Appl. Phys. Lett. 35, 799 (1979).

16. J. R. Patel and A. R. Chandhuri, J. Appl. Phys. 34, 2788 (1963).

17. J. E. Lawrence, Brit. J. Appl. Phys. <u>18</u>, 405 (1967).

18. A. A. Tranmanesh and R. F. W. Pease, paper presented at the Electrochem. Soc. Meeting, Montreal, Quebec, Canada (May 9-14, 1982).

CHARACTERISTICS OF LASER IMPLANTATION DOPING

K G IBBS AND M L LLOYD
The General Electric Company, p.l.c., Hirst Research Centre, Wembley, England, HA9 7PP

ABSTRACT

UV laser photochemical dissociation and laser enchanced thermal dissociation have been used to generate free metal dopant species from a variety of organometallic molecules near a semiconductor substrate surface. Simultaneous laser annealing via a localised melt phase allows diffusion driven implantation of the metal atoms and subsequent electrical activation in the regrowing material. High levels of dopant concentration and activation are readily achieved in this way.

Results will be presented on doping of silicon by boron using an ArF laser. These will include data on junction depths, number density and carrier density as a function of depth and interpretation of the data in terms of calculated temperature profiles.

The possibility of tailoring junction characteristics by control of laser and gas flow parameters will be considered with preliminary experimental data.

INTRODUCTION

The development of laser materials processing to semiconductor device technology now encompasses such diverse effects as direct thermal processing for annealing ion implant damage [1], enhancement of CVD reactions at the substrate surface (laser enhanced CVD - LCVD) [2,3], and laser photochemistry for the selective generation of materials from the vapour phase (laser photochemical deposition/doping - LPD) [4,5,6]. We have primarily been interested in single step laser doping of silicon by Boron, formed by photolysis and pyrolysis of Triethyl Boron (TEB), using a 193 mm ArF laser [7]. In single step doping the laser is used to simultaneously generate free dopant species, and to rapidly heat the substrate at the irradiated site to produce a localised melt zone in which the dopant may diffuse [8]. The substrate material then cools and regrows epitaxially from the surrounding single crystal phase, incorporating the dopant on electrically active sites with essentially 100% efficiency in analogy with pulsed laser annealing of ion implants.

Single step doping combines the advantages of the very short thermal cycling times found in pulsed laser annealing (~100 nS) with the localised in situ generation of dopant material to produce a processing facility that may be used for maskless writing of device structures [9]. Such IC laser fabrication places very stringent requirements on the dopant precursor materials and the source laser, as will be discussed.

EXPERIMENT

The experimental apparatus consists of a Lambda Physik EMG 101 rare gas halide laser with unstable resonator optics, giving a typical average output pulse energy of 50 mj with a reproducibility of ~10%. After spatial filtering the laser passes through an attenuator and GEC model TF energy meter modified for use in the UV. The output from the energy meter is focussed into a stainless steel vacuum cell containing the silicon substrate in an atmosphere of TEB at typically 0.01 to 1.0 torr pressure. The cell may be translated with respect to the beam using an Ealing microprocessor controlled X-Y stage. The substrate material used in all of the work presented here is (100) oriented high resistivity n type (~2.10^{15} p.cm^{-3}) silicon wafers.

RESULTS

A typical laser implanted junction is shown in Figure 1. In this case 10 laser pulses of average energy 17 mj were used to implant from an ambient TEB vapour pressure of 0.32 torr over an area of 0.5 x 3 mm, after which the sample was bevelled at an angle of 1° and stained with copper. The doped region is clearly visible as a white, unstained, trough of p type material beneath the oxide layer, showing that the depth of the junction varies from zero at the edges to a maximum of typically 0.4 μm in the centre, corresponding to variations in the peak energy density across the laser leading to variations in melt depth of the silicon. By control of attenuation and beam focus we have identified junctions with maximum depths of as little as 0.05 μm and as much as 0.8 μm before the onset of visible surface damage. Because of the shape of the energy profile of this particular laser, it is not possible to unambiguously assign a specific energy density to a particular implant depth. However, using the melting model program devised by Godfrey [10] with silicon parameters from Philipp [11] we have calculated that the energy threshold for melting occurs at some 0.45 J.cm^{-2}. With increasing energy the depth of melt increases until surface damage; but for typical junction depths of 0.4 μm the calculated local laser energy density must be ≈1.6 J.cm^{-2}, a value comparable to that used for long wavelength pulsed laser annealing - despite the vastly increased room temperature absorption coefficient of silicon at 193 nm.

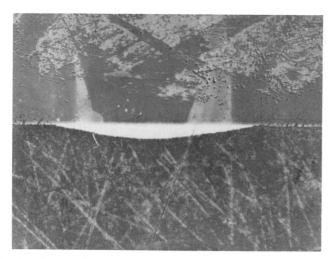

Figure 1 Bevel and stained junction showing the shape of the implant

In order to determine the electrical characteristics of the implanted material as a function of depth, a two point spreading resistance probe has been used to step down the bevelled surface in steps of 5 μ. A series of such results on three samples is shown in Figure 2, where the vapour pressure of TEB has been changed for each sample, and the spreading resistance data deconvoluted to give the concentration of activated dopant directly. The high surface concentration of dopant persists to some depth below the surface before falling rapidly to a level given by the residual spreading resistance of the starting material. This junction profile is consistent with the melting model of pulsed laser annealing where the dopant is evenly distributed throughout the melt zone due to rapid liquid phase diffusion, but falls very quickly at the melt/crystal interface where the diffusion rate is much reduced.

The effect of our inconsistent pulse energy is clearly shown up by two features of Figure 2. Firstly, although the three regions were implanted using nominally identical conditions, the melt depth is different in each case, being given by the maximum laser pulse energy occurring during the processing. Secondly, the fall off in dopant concentration of the melt/crystal interface is not as sharp as that obtained in annealing experiments where the laser pulse energy is typically more reproducible. A third feature of Figure 2 not clearly shown here, is that the spreading resistance values corresponding to the dopant profiles should produce a singularity at the junction itself where there is either complete compensation and therefore effectively infinite resistance or else one probe on either side of the junction where rectification should prevent a current flow across the junction, again producing infinite resistance. This is often not the case with laser implanted material, due to leakage effects. It is not yet clear what is causing the leakage, but an obvious possibility is a high defect concentration at the junction produced, perhaps, by a high concentration of impurities – as discussed later.

The three samples shown in Figure 2 demonstrate that the vapour pressure of TEB in the cell governs the context of doping as measured by the peak dopant concentration at the silicon surface. In Figure 3 these peak concentrations are plotted as a function of the TEB vapour pressure over the range 10^{-2} to 1 torr. For relatively high TEB pressures of 0.1 torr or more the peak dopant concentration in linearly related to the pressure, but below about 0.1 torr the concentration becomes progressively independent of pressure. This effect is due to surface adsorbed TEB; which would prohibit this precursor from being useful for low level doping, without the additional problems of high substrate temperatures or long pumping times to reduce the degree of adsorption. We have yet to determine whether other precursors will provide a more suitable supply of dopant over a greater range of pressures.

The selection of precursors will become a principal problem for those engaged in controlling single step laser doping for real devices, not only because of the surface adsorption characteristics, but also because of the dissociation products. The metal alkyls tend to be both thermally and photochemically unstable in forming free metal – a property that allows them to be used in both LCVD and LPD processing – so that in the case of UV laser implantation both thermal and photochemical dissociation mechanism will contribute to the formation of the dopant material. In order to isolate the two effects we have performed implantation of Boron of the two wavelengths indicated in Figure 4. The lower trace of Figure 4 corresponds to the surface spreading resistance across an implanted area using the ArF laser as already discussed. The lowest spreading resistance value produces a calculated number density of activated dopant of some 10^{20} cm^{-3} for a TEB vapour pressure of 1 torr. This compares well with the data in Figure 2. The upper trace of Figure 4 represents the spreading resistance across the surface of an implant formed by an XeF laser of wavelength 351 nm, where TEB has no measurable absorption. The junction formed by the XeF laser has an order of magnitude higher spreading resistance than that formed with ArF, indicating that the efficiency of Boron formation is enhanced by excitation with the shorter wavelength source. It is not, however, obvious from the data whether either of the two mechanisms is more suitable for producing device structures. A completely thermal process may have the advantage of producing only surface reactions that limit the diffusion of dissociation products from the irradiated reaction site.

In both photolytic and pyrolytic dissociation of the metal alkyls, there are inevitably hydrocarbons formed as dissociation products along with the desired metal dopant, which are also available to diffuse with the silicon melt zone. In Figure 5, we show an Auger electron analysis depth profile of a typical high laser energy Boron implant showing levels of Boron, Carbon and Oxygen. The high surface levels of carbon and oxygen are due to atmospheric contamination – but the carbon signal persists to a depth of 0.6 µm into the silicon substrate indicating that a high level of hydrocarbon has been implanted along with the Boron. It is possible that these hydrocarbons are responsible for the high defect formation that induces the leakage of the junction discussed earlier, effectively preventing the formation of device quality material by direct laser implantation from such metal alkyl precursors.

CONCLUSION

We have shown that single step pulsed laser implantation by photolysis and pyrolysis of metal alkyls can produce high activated levels of dopant in silicon over a wide range of dopant concentrations and junction depths. It is expected that careful control of dopant precursor vapour pressure/surface adsorption, and laser energy density will lead to the feasibility of forming multilayer p-n structures. There are however considerable problems arising from the use of metal alkyl precursors for single step implantation that will require the development of new precursors or a multistep doping procedure requiring separate dissociation and implantation/annealing steps.

REFERENCES

1. B. R. Appleton and G. K. Celler, (Eds) Laser and Electron Beam Interactions with Solids. Proc. Materials Research Society 4 November 1981. Elsevier Science Pub. Co. Inc. (1982)

2. S. D. Allen, J. App. Phys., 52(11), 6501, (1981)

3. P. K. Boyer, G. A. Roche, W. H. Ritchie and G. J. Collins, App. Phys. Lett., 40(8), 716, (1982)

4. J. Y. Tsao, D. J. Ehrlich, D. J. Silversmith and R. W. Mountain, IEEE Electron Device Letts., 3(6), 164, (1982)

5. W. E. Johnson and L. A. Schlie, App. Phys. Lett., 40(9), 798, (1982)

6. R. W. Andreatta, C. C. Abele, J. F. Osmundsen, J. G. Eden, D. Lubben and J. E. Greene, App. Phys. Lett., 40(2), 183, (1982)

7. K. G. Ibbs and M. L. Lloyd, Optics and Laser Technology – to be published February 1983

8. T. F. Deutsch, D. J. Ehrlich, D. D. Rathman, D. J. Silversmith and R. M. Osgood, App. Phys. Lett., 39(10), 825, (1981)

9. D. J. Ehrlich, R. M. Osgood and T. F. Deutsch, App. Phys. Lett., 36(11), 916, (1980)

10. D. J. Godfrey, A.C. Hill and C. Hill, J. Electrochem. Soc., 128(8), 1798, (1981)

11. H. R. Philipp and E. A. Taft, Phys. Rev. 120(1), 37, (1960).

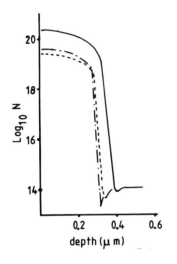

Figure 2 Two point probe spreading resistance plots of dopant concentration as a function of depth for TEB vapour pressures

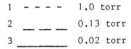

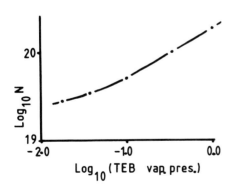

Figure 3 Maximum dopant concentration as a function of TEB vapour pressure

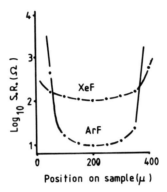

Figure 4 Surface spreading resistance across laser implants using ArF (193 nm) and XeF (351 nm) wavelengths

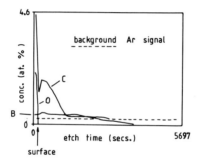

Figure 5 Auger electron depth profile showing the real surface and depth profiles of boron and carbon. The boron signal overlaps that from the argon etchant

Figures 4 and 5 reprinted from 'UV laser doping of silicon' by K G Ibbs and M L Lloyd in Optics and Laser Technology, vol 15 (February 1983), with permission from Butterworth Scientific Limited, Guildford, Surrey.

USING OPTICAL FIBERS IN LASER PROCESSING

L.D. LAUDE, L. BAUFAY and A. PIGEOLET
Université de l'Etat, Faculté des Sciences, 7000 Mons, Belgium.

ABSTRACT

Phase transformation occuring upon CW laser irradiating through optical fiber polymetallic, multilayered films deposited on insulating substrates is shown to provide a simple and versatile way to optically micro-print pre-determined patterns. The technique allows both further reduction to the Rayleigh limit and simultaneous multiplication of the patterns.

INTRODUCTION

Several attempts have been made in the past few years to "optically" print an encoded information in an irreversible and permanent manner. Such attempts were part of an overall effort towards developing mass memories of considerable capacity. In such instances, two requirements are of complementary importance : i) the physical process on which the "printing" is based has to be sufficiently rugged as to accomodate a rather large range of technical uncertainties in its application; and ii) such a process should be versatile to allow miniaturization and duplication. To some point, these requirements oppose each other and the success (or the limits) of the technique is essentially controlled by some compromise to be found between versatility and simplicity.

The object of this paper is to describe some of the aspects of a new technique which has been tested to provide a rather easy way to inscribe permanently digitized signals in a metallic film deposited on an insulating substrate, for instance glass. This technique utilizes the phase transformation produced by a laser beam of a given profile impinging the surface of a multi-layered metallic film formed by a stack of individual layers, each being made of atoms alternatively belonging to the IIIrd (or IInd) and Vth (or VIth) columns of the periodic table in stochiometric amounts [1,2] . It has been shown [3] that, under certain conditions (energy density in the beam, power delivered to the film, etc.), the III-V (or II-VI) semiconducting compound is formed upon lasing the layered structure. This changes abruptly all physical properties of the material, in particular optical absorption. Whilst parts of the film which are not irradiated remain opaque to visible and IR light, irradiated regions become transparent down to a wavelength corresponding to the band gap energy of the compound. This laser-induced effect is shown here to be finely confined when the laser beam travels through the core of a single-mode optical fiber before reaching the film. Scanning this beam onto the film provides a simple way to optically "write" in the film any coded signal. Various parameters entering the process are discussed. Its advantages and limits are further outlined in view of possible large scale applications in the optical printing technology.

EXPERIMENTAL

Details of the layered film preparation have been presented elsewhere [1] , as well as the conditions under which the compound formation is obtained as a function of laser parameters [3] . Attention is focussed on the optical components of the technique and on the scanning procedure which have been experimented in this work. Extrapolation of the described setting to any other alternative (different laser source, optical fiber, scanning, or else metallic films) will appear to be obvious to the reader. In this work, such layered films are deposited on glass and, therefore, dissipation of the laser energy through the film/substrate interface has to be taken into account when defining the energy balance of the system. Under such conditions, it has been shown that phase transformation occurs at and above a critical power level P_c at the laser source which depends on the material being treated. In this work, a Nd-YAG laser is used which provides for 2.5 W in CW regime, all lines, distributed over a beam diameter of 3 mm^2, at a wavelength of 1064 nm. Additional concentration via a lens is therefore required before entering the fiber. The experimental step-index fiber has a Ge doped silica core of 8μ diameter, and a silica cladding of 125μ diameter. Numerical aperture of the fiber is 0.1 which provides for single mode operation at λ = 1064 nm. For this particular application however, there is no restriction to a multi-mode operation (at $\lambda < 1000$ nm). Attenuation along the fiber core is 0.9 dB/km, equivalent to some 19% loss per km. Actual experiments were carried out, for instance, with a fiber length of 300 m (i.e. a few % loss between entrance and exit). In order to maintain a stable laser output, adjusting the power delivered to the film via the fiber is performed not by tuning the laser source itself but by manualy displacing the fiber entrance along the lens axis, in the **vicinity** of its focus (see Fig. 1) and further, by controlling the fiber output with a powermeter, prior irradiating the film. In this configuration, the concentrated laser beam enters core and cladding. Given the diameter of the core, one could consider the portion of the beam entering the core to have a nearly constant profile.

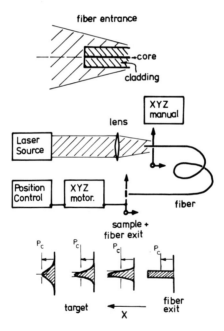

Fig. 1 Schematic of the experimental set-up used in this work. At the bottom is shown the actual progressive spread of the beam between the fiber exit and the target film.

A radial energy gradient would be effective in the cladding only, but such part of the beam entering the cladding does not propagate within the latter over more than ~20 cm. The actual light source at the fiber exit has therefore a nominal diameter equal to the core diameter, or 8µ with this fiber, and power density adjusted at values exceeding 5 mW cm^{-2}. Between fiber exit and target, the beam tends to disperse in air. This dispersion is defined by the numerical aperture (NA) of the fiber. With NA =0.1, dispersion would be around 10µ at a distance x = 100µ from fiber exit. Although such dispersion is not linear, the beam spread enlarges the irradiated area of the film when increasing x. However, since the synthesis of the compound in the film requires a given level of power density (Fig. 1), it is clear that the actual area over which the power density would be larger than P_c shrinks below 8µ diameter at increasing distances x from fiber exit, down to nothing at distances where the maximum power level in the spread off beam drops below P_c, obliterating any phase transformation. Therefore, the lower the power density at the fiber exit, the shorter the distance x between film and fiber would be.

An additional effect is to be considered here. The core exit plays the role of a diaphragm on the laser beam. Diffusion of the coherent light through this diaphragm produces the known speckle effect or granulation of the beam which disturbs its gaussian profile. The average cross-dimension of a speckle spot of light is given by $\Delta = \frac{\lambda}{tg\theta} = \frac{\lambda x}{D}$ where θ is the angle under which the core diameter D is seen from any site of the irradiated film at x. Given the actual values of λ and D, the gaussian profile of the laser beam (Fig. 1) is not affected by speckling for $x \geq 60µ$. This argument opposes the previous one about the spread of the gaussian profile with x. A simple way to find a compromise is to increase the power density delivered to the sample well above P_c (for instance, 3 or 4 times P_c). Note that speckling would eventually produce a distribution of large crystallites (~10µ) which develop laterally to the beam path, thus affecting the homogeneity of the transformed path.

The distance x being set at $x \simeq 100µ$, the film is now displaced in the YZ plan, perpendicularly to the fiber axis, using two step-motors (in the Y and Z directions, respectively) which are controled via a mini-computer. A given path is programmed which activates the automatic displacement of the film in front of the fiber exit. In present tests, the scanning procedure ran at a constant speed of 200µ sec^{-1}, with 0.1µ step, i.e. actual irradiation progressed spot by spot, every tenth of a micron at 0.5 msec intervals. At such a low speed, the edge definition of the transformed path is well below 1µ, which assimilates this scanning to a semi-continuous process. At much higher speeds, the path edge deteriorates. Another application of the technique is most evident. By interrupting (electromechanically, for instance) the beam at the fiber entrance and, simultaneously, displacing the film as above, it is possible to interrupt the printed path. This interruption can be repeated systematically. Depending on the characteristics of the shutter in front of the fiber and of the scanning program of the film, coded signals can be deposited in the film. This occuring via an irreversible transformation of matter which is further miniaturized by using fibers of low core diameter, a number of spots and dashes can be alined on the target film, over several lines the width of which is essentially controlled by the core diameter of the fiber.

In addition, instead of one single fiber, a single mode fiber array can be picked in the focussed laser beam to provide for a number of individual intense light sources equal to the number of fibers in the array. This provides the easy multiplication of the desired path a) on an equivalently large number of films mounted at once on the same Y-Z table, or b) on one single large film on which all fibers are pointing in an array.

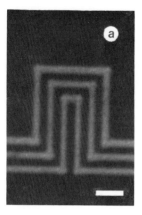 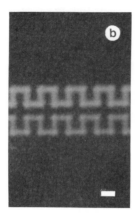 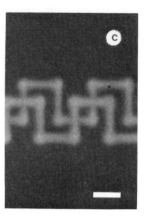

Fig. 2 Various paths which have been "printed" in Cd-Te metallic films. The light paths consist of the semiconducting CdTe compound, whilst the rest of the film, being non-irradiated, remains metallic. The bars are 40µ long.

EXAMPLES

The above described technique is exemplified here in its semi-continuous version. In Fig. 2, several printed patterns are shown in transmission photographs obtained through a microscope. They were obtained by scanning a Cd-Tc film in front of a 8µ core diameter single mode fiber delivering a nominal power of 10 mW. The film was positioned at ~100µ from fiber exit, in a YZ plan perpendicular to the fiber exit axis. In Fig. 2a, the three paths were monitored to give, successively : 100 x 100µ , 100 x 60µ and 100 x 20µ imbricated loopholes. The lighter traces consist of the compound CdTe, the darker parts remaining metallic, i.e. opaque to white light. The CdTe path itself is 8 to 10µ wide and the distance between adjacent paths is 10µ . In Fig. 2b, loop-hole paths are traced at 40µ distance from each other; the darker center part is metallic, the lighter being again semiconducting. In Fig. 2c, the two traces of Fig. 2b have been displaced to overlap. Quite noticeable, is the fact that upon such a scanning, metallic dots (~10µ diameter) can be isolated in a semiconducting environment. Given the 0.1µ resolution of the step-motor translations, it is obvious that such printed paths can be further reduced by using core diameters much smaller than the ones used here to demonstrate the ability of the fiber-guided technique, ultimate reduction being solely confined to the Rayleigh limit.

CONCLUSIONS

In this paper, phase transformation occuring upon CW laser irradiating through optical fibers polymetallic, multilayered films deposited onto insulating substrate is shown to provide an easy and versatile mean to optically and permanently inscribe any desired pattern. The technique extends the printing resolution to the core diameter of single mode fibers. It allows further reproduction of the signal by using fiber arrays. Extrapolation of this process to encoding minute and digitized signals into films is outlined.

ACKNOWLEDGMENTS

The authors thank R. Helvenstein, M. Lamquin and M. Morand for access to their equipment and useful discussions. This work has been performed under ProjectIRIS and the Energy Program of the Belgian Ministry for Science Policy, Brussels.

REFERENCES

1. R. Andrew, M. Ledezma, M. Lovato, M. Wautelet and L.D. Laude, Appl. Phys. Letters 35, 418 (1979).

2. L. Baufay, D. Dispa, A. Pigeolet and L.D. Laude, J. of Crystal Growth, 59, 143 (1982).

3. R. Andrew, L. Baufay, A. Pigeolet and L.D. Laude, J. Appl. Phys., 53, 4862, (1982).

SECTION VIII
NOVEL PROCESSES

LASER-PULSED PLASMA CHEMISTRY: SURFACE OXIDATION OF NIOBIUM

R.F. Marks, R.A. Pollak, and Ph. Avouris
IBM T.J. Watson Research Center, Yorktown Heights, NY 10598

Laser irradiation of a solid surface under an oxidizing ambient gas can activate localized, heterogeneous chemical reactions which modify the surface. Under suitable conditions, the laser initiates a reactive plasma near the gas/solid interface. This plasma mechanism is proposed as the basis for a new surface chemical technique which we denote laser-pulsed plasma chemistry (LPPC). LPPC experiments on niobium metal under one atmosphere of oxygen employed a pulsed CO_2 laser and displayed single-pulse, self-limiting, oxide growth. Product oxide thickness increased with optical intensity. Surface layer thickness and chemical composition were determined for oxide layers between 1 nm and 5 nm thick using x-ray photoelectron spectroscopy (XPS or ESCA). Composition of these niobium oxide ($Nb_2O_{5-\delta}$) surfaces was similar to the composition produced by RF plasma oxidation, but the valence defect, δ, for LPPC oxides was approximately two to five times lower. At high laser intensity ($\gtrsim 4 \times 10^6$ W/cm^2), direct optical heating or plasma-mediated thermal coupling to the solid activates interdiffusion at the oxide/metal interface.

I. Introduction

As part of a program to study the physics and chemistry of very thin surface layers on solids we wish to understand in detail processes which lead to surface film growth. Surface layers of less than 10 nm thick have important applications in microelectronics including fabrication of Josephson junctions and field effect devices. Initial efforts focused upon optically-driven surface oxidation employing pulsed infra-red radiation from a CO_2 laser incident on niobium surfaces in a pure oxygen ambient. Results point to a mechanism of heterogeneous chemistry in which a localized plasma is generated by the laser near a metal surface where the plasma provides excited reactants which combine with metal atoms to form overlayers 1-5 nm thick, depending upon laser intensity. This process which we denote laser-pulsed plasma chemistry[1] (LPPC) may prove valuable as a new technique for chemical modification of surfaces under highly controlled conditions. LPPC observations will be contrasted and interpreted with respect to experiments[2] which employed near ultra-violet pulses from a XeCl excimer laser to stimulate laser-pulsed thermal chemistry (LPTC). Composition and structure of the surface layers resulting from these distinct processes can be characterized by x-ray photoelectron spectroscopy (XPS or ESCA). Figure 1 depicts LPPC and LPTC schematically along with XPS spectra of samples before laser exposure (room temperature thermal oxidation only) and following IR and UV irradiation under one atmosphere of oxygen. Note the formation of intermediate oxidation states of Nb following UV exposure. This is characteristic of high temperature oxidation and consequent interdiffusion at the oxide/metal interface.

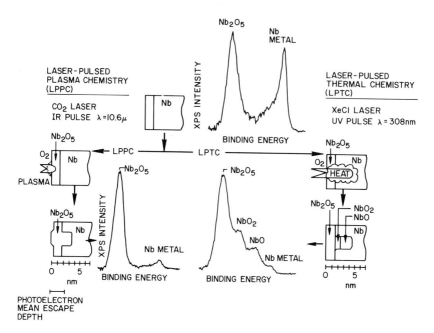

Fig.1: Comparison of LPPC and LPTC oxidation processes. Schematic representation of LPPC shows an infra-red laser pulse which produces a reactive plasma near the surface resulting in well defined oxide stoichiometry and a sharp oxide/metal interface. By contrast, LPTC employs UV laser heating and results in graded product composition represented by three oxide layers of different stoichiometry. Initial and product XPS spectra illustrate these processes. To simplify interpretation, the spectra show only the Nb $3d_{5/2}$ spin components for each chemical species.

Technologically important materials including Si, Al and Nb react in air at room temperature to form thin surface oxide layers. This oxidation proceeds only to a limited depth due to an activation barrier for diffusion which can be overcome by thermal excitation or, in the case of mobile ionic reactants, by supplying an electrical potential to bias the metal/oxide and solid/adsorbate interfaces. The latter method effectively supplements the Mott potential[3] which is equal to the difference between the electron affinity level of the adsorbate and Fermi level of the solid. Plasma oxidation[4] is a low temperature process which has been employed for some time in Josephson junction fabrication.[5] We shall see that oxides produced by laser-pulsed plasma chemistry have composition similar to films produced by plasma oxidation;[6] moreover, analysis by XPS indicates that LPPC oxides of niobium, $Nb_2O_{5-\delta}$, are more fully oxidized (smaller valence defect δ) than those formed by plasma oxidation.

Laser-ignited plasmas in air[7] occur above a threshold irradiance of $\sim 10^9$ W/cm^2 which is reduced to $\sim 10^6$ W/cm^2 when the laser is incident upon a metal surface. The interaction of the leading edge of the laser pulse with the surface frees electrons from the solid which accelerate by absorbing photons during collisions with ions and neutrals in the gas ambient (inverse bremsstrahlung). The accelerated electrons multiply by impact ionization of the gas, creating a plasma which absorbs much of the incoming radiation and largely shields the surface from the incident photon flux (see Fig. 1). Although these processes have been well studied,[7-9] the chemical effects of the plasma on the surface have not. To date, heterogeneous laser photochemistry of Cr,[10,11] Si[12] and GaAs[13] surfaces has been described as thermally-activated reaction, i.e., as LPTC.

In the present work, we have observed dramatically different composition depth profiles for LPPC and LPTC oxides of niobium. Whereas LPTC produces diffuse oxide/metal interfaces, it may be useful for creating films up to 200 nm thick[14] by repeated laser irradiation. Laser-pulsed plasma chemistry produces niobium oxide films less than 5 nm thick but with sharp oxide/metal interfaces in a process which is single-pulse self-limiting. Both techniques may offer advantages inherent in laser-induced chemistry including highly localized surface modification and capability to activate heterogeneous reaction from outside a sealed, well controlled chemical environment.

II. Experiment

Niobium foil samples (MRC Marz grade) 0.13 mm thick were cut to 10 mm x 7 mm and spotwelded to 0.51 mm diameter Ta wire supports. This sample assembly was washed in 11M HNO_3, distilled water and ethanol. Dried samples were installed in a bakeable UHV ($\leq 10^{-8}$Pa) preparation chamber and further cleaned by electron beam heating to 2000 C prior to oxygen and laser exposure. A bellows mechanism permitted samples to be transferred directly into the HP 5950A ESCA spectrometer. Measured sample area could be limited to 1 mm x 1 mm by reducing the photoelectron detector window to 10%.

The CO_2 laser (Tachisto Tach II) was operated with a totally reflective rear mirror at 10.6 μ, $\leq$ 1 Hz. A Lumonics 20D175 pyroelectric detector was used to measure laser pulse energy. The CO_2 laser was visually targeted on the samples using a collinear beam from a HeNe laser. The beam was focused by a 500 mm focal length biconvex BaF_2 lens through a NaCl window into the preparation chamber and onto the target at normal incidence. Irradiance at the sample was varied by translating the lens along the optical axis or by adjustment of CO_2 laser discharge voltage and the use of a silicon attenuator. The illuminated sample area was estimated from laser "burn" patterns on a Nb thin film sample exposed in air. All irradiances and fluence values have been corrected for aperture and reflective losses in the optical system and refer to energy incident at the sample; reported irradiances are average values over the 200 nsec (FWHM) pulse duration.[15] Visible laser-induced luminescence was observed at 60° to target normal through an IR absorbing filter.

III. Data Analysis

The interpretation of XPS spectra of oxidized niobium is somewhat complex since niobium oxides occur in a range of composition between Nb_2O_5 and Nb metal.[16] Niobium 3d core level chemical shifts permit quantitative study of the metal oxidation states, thus providing some information on the oxygen concentration depth profile in the oxide and at the oxide/metal interface. The range of Nb $3d_{5/2}$ chemical shifts is 5.2 eV which is comparable to the 2.73 eV $3d_{5/2}$ to $3d_{3/2}$ spin-orbit splitting. Using this fixed spin-orbit interval and the statistical 3:2 intensity ratio for $3d_{5/2}:3d_{3/2}$ spectral features, redundant information can be eliminated and analysis of data simplified by processing each spectrum to show only features corresponding to the 5/2 spin-orbit component.[6] Characteristically for 1 to 5 nm thick oxides, a large peak corresponding to Nb^{+5} in Nb_2O_5 is observed at 207.5 eV binding energy and a smaller peak from the underlying metal at 202.3 eV (see initial thermal and LPPC oxide spectra in Fig.1). Relatively weak emission between these two peaks originates from Nb atoms with intermediate oxidation states between +5 and 0. To facilitate the discussion and interpretation of the data, we decompose the Nb $3d_{5/2}$ photoelectron band into four distinct bands which we label $Nb^°$, Nb^{+2}, Nb^{+4}, and Nb^{+5}, and associate them with spectral areas centered around 202.3, 204, 206, and 207.5 eV, respectively. These are shown most strikingly in the LPTC oxide spectrum of Fig.1. To obtain quantitative results from XPS spectral areas, we employ a photoelectron attenuation model[1] which treats the LPPC oxide as three layers: Nb metal/"NbO"interface/$Nb_2O_{5-\delta}$ oxide. Nb atoms at the metal/oxide interface that are coordinated from below by metal and from above by oxide are denoted by "NbO".

Three possible sources of the Nb^{+4} signal are: (1) incompletely oxidized Nb atoms within the Nb_2O_5 oxide layer which signal the existence of inhomogeneously mixed valence ($\delta > 0$), (2) surface atoms which have shifted core level binding energies, or (3) Nb atoms above the metal/oxide interface but within the chemical potential gradient between $Nb^°$ and Nb^{+5}. For LPPC oxides, we attribute the Nb^{+4} signal mostly to (1). This assignment is consistent with the nature of $Nb_2O_{5-\delta}$ compounds which have a special degree of structural freedom resulting from the possibility of forming crystallographic shear planes[17] and thus accommodate a wide range of niobium/oxygen stoichiometry.

IV. Results and Discussion

An initial objective in this study was to characterize conditions for laser-activated oxide growth and oxide thinning. Oxide thinning was determined to occur above ~0.9 J cm^{-2} per pulse. CO_2 laser-activated thinning experiments were carried out under UHV conditions and were accompanied by a pressure rise of $\gtrsim$ 50% during the first laser pulse and by visible laser-induced luminescence which was spectrally resolved and detected using an optical multichannel analyser (PAR OMA II). Analysis showed banded emission, predominantly from electronically excited NbO, which is similar to that observed in experiments employing an ArF excimer laser.[14]

All laser-activated oxidation experiments were carried out below the 0.9 J cm^{-2} per pulse threshold for oxide thinning. Experiments to determine the dependence of laser-initiated plasma oxidation upon ambient pressure showed no evidence of surface modification in the range 10^{-6} to 10^{-1}Pa (10^{-8} to 10^{-3} torr). For effective CO_2 laser-pulsed plasma chemistry, the present study has employed oxygen pressure of approximately one atmosphere.

Results from eight niobium oxide LPPC films are tabulated in Table I. XPS integrated intensities are normalized to $I(Nb^{+5}) = 100$. The first two entries are from 1.6 nm thick native oxides before laser irradiation. The following six entries are from 1.8 to 4 nm thick LPPC oxides each formed by a single pulse. The dependence of oxide layer thickness upon laser fluence in single-pulse experiments is summarized in Figure 2. Squares represent $Nb_2O_{5-\delta}$ and triangles "NbO" layer thicknesses. The diameter of the area oxidized was ~1 mm compared with the 2.4 mm laser beam 1/e diameter. The striking increase in nominal Nb^{+2} thickness for fluences above 0.6 J cm^{-2} per pulse is indicative of some diffusion at the oxide/metal interface, possibly due to optical heating of Nb_2O_5 [18,19] or to plasma-mediated thermal coupling[7] whereby heat from the adjacent plasma is transferred to the solid. The formation of interface suboxides is characteristic of interface heating and is also observed after UV laser oxidation by LPTC.[1]

TABLE I

SINGLE PULSE CO_2 LASER-ACTIVATED OXIDATION

Fluence J/cm^2	$I(Nb^\circ)$	$I(Nb^{+2})$	$I(Nb^{+4})$	t_2 (nm)	t_{4+5} (nm)	δ	volume number	spectrum number
--	69.6	16.1	15.6	0.2	1.6	0.135	103	4
--	64.0	20.4	13.5	0.3	1.6	0.119	103	13
0.24	51.7	19.0	12.9	0.4	1.8	0.114	103	5
0.47	34.6	13.0	7.3	0.4	2.1	0.068	103	8
0.49	24.1	9.9	4.6	0.4	2.5	0.044	103	2
0.75	5.9	9.9	3.8	1.1	3.4	0.037	101	97
0.77	2.2	6.3	2.4	1.5	4.2	0.023	103	1
0.79	1.8	7.8	2.3	1.8	4.0	0.022	103	11

Notes: (a) $I(Nb^\circ)$, $I(Nb^{+2})$ and $I(Nb^{+4})$ normalized to $I(Nb^{+5}) = 100$.

(b) $\delta = \dfrac{I(Nb^{+4})}{I(Nb^{+4}) + I(Nb^{+5})}$

(c) t_2 is thickness of "NbO" interface layer.

(d) t_{4+5} is thickness of $Nb_2O_{5-\delta}$ oxide.

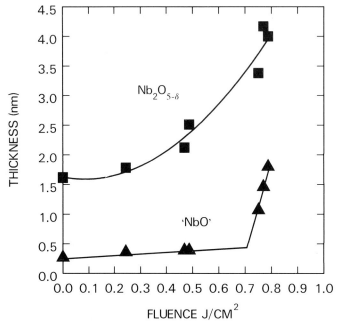

Fig.2: Niobium oxide thickness as a function of single CO_2 laser pulse fluence. The upper trace denotes the $Nb_2O_{5-\delta}$ surface layer. The fluence dependence of the NbO interface layer thickness (lower trace) indicates sharply increasing oxide/metal interdiffusion above 0.7 J cm^{-2}.

We have noted that single-pulse laser-activated oxidation produces thicker films than multiple-pulse experiments employing up to 700 pulses at comparable irradiance, and believe that this results from opposing effects due to two distinct physical processes occurring at ~10^6 W/cm^2: LPPC oxidation versus surface oxide heating. In multiple pulse experiments, the thicker $Nb_2O_{5-\delta}$ film resulting from the first pulse may impede subsequent plasma initiation by reducing electron tunneling from the metal to the gas/solid interface while increasing surface heating and evaporation of the oxide film due to increased absorption of the CO_2 laser radiation by the oxide.

The valence defect δ in $Nb_2O_{5-\delta}$ is a measure of incomplete oxidation. We define $\delta = I(Nb^{+4})/[I(Nb^{+4})+I(Nb^{+5})]$ where the I's are the spectral peak areas described above. δ can be thought of as the fraction of Nb atoms which are incompletely oxidized, i.e., in the Nb^{+4} oxidation state. The valence defect decreases monotonically with oxide thickness (Table I) as it did for a series of RF plasma oxides.[6] However, δ for a given LPPC oxide thickness is three to five times smaller than δ for the corresponding RF plasma oxide.

263

The observed non-zero values of δ in thin $Nb_2O_{5-\delta}$ films may help to explain the tunnel barrier characteristics of these films. Incomplete oxidation of niobium creates Nb^{+4} sites which have valence electron density that does not participate in Nb-O bonds. This non-bonding electron density may lead to impurity bands and/or localized states which can effect the magnitudes of Josephson and excess currents in tunnel junctions. If so, it would be desirable to determine oxidation conditions which kinetically and thermodynamically favor low δ oxide formation in the thickness range required for tunnel junctions.

The oxidation-state distribution observed by XPS after CO_2 laser-activated oxidation is in sharp contrast with experiments[1,2] employing a XeCl excimer laser (λ = 308 nm, pulse FWHM = 32 ns) to initiate oxidation. The XeCl laser promotes formation of niobium suboxides (Nb^{+2} and Nb^{+4}) far more than does the CO_2 laser (see Fig. 1). Similar results were obtained for XeCl fluence up to 0.71 J cm^{-2} per pulse. We believe that this may reflect the higher, and thus unattained, plasma-initiation threshold at 308 nm[7] as well as the optical absorption characteristics of the surface layers. Whereas Nb metal is almost totally reflective at 10.6 μ,[20] at 308 nm absorptivity is $\geq$ 0.55. Absorption by Nb_2O_5 surface films up to 5 nm thick would be $\lesssim$ 8% at 308 nm.[21,22] It is likely that the primary coupling mechanism between the XeCl laser and the solid is absorption by the metal thus resulting in heating of the oxide/metal interface to 1000 to 1500 C over the fluence range studied to date. Hence, it is not surprising that exposure of thin native oxides of niobium to 308 nm radiation induces significant interdiffusion at this interface.

The oxide thickness resulting from LPPC is very small, ranging from 1.8 to 4.0 nm for fluences between 0.24 and 0.79 J cm^{-2} per pulse, respectively. Under most circumstances, such thin surface films might be considered insignificant or be too thin to detect and thus be ignored. However, this range of thickness control is essential for fabrication of tunnel barriers in tunneling devices. Hence, LPPC may offer a versatile method of achieving well-defined, very thin dielectrics which are difficult to produce by conventional chemical means. Thicker oxides may possibly be produced by LPPC if, by analogy to plasma anodization,[23] a bias is applied to the sample during laser exposure.

V. Conclusions

A pulsed CO_2 laser has been employed to activate heterogeneous chemistry (oxidation) at a metal surface. The laser-induced plasma results in single-pulse self-limiting oxidation which can be quantitatively controlled by varying the fluence of the incident laser pulse to yield product oxide films from 1.6 to 4.5 nm thick. Laser-pulsed plasma chemistry initiated by a CO_2 laser is distinguished from laser-pulsed thermal chemistry resulting from irradiation by a XeCl UV excimer laser which generates oxide composition characteristic of a high temperature process. Very thin niobium oxides prepared by thermal, RF plasma, and LPPC oxidation are all found to be incompletely oxidized. However, XPS studies show that the LPPC oxides have the smallest valence defect δ. We propose that incomplete Nb oxidation (high δ) may contribute to observed nonideal tunneling behavior of conventionally prepared $Nb/Nb_2O_5/Nb$ Josephson junctions. The CO_2 laser has also been employed to generate atomically-clean niobium metal surfaces under ultra-high vacuum.

Pulsed laser-activation promises versatile techniques for heterogeneous chemistry. Special features of LPPC include: (a) a localized reaction zone defined by the size of the laser beam, (b) product layer thickness control by controlling the laser irradiance and (c) stoichiometry control.

References

[1] R.F. Marks, R.A. Pollak, Ph. Avouris, C.T. Lin, and Y.J. Théfaine, to be published in J. Chem. Phys.

[2] R.F. Marks, R.A. Pollak, unpublished

[3] F.P. Fehlner, N.F. Mott, Oxidation **1**, 59 (1970).

[4] J.L. Miles, P.H. Smith, J. Electrochem. Soc. **110**, 1240 (1963)

[5] A.T. Fromhold, Jr., J.M. Baker, J. Appl. Phys. **51**, 6377 (1980).

[6] R.A. Pollak, H.J. Stoltz, S.I. Raider, and R.F. Marks, unpublished.

[7] J.A. McKay, J.T. Schriempf, IEEE J. of Quant. Electronics QE-17, **10**, 2008 (1981), and refs. therein.

[8] D.C. Smith, J. Appl. Phys. **48**, 2217 (1977).

[9] G. Weyl, A. Pirri, R. Root, AIAA J., **19**, 460 (1981)

[10] S.M. Metev, S.K. Savtchenko, K.V. Stamenov, J. Phys. D: Appl. Phys. **13**, L75 (1980).

[11] S.M. Metev, S.K. Savtchenko, K.V. Stamenov, V.P. Veiko, G.A. Kotov, G.D. Shandibina, IEEE J. Quantum Electronics QE-17, 2004 (1981).

[12] Yung S. Liu, S.W. Chiang, F. Bacon, Appl. Phys. Lett. **38**, 1005 (1981).

[13] M. Matsuura, M. Ishida, A. Suzuki, K. Hara, Japanese J. of Appl. Phys. **20**, L726 (1981).

[14] C.T. Lin, Ph. Avouris, Y.J. Théfaine, R.F. Marks, R.A. Pollak, unpublished.

[15] Ph. Avouris, I.Y. Chan, M.M.T. Loy, J. Chem. Phys. **70**, 5315 (1979).

[16] D. Simon, C. Perrin, P. Baillif, C.R. Acad. Sci. Paris **C241**, 283 (1976).

[17] A.D. Wadsley, Sten Andersson, in Perspectives in Structural Chemistry, Vol. 3, eds. J.D. Dunitz, J.D. Dunitz, J.A. Ibers, J. Wiley and Sons, 1970, p. 1.

[18] S.I. Alyamovskii, G.P. Shveikin, P.V. Gel'd, Russian J. of Inorg. Chem. **12**, 915 (1967).

[19] F.P. Emmenegger, M.L. A. Robinson, J. Phys. Chem. Solids **29**, 1673 (1968).

[20] J.H. Weaver, D.W. Lynch, C.G. Olson, Phys. Rev B**7**, 4311 (1973).

[21] W.M. Graven, R.E. Salomon, G.B. Adams, J. Chem. Phys. **33**, 954 (1960)

[22] W.M. Graven, J. Chem. Phys. **35**, 1526 (1961)

[23] J.F. O'Hanlon, J. Vac. Sci. and Tech. **7**, 330 (1969).

PHOTOELECTROCHEMICAL DEPOSITION OF METAL PATTERNS ON SEMICONDUCTORS

TIMOTHY L. ROSE, RONALD H. MICHEELS, DAVID H. LONGENDORFER AND R. DAVID RAUH
EIC Laboratories, Inc., 111 Chapel Street, Newton, MA 02158, USA

ABSTRACT

Microscopic metal patterns may be produced on p-type semiconductors using a maskless photoelectrochemical procedure in which electroplating is induced by minority carriers in illuminated portions of a semiconductor electrode. Resolution exceeding 10µ has been achieved for deposits of Au on p-GaAs and Cu on p-Si. "Electroless" imaging and negative photoelectrochemical imaging are also discussed.

INTRODUCTION

Photoelectrochemical imaging is a versatile technique for pattern generation on semiconductor surfaces [1,2]. Images are formed in a one-step process, in which a light pattern projected onto the surface of a semiconductor electrode becomes replicated on the surface as an electrochemical product. This product can be an insulating oxide, a polymer "resist", soluble ions from the semiconductor itself (etching), a colored "photoelectrochromic" compound, or a metal. Photoelectrodeposition of metals onto Si and GaAs is discussed in this article, as it represents an area of current interest [3,4]. Its potential applications include single step production of both ohmic and rectifying metal-semiconductor contact patterns, and arrays for fabrication of solar cells, imagers, and other electronic devices.

For the direct, maskless, photoelectrochemical deposition of spatially resolved metal patterns, a p-type semiconductor substrate is required. The semiconductor is used as one electrode in an electrochemical cell. As shown in Figure 1, the semiconductor is irradiated through a front window of high optical quality. The cell also contains a counter electrode, which undergoes an oxidation reaction to balance the cell current (for some applications dissolution of the same metal being plated), and a reference electrode, such as standard calomel (SCE), to monitor or control the potential of the semiconductor. The electrolytes employed are commercial or conventional plating baths which are attainable for many metals - Cu, Ag, Au, Pd, Ni, Zn, etc.

A rectifying junction is formed at the semiconductor-electrolyte interface when the semiconductor is back-biased by an external power supply through an ohmic contact. For a p-type semiconductor, biasing to negative potentials increases the downward bending of conduction and valence bands. Electrons and holes produced by irradiating the junction with light of energy greater than the band gap will be separated by the space charge field. Minority carriers - conduction band electrons in this case - are drawn to the surface, while majority carriers are swept into the bulk and out through the circuit to the counter electrode. If the electrons at the semiconductor surface are energetic enough, they can react with reducible species in solution. In plating baths, the species are metal ions which are reduced to produce the desired metal deposits. Because minority carriers are generated only in irradiated areas of the electrode, complex metal replicas of projected images may be formed. Since this deposition is fundamentally a quantum process, efficiency can approach one atom-equivalent of metal deposited per photon absorbed. The deposition requires only low light fluxes and mild conditions, ideal for chemically sensitive surfaces.

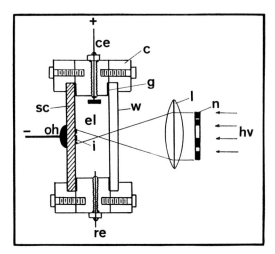

Fig. 1. Cell for photoelectrochemical deposition. Key: SC, semiconductor; W, window; ℓ, focusing lens; n, negative transparency; oh, ohmic contact; ce, counter electrode; re, reference electrode; el, electrolyte; c, cell body, held together with screws; g, silicone rubber gasket; i, metallic image.

RESULTS AND DISCUSSION

Selection of electrolyte

In order for imaging to occur, the semiconductor must show rectifying behavior in contact with the electrolyte of choice. The current-voltage characteristics of p-Si in several acceptable plating electrolytes are shown in Figure 2. The metal plating potentials associated with these electrolytes are rather negative, ranging from -0.18V vs. SCE for Au to -0.42V for Ni. These potentials are well negative of the flat band potential range of p-Si in acidic to neutral pH (∼0.1V vs. SCE)[5]. Thus, the metal deposition is only slightly observed in the dark (due to leakage currents arising from electrical imperfections in the semiconductor surface), and is greatly enhanced in the light. Figure 3 shows p-Si in contact with a Cu plating bath containing Cu in an uncomplexed form, thus plating at a more positive potential than the pyrophosphate bath. Here, we observe a relatively large dark plating current, probably due to injection of electrons from the valence band at potentials positive of flat band. Poor resolution would be expected from this electrolyte. In general, electrolytes with negative lying plating potentials give the most satisfactory results.

Images using constant current

A large number of metal patterns have been produced on p-Si and p-GaAs using a variety of plating baths and conditions. As seen in Figure 2, the greatest enhancement of light over dark current is observed at negative bias potentials. In general, more reproducible images were achieved if this negative bias was maintained employing a constant current power supply while ensuring that the injected electron density is well within the bounds defined by the photon flux.

In theory, the growth of the deposit should be dependent on the type of bias control employed. After the initial monolayers of metal are deposited, the

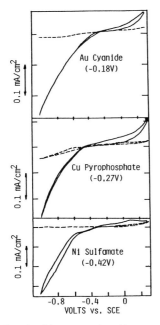
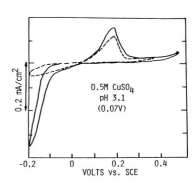

Fig. 2. Cyclic current-voltage curves on p-Si (0.1 Ω-cm, (100) face) in the dark and under 50 mW/cm² tungsten-halogen lamp illumination, in Au, Cu and Ni plating electrolytes. Plating potentials on like-metal substrates are shown in parentheses. Sweep rate: 0.1V/sec.

Fig. 3. Cyclic current-voltage curves on p-Si, as shown in Fig. 2. Uncomplexed Cu^{+2} electrolyte gives rise to plating at a relatively positive potential (0.07V), near the p-Si flat band potential, resulting in high dark currents and ohmic-type stripping behavior.

metal-semiconductor contact should determine the rectifying and electrochemical properties of the interface. The possibilities are illustrated in Figure 4. If photoelectrodeposition is carried out at constant voltage, thickening of the deposit will depend on the degree of band bending at the metal-semiconductor contact. If the contact is ohmic, separation of light-generated electron-hole pairs will cease, and the deposit will fail to grow. Under constant current conditions, however, growth may continue in the dark on top of the like-metal ohmic contacts, due to their reduced overpotential. Conversely, under conditions where the deposited metal forms a rectifying contact, growth will continue as long as light can penetrate to the interface. Under constant voltage, all deposition will then cease. Under constant current, the voltage may increase sharply at this point, giving rise to minority carrier injection into dark areas, and loss of resolution.

It is also found that the resolution of the deposits is influenced by deposition conditions similar to those commonly affecting morphology in electroplating technology [1]. Both flowing and heating the electrolyte enhanced the quality of an image projected from a USAF-1951 resolution target using a Canon f/1.8, 55 mm camera lens. Optimal results, with resolution better than 10μ, were

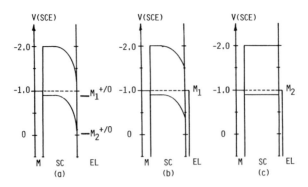

Fig. 4. Band bending in p-Si accompanying photoelectrochemical deposition of low (M_1) and high (M_2) work function metals. Applied voltage is -1.0V vs. SCE in neutral aqueous electrolyte: (a) before deposition; (b) after deposition of rectifying contact; (c) after deposition of ohmic contact.

obtained for Cu on p-Si, using a pyrophosphate plating bath, and for Au on p-GaAs, using a commercial cyanide bath (Technic, Orotemp 24). Heating the Au electrolyte and flowing it over the electrode surface had positive effects on the hardness, adherence and resolution of the final deposit [1]. A photomicrograph of the Au deposit on p-GaAs is shown in Figure 5. In Figure 6, a high magnification of one of the numerals shows that resolution is yet limited by the deposit nucleation behavior. Similar resolution was achieved with a focused laser spot scanned across the electrode surface. In our view, etching or pre-coating procedures which render the surface electrically homogeneous will be necessary to improve the resolution further.

Negative imaging

Imaging of metal patterns has also been observed on n-type semiconductors. Employing n-GaAs and a nickel sulfamate plating bath (Technic,Nickel S), negative images, i.e., plating only on the dark regions, were recorded at 25 $\mu A/cm^2$ constant cathodic current and ~50 mW/cm^2 tungsten-halogen illumination. However, at 100 $\mu A/cm^2$ plating was observed over the entire surface but was enhanced in illuminated regions. We suspect the plating in the illuminated region is due to a photoelectrochemical mechanism, rather than a photochemical or photothermal process, because of the low illumination levels used.

A possible mechanism is illustrated in Figure 7, using hypothetical current-voltage curves for an n-type semiconductor in an aqueous plating electrolyte in the dark and in the light. At positive potentials (region I), no current is observed in the dark, but a large minority-carrier induced oxidation current is observed in the light due to electrode decomposition (etching). Thus, if a pattern were projected onto the electrode held at a potential in region I, an etched image would result. At the more negative potentials of region II, a cathodic dark current will be observed, resulting from thermionic emission and tunneling of majority carriers through the space charge region. This dark current will co-exist with a net anodic etching current in the lighted portions of the electrode. Thus, in region II we might observe plating in the dark regions and etching in the illuminated regions of the electrode. At the potential dividing regions II and III, no current flows in lighted portions, and

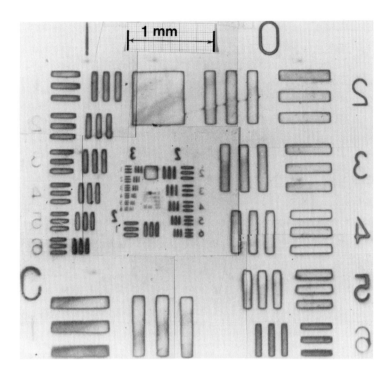

Fig. 5. Photomicrograph of a photoelectrochemical Au deposit on p-GaAs, produced from the projected image of a USAF-1951 resolution target.

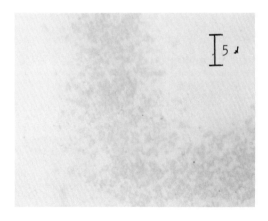

Fig. 6. High resolution photomicrograph of one of the numerals in Fig. 5, showing inhomogeneous metal nucleation.

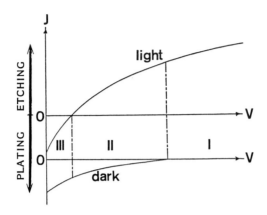

Fig. 7. Hypothetical current-voltage curves for a n-type semiconductor in the dark and light, showing overlapping regions of photo and dark current. The axis for the dark current has been offset for clarity.

plating occurs in the dark. This potential is the ideal value for negative imaging. In region III, which is negative of the flat band potential, majority carrier currents occur in both the light and dark portions of the electrode. At the more positive end of III, the current density in the dark is still higher than in the light. However, at more negative potentials, majority carrier current density in <u>illuminated</u> areas becomes higher, the photoconductivity effect. Thus, positive metal images over a plated-metal background may be observed at these potentials, as we observed at the higher current densities for n-GaAs.

Electroless imaging

Recent experiments have been aimed at eliminating the use of an electrochemical cell configuration in the imaging process. Here, the crystal is simply immersed in the electrolyte bath and irradiated, with no external electrical connections. Complementary oxidation and reduction reactions take place on illuminated and dark areas. Hence, polymeric or gelatinous ion conductive coatings might be developed containing appropriate redox reagents. These would be applied to the crystal surface. Projection of an image onto the coated surface could yield a positive or negative pattern of oxide, polymer, metal or etched relief, depending on the redox reactions employed.

Electroless production of Au and Cu patterns on p-GaAs and p-Si were demonstrated [1], although the deposition rates were an order of magnitude lower than those produced at optimum electrode potentials. Recent experiments show, however, that very rapid light-localized electroless plating of electropositive metals (Zn, Cd, etc.) is achieved on p-Si and p-GaAs [6]. This is accomplished by first incorporating some of the metal onto a portion of the crystal away from the area of interest. This fixes a band bending at the semiconductor-electrolyte interface. For p-type semiconductors, metals with negative redox potentials are favored for large band bending, and hence efficient separation of optically produced electrons and holes. Highly photosensitive surfaces of p-type semiconductors are obtained using Zn and Cd as internal bias agents. In Figure 8, the experimental arrangement for metal deposition is shown, employing a 50 μm He-Ne laser spot (∿50 mW/cm^2 intensity) scanned across a p-Si substrate immersed in a 0.1M ZnSO$_4$ electrolyte. A layer of Zn had been plated onto one edge of the Si. Following deposition, the Zn was exchanged for Au by dipping the crystal into a Au plating solution in order to enhance the contrast of the plated regions. A photomicrograph showing the deposit is reproduced in Figure 9.

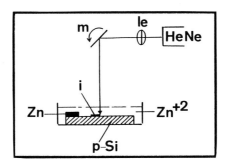

Fig. 8. Experimental arrangement for electroless photoelectrochemical deposition of fine lines of Zn on p-Si. A He-Ne laser is used, focused to a 50 μm spot with a convex lens (le), and scanned over the crystal surface with a rotating mirror (m) (General Scanning Corp.). The p-Si has some Zn plated on one end, and is immersed in a Zn^{+2} electrolyte. The developing image is shown as region i.

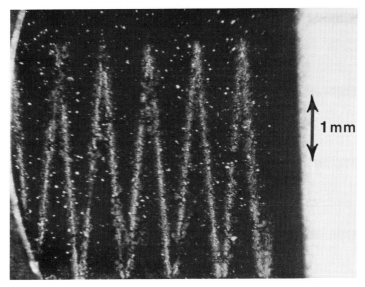

Fig. 9. "Electroless" metal deposit produced by a scanned 50 μm He-Ne laser spot across a p-Si surface in a 0.1M ZnSO$_4$ electrolyte. The p-Si is internally biased by a layer of Zn plated on one edge. The original Zn line was exchanged for Au by dipping in an Au plating bath.

CONCLUSIONS

We have shown in this article that photoelectrochemistry can be employed to generate metal patterns on surfaces of semiconductors of technological importance. In principle, the process is general, allowing imaging on all p- and n-type semiconductors. The ultimate resolution of photoelectrochemical imaging is limited by the lateral diffusion length of minority carriers at the semiconductor/electrolyte interface [7]. This spreading is expected to be small for carriers generated by short wavelength irradiation which are produced within the space charge region and rapidly consumed by electrochemical reaction at the interface. The drift velocity of these minority carriers towards the surface which is driven by the space charge field is very much greater than the diffusion velocity parallel to the surface. Diffraction gratings with about $\sim 0.25\mu$ spacings have been produced on semiconductors by photoelectrochemical etching [8]. For photoelectrochemical deposition of metals, therefore, it is likely that the practical resolution will be limited by surface morphology, dendritic growth, and the diffraction limit imposed by the wavelength of the light.

The very low power requirements and high theoretically achievable resolution of photoelectrochemical deposition distinguishes it from techniques requiring localized heating effects to promote deposition [4]. It is also simpler to use and can be applied to a wider variety of deposited materials than gas phase photodissociative laser deposition [3]. However, unlike the other methods, photoelectrochemical deposition requires electrical conductivity and is strongly dependent on initial surface preparation and the doping type of semiconductor. Nevertheless, its versatility as a maskless method for photo and laser processing make it worthy of consideration for fabrication of conducting elements onto new semiconductor materials and devices.

ACKNOWLEDGMENT

This work was supported by the Office of Naval Research.

REFERENCES

1. R. H. Micheels, A. D. Darrow and R. D. Rauh, Appl. Phys. Lett. 39, 418 (1981).

2. T. Inoue, A. Fiyishima and K. Honda, J. Electrochem. Soc. 127, 1582 (1980).

3. (a) T. F. Deutsch, D. J. Ehrlich and R. M. Osgood, Appl. Phys. Lett. 35, 175 (1979); (b) D. J. Ehrlich, R. M. Osgood and T. F. Deutsch, Appl. Phys. Lett. 38, 946 (1981).

4. (a) R. F. Karlicek, V. M. Donnelly and G. J. Collins, J. Appl. Phys. 53, 1084 (1982); (b) R. J. von Gutfeld, E. E. Tynan, R. L. Melcher and S. E. Blum, Appl. Phys. Lett. 35, 651 (1979).

5. M. J. Madou, B. H. Loo, K. W. Frese and S. R. Morrison, Surf. Sci. 108, 135 (1981).

6. T. L. Rose, D. H. Longendorfer and R. D. Rauh, Appl. Phys. Lett., in press.

7. L. V. Belyakov, D. N. Goryachev, S. M. Ryvkin and O. M. Sreseli, Sov. Phys. Semicond. 12, 1334 (1978).

8. Zh. I. Alferov, D. N. Goryachev, S. A. Gurevich, M. N. Mizerov, E. L. Portnoi and B. S. Ryvkin, Sov. Phys. Tech. Phys. 21, 857 (1976).

ANALYSIS OF LASER-ENHANCED ADSORPTION/DESORPTION PROCESSES ON SEMICONDUCTOR SURFACES VIA ELECTRONIC SURFACE STATE EXCITATION

WILLIAM C. MURPHY, A. C. BERI AND THOMAS F. GEORGE
Department of Chemistry, University of Rochester, Rochester, New York 14627 USA

and

JUI-TENG LIN
Laser Physics Branch, Optical Sciences Division, Naval Research Laboratory, Washington, D.C. 20375 USA

ABSTRACT

Electronic surface states in semiconductors often lie between the valence and conduction bands and give rise to charge densities confined to the surface region. Laser radiation of frequency less than the energy gap can excite electrons from delocalized valence band states to these localized surface states leading to large changes in the charge distribution at the surface. Selective enhancement of adsorption/desorption processes involving ionic or polar adspecies can result from such a charge redistribution. Using a one-dimensional model for silicon, the cross-section for the laser-induced electronic transition to surface states is shown to be large. The interaction energy of an adspecies with the surface changes significantly with direct excitation of surface states in a semiconductor. For a one-dimensional metal, however, direct transitions between bulk and surface states are not allowed, but phonon-mediated transitions coupled with laser radiation lead to substantial charge transfer as for semiconductors.

INTRODUCTION

Much effort has been devoted to the study of the effects of laser radiation on the phonons in solid surfaces. Both theoretical [1] and experimental [2] works have relied on the laser to excite these vibrational modes of the system in order to enhance surface processes.
On the other hand, photo-induced surface reactions can occur through electronic excitation. Synchrotron radiation studies [3] on metal surfaces have shown induced desorption due to the shift of electronic charge in the surface region [4].
For a semiconductor, states with charge localized in the surface region exist in addition to the bulk conduction and valence bands states [5]. In the following, we will demonstrate the use of a laser for exciting charge into these surface states and discuss the effect on surface processes.
For a truncated one-dimensional chain of length L and lattice constant a, the solutions of the Schrödinger equation can be obtained within the nearly-free-electron approximation [5]. The energy for the bulk electronic states is

$$E_k = \frac{1}{4}\{[k^2+(k-g)^2] \pm \sqrt{[k^2-(k-g)^2]^2 + 4E_g^2}\} \quad (1)$$

where k is the wavenumber of the electron, $g = 2\pi/a$ is the reciprocal lattice vector and E_g is the band gap energy. The results for the valence band (negative branch) and conduction band (positive branch) are illustrated in figure 1. The wavefunctions are constructed from sums of plane waves [6]. For

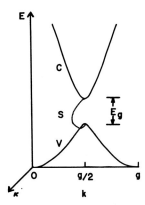

Figure 1. Dispersion relationship in complex crystal momentum space (k+iκ) for a finite linear chain. The valence, surface and conduction bands are labeled V, S and C, respectively.

example, at the top of the valence band we have

$$\psi_k(z) = \frac{2}{L^{1/2}} \sin[(g/2)(z-a/2) + \theta] \quad (2)$$

for inside the chain and

$$\psi_k(z) = \frac{2}{L^{1/2}} \sin\theta \, e^{-q(z-\frac{a}{2})} \quad (3)$$

for outside the chain. The phase factor, θ, is determined by the continuity condition and $q = (2W-k^2)^{1/2}$, where W is the work function [6].

Since we have a truncated chain, in addition to the above solutions of the Schrödinger equation, we can have solutions with complex crystal momentum [5].

$$k = g/2 + i\kappa. \quad (4)$$

Inserting this into our energy, equation (1), we obtain

$$E_\kappa = \frac{1}{2}\{(\frac{g}{2})^2 - \kappa^2 \pm \sqrt{E_g^2 - \kappa^2 g^2}\}. \quad (5)$$

Likewise using equation (2), we obtain the wavefunction

$$\psi_\kappa(z) = C_S \sin[(\frac{g}{2})(z-\frac{a}{2})+\theta] e^{-\kappa(z-\frac{a}{2})} \quad (6)$$

where C_S is a normalization constant. The external wavefunction will have the same form as equation (3). Here we have disregarded the contribution to the wavefunction at the far surface (z = a/2-L). The energy, equation (5), is also illustrated in figure 1 by the band labeled S. These are surface states since the charge density associated with them is localized in the surface region due to the exponential factor in equation (6). The bulk states, equation (2), however, have charge more or less uniformly distributed throughout the system.

Consequently, if we excite electrons from the valence band to the surface band, we can transfer charge from the bulk of our crystal to the surface. The resultant Coulombic effect could have significant effect on surface processes. To explore this concept, we first wish to see how well laser radiation can excite charge into the surface states.

SURFACE STATE EXCITATION

Laser induced transitions to the surface states will be governed by the integral

$$H_{\kappa k}(t) = <\kappa|\vec{A}\cdot\vec{p}|k>, \tag{7}$$

where $\vec{A}$ is the vector potential of the laser radiation and $\vec{p}$ is the momentum operator of the electron. If we use a laser that is polarized parallel to the chain and exploit the periodicity of the functions contained in our wavefunction [6], we obtain

$$H_{\kappa k}(t) = -i\left(\frac{2\pi I}{137}\right)^{1/2} \frac{e^{-i\omega t}}{\omega} S <\kappa|\frac{d}{dz}|k>_0, \tag{8}$$

where I is the intensity of the laser, ω is the frequency and the subscript zero indicates integration over the first unit cell. The sum, S, is given by

$$S = \sum_{\ell=0}^{N-1} e^{i(g/2-k)\ell a} e^{\kappa \ell a}, \tag{9}$$

where N is the number of atoms in our chain. To obtain the transition probability, we would take the square modulus of equation (8). If we assume that N is very large [6], the sum squared can be approximated by

$$|S|^2 \approx \frac{2\pi}{a} \frac{\delta(k-g/2)}{1-e^{2\kappa a}}, \tag{10}$$

where $\delta(k-g/2)$ is the Dirac delta function. Consequently, the transition from the bulk to a surface state is only permitted if the real part of the crystal momentum remains unchanged. This relationship is not too surprising since it is an exact restriction of laser-induced transitions between bulk bands [7]. Furthermore, for our model, it confines us to the top of the valence band, where the density of states is a maximum (infinite) and the laser frequency needed for a transition is a minimum.

To first order, the transition rate from the valence band to the surface band is

$$T = \left(\frac{2\pi}{t}\right) \sum_{\kappa} \sum_{k} \left|\int_0^t dt' H_{\kappa k}(t') e^{i\omega_{\kappa k} t}\right|^2, \tag{11}$$

where $\omega_{\kappa k} = E_\kappa - E_k$. Using equations (8) and (10) in this expression, after evaluating the sums and time integral the transition rate becomes

$$T = \frac{8\pi}{137} \frac{Ig_L^2}{E_g \omega^2} \frac{|<\kappa|\frac{d}{dz}|g/2>_0|^2}{1-e^{2\kappa a}} \left|\frac{dk}{dE_\kappa}\right|, \tag{12}$$

where κ now refers to the state obeying the resonance condition

$$\omega = \frac{1}{2}[E_g - k^2 \pm (E_g^2 - g^2\kappa^2)^{1/2}]. \tag{13}$$

The integral over the wavefunctions and the energy derivative can be readily evaluated [6]. Finally, we obtain the cross section, σ, from the relationship,

$$\sigma \equiv \frac{\omega T}{I}. \tag{14}$$

Although the complete expression for σ is quite complicated [6], we can make some simple observations.

If the exciting laser radiation is at a frequency near $0.5\ E_g$, the energy derivative will vanish and

$$\sigma_{\omega \approx 0.5\ E_g} = 0. \qquad (15)$$

This is exactly what one would expect since this mid-gap energy is a branch point at which no surface state exists.

If the laser radiation is near a frequency 0 or E_g, the cross-section becomes

$$\sigma_{\omega \to 0, E_g} \sim \left|\frac{1}{\kappa}\right|. \qquad (16)$$

At both extremes κ goes to zero and σ diverges. This occurs because at the surface band edges the charge associated with the surface states becomes more and more delocalized throughout the lattice, until at κ = 0 the charge is completely delocalized. At this point the surface states become bulk states, and instead of cross-sections, one should consider absorption coefficients.

Figure 2 depicts the behavior of the cross-section over the entire frequency range. The values for the lattice constant, a = 2.35Å, and the energy gap, E_g = 1.17 eV, are typical of silicon [8].

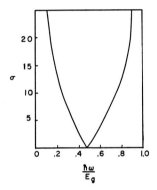

Figure 2. Absorption cross-section for surface states, σ, in Å^2 versus the frequency of the exciting laser radiation.

To illustrate what laser intensity is required for a certain absorption rate, we consider exciting a surface state at $0.4\ E_g$. This corresponds to a laser frequency of about 10^{15} Hz which falls in the infrared. From figure 2, the cross-section is about 3Å^2. If we assume our laser intensity is 1 W/cm^2, the transition rate is about 4 x 10^{-5} photons absorbed per second. Since an electron is excited for each photon absorbed and the effective charge depth for the surface state is about 8 atomic layers, the transition rate is about 5 x 10^{-6} electrons per surface atom per second. To obtain the number of transitions per unit surface area, we divide by the surface area of the end atom, whereby we obtain 10^{10} photons absorbed per cm^2 per second. This value is quite large considering the low power of the laser. Consequently, using such a laser can lead to appreciable charge excitation in the surface region.

Since the charge depth increases as we move away from the mid-gap region, we wish to excite surface states near 0.5 E_g to obtain the greatest effect on surface charge. From figure 2, we see that in this region the cross-section is quite substantial. Consequently, we would expect a laser tuned to a frequency near 0.5 E_g to be an effective controller of surface charge.

ADSPECIES-SURFACE INTERACTION

To examine the effect of this surface charge on adspecies, we must first determine the charge profile in the surface region. For the unexcited system, the electron density is

$$n_0(z) = \frac{2L}{\pi^2} \int_0^{k_F} dk (E_F - E_k) |\psi_k(z)|^2 \tag{17}$$

where the subscript 0 indicates ground state and E_F is the Fermi energy with crystal momentum k_F. If the semiconductor is now exposed to a laser with an energy less than the energy gap, an electron will be excited from state $k = g/2$ to a surface state indicated by κ. The new density will be the sum of the ground state density and the surface state density less the charge associated with the excited bulk state. However, the bulk state is delocalized throughout the system and its effect on the density will be negligible. Therefore, the excited system will have a density

$$n(z) = n_0(z) + |\psi_\kappa(z)|^2. \tag{18}$$

We have evaluated the densities for silicon and the results are depicted in figure 3. The solid line is the ground state charge density. The oscillations of the charge as one goes into the bulk of the crystal is due to the concentration of charge around the ions. The dashed line represents the density for the system with the excited surface state of $\kappa = 0.5\ E_g/g$ in the lower branch. As can be seen by this plot, the charge in the excited surface state produces a total electronic charge in the surface region that is twice as great as the bulk average. If one excites surface states closer to the branch point near the gap center, the charge concentration in the first few layers of the surface will increase up to about thrice the average density.

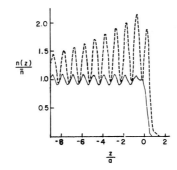

Figure 3. Electron density distribution at the surface. The solid line represents the ground electronic state, and the dashed line represents the system with the excited surface state $\kappa = 0.5\ E_g/g$ in the lower branch.

If a charged adspecies is above the surface, this excess charge in the surface region can produce a marked effect on the adspecies surface interaction. This interaction can be written classically as

$$U(z_I) = -\int d\vec{r}\, n(z) v(r), \qquad (19)$$

where $v(r)$ is the electron-ion potential of the adspecies at z_I. We have assumed that the charge density is uniform in the x and y directions. If we take $v(r)$ to be Coulombic with Thomas-Fermi screening [9], we can readily evaluate the integrals over x and y to obtain

$$U(z_I) = -\frac{2\pi Z}{\lambda} \int_{-\infty}^{\infty} dz\, n(z) e^{-\lambda|z-z_I|}, \qquad (20)$$

where λ is the Thomas-Fermi screening parameter:

$$\lambda^2 = \frac{6\pi \bar{n}}{E_F}. \qquad (21)$$

Using our density expression, equation (18), we obtain

$$^sU(z_I) = \frac{2\pi Z}{\lambda} \int_{-\infty}^{\infty} dz\, |\psi_\kappa(z)|^2 e^{-\lambda|z-z_I|}. \qquad (22)$$

Since we are not concerned with the interaction of adspecies with the semiconductor in the ground state, we only consider the surface contribution to the potential (superscript s) in equation (22). If we now insert the expression for the surface wavefunction in equation (22), we will obtain

$$\frac{^sU(z_I)}{Z} = e^{-\lambda z_I} A(\kappa) - e^{-2qz_I} B(\kappa) \qquad (23)$$

where the coefficients $A(\kappa)$ and $B(\kappa)$ are given elsewhere [10]. The potential in equation (23) is exponentially damped as one moves away from the surface. In the vicinity of the surface the effect on the total potential can be quite

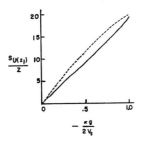

Figure 4. The magnitude of the surface interaction potential (in millihartrees) at a distance $z_I = a$ for the system with various excited surface states. The solid line represents surface states in the lower energy branch; the dashed line, the upper energy branch.

substantial. To illustrate this for various surface states, we have plotted the change in potential at $z_I = a$ for all surface states in figure 4. The upper branch states are at a higher energy than the lower branch states. Therefore, the exponential tail of the charge density and, subsequently, the interaction is slightly greater.

Our contention that lasers can control surface charge density in semiconductors and, subsequently, enhance surface processes has been confirmed. Since metals also play an important role in catalysis, the effect of lasers on metal surfaces will also be examined via a simple model.

ELECTRON-PHONON COUPLING

If we model a metal as a truncated one-dimensional chain, we will obtain expressions for the bulk and surface wavefunctions and their associated energies which are the same in form as those for the one-dimensional semiconductor. However, whereas the lower band in a semiconductor is completely filled (see figure 1), in a metal this band is only partially filled. For example, in the case of sodium [8], the top of the lower band lies at 3.8 eV but the band is only occupied up to 3.1 eV in the ground state.

If we shine a laser on our metal, we cannot directly excite electrons from the bulk to the surface. This is due to our selection rule [see equation (10)] which says that we can only excite bulk states with $k = g/2$. In a metal, there are no occupied bulk states with real momentum at or near this crystal momentum. To overcome this problem, the electrons can be excited to the $k = g/2$ state with the phonons of the crystal before excitation into the surface states by the laser photons. Thus photons would supply the energy needed for the transition and phonons would supply the needed crystal momentum. Figure 5 illustrates the bands in a metal and the suggested pathway for exciting surface states.

Since the first-order transition probability will vanish since neither crystal momentum nor energy are conserved, we can write the transition probability of state k" to k via intermediate state k' as

$$M = 2\pi\delta(\omega_{kk''}-\omega_f-\omega_p)\left\{\sum_{k'}\frac{H^f_{kk'}H^p_{k'k''}}{\omega_{k'k''}-\omega_p}\right\}^2 \quad (24)$$

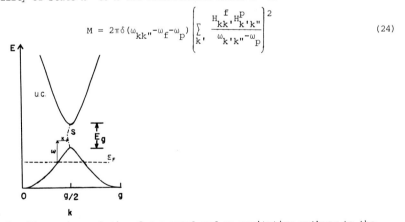

Figure 5. Dispersion relation for a metal and an excitation pathway to the surface states(s). The vertical arrow represents a photon of frequency ω; the horizontal arrow, a phonon of momentum K. UC is an upper conduction band.

where the super- and subscripts f and p refer to the laser field and the phonons respectively. The matrix element $H^f_{kk'}$, is equivalent to equation (7) with the time exponential factored out. The phonon matrix element can be written [7],

$$H^p_{k'k''} = -i\left(\frac{1}{NM}\right)^{1/2} \frac{Kv(K)}{2\omega_p}[a(K) + a^\dagger(K)] \quad (25)$$

where M is the mass of the lattice atom, $a(K)$ and $a^\dagger(K)$ are the annihilation and creation operators of the phonon, $v(K)$ is the form factor, and the crystal momentum of the phonon, K, must equal $k'-k''$.

If we insert equations (7) and (25) into equation (24) and average over the phonon number states, $|n(K)\rangle$, we obtain the transition probability. If we now sum over all initial and final states, we will obtain the second-order transition rate

$$T = \left(\frac{L}{NM\pi}\right) \int dk'' \frac{K^2 v(K)^2 [2n(K)+1]}{2\omega_p (\omega_{g/2,k''} - \omega_p)^2} T^{(1)}(\kappa, g/2), \quad (26)$$

where $K = g/2-k''$. $T^{(1)}(\kappa, g/2)$ is the first-order transition rate between bulk state $g/2$ and surface state κ induced by the laser field and is given by equation (12). We can convert this expression into an integral over energy. If we then assume a thermal distribution of phonons and electrons, we need only consider the integral within an interval $k_B T_L$ around the Fermi energy where T_L is the lattice temperature. At room temperature, this interval is small and the integrand can be considered a constant:

$$T = \left(\frac{ak_B T_L}{2\pi M}\right)\left(\frac{k_F}{2E_F}\right) \frac{K^2 v(K)^2 [2n(K)+1]}{\omega_p (\omega_{g/2,k_F} - \omega_p)^2} T^{(1)}(\kappa, g/2) \quad (27)$$

where $K = g/2-k_F$.

For sodium we can readily evaluate equation (26):

$$T = 2.38 \times 10^{-4} T^{(1)}(\kappa, g/2). \quad (28)$$

Since the various physical constants for sodium are not significantly different from those of silicon, we would expect the first-order rates to be roughly comparable. From the previous section, we saw that a significant photon absorption in silicon could be induced with a low power laser (1 to 10 W/cm^2). Therefore, we would expect to produce a similar effect in sodium with a moderate power laser (10 to 100 kW/cm^2). Consequently, as with semiconductors, we would expect a laser to act as an efficient controller of surface charge in a metal. Subsequent interactions would likewise be effected.

CONCLUSION

Using a laser to localize electronic charge in the surface region of a semiconductor or a metal can produce an appreciable effect on adspecies-surface interaction. For a negatively charged adspecies, desorption can be induced; if positively charged, adsorption is enhanced. In a more realistic model with both occupied and empty surface states, the laser could excite holes as well as electrons and thus selectively enhance adsorption or desorption for the same charged adspecies.

Of course, this same formalism would apply to a polar adspecies. The positive end of a molecule would be attracted to a negatively charged surface. Thus, in addition to enhancing adsorption or desorption, the laser will cause the adspecies to line up in a desired orientation.

Furthermore, since the charge distribution of an adspecies is a function of its electronic state, our laser controlled surface could select the desired state. Finally, once molecules are adsorbed on the surface, new energy bands could be introduced through which the laser could enhance surface processes. To improve our understanding of the adspecies-surface system, the dielectric screening problem would have to be addressed in more detail.

Because the concentration of charge is so large in the surface region, it is conceivable that a lattice rearrangement could be induced in the surface area. Such an effect could lower the charge in the surface. On the other hand, the new surface states would probably be more stable and, subsequently, have a larger lifetime. To study these effects, a self-consistent-field calculation would have to be performed.

The major limitation of the above model, however, is its one-dimensionality. The three-dimensional interaction potential may be quite complex depending not only on the distance from the surface but also on the position of the adspecies with respect to the plane of the surface. Finally, in a real metal or semiconductor, the surface states are not necessarily confined to the gap between the valence and conduction bands.

Nonetheless, we have clearly demonstrated that lasers can be used to control surface charge in both metals and semiconductors. Such charge, in turn, can lead to enhanced surface processes. The effects on these processes of adspecies-surface dynamics and higher dimensions are the subject of continuing research.

ACKNOWLEDGMENTS

This work was supported in part by the Office of Naval Research, the U.S. Army Research Office and the Air Force Office of Scientific Research (AFSC), the United States Air Force, under Grant AFOSR-82-0046. The United States Government is authorized to reproduce and distribute reprints for governmental purposes notwithstanding any copyright notation hereon. TFG acknowledges the Camille and Henry Dreyfus Foundation for a Teacher-Scholar Award (1975-84).

REFERENCES

1. J. Lin, A. C. Beri, M. Hutchison, W. C. Murphy and T. F. George, Phys. Lett. 79A, 233 (1980).

2. T. J. Chuang, J. Chem. Phys. 74, 1453 (1981).

3. D. P. Woodruff, M. M. Traum, H. H. Farrell, N. V. Smith, P. D. Johnson, D. A. King, R. L. Benbow and Z. Hurych, Phys. Rev. B 21, 5642 (1980).

4. M. L. Knotek and P. J. Feibelman, Phys. Rev. Lett. 40, 964 (1978).

5. S. Lundqvist, in Surface Science, Vol. 1 (International Atomic Energy Agency, Vienna 1975), p. 331.

6. W. C. Murphy and T. F. George, Surface Sci., <u>114</u>, 189 (1982).

7. See, e.g., J. Callaway, <u>Quantum Theory of the Solid State</u> (Academic Press, New York 1976) p. 521 ff; p. 576 ff.

8. C. Kittel, <u>Introduction to Solid State Physics</u>, 4th ed. (Wiley, New York 1971) pp. 38, 364, 338.

9. See, e.g., C. Kittel, <u>Quantum Theory of Solids</u> (Wiley, New York 1963) p. 105.

10. W. C. Murphy and T. F. George, J. Phys. Chem., in press.

FORMATION OF CdO AND Cu$_2$O FILMS BY LASER IRRADIATION OF THE CORRESPONDING METALLIC FILMS IN AIR

ROD ANDREW, LUC BAUFAY, ANDRE PIGEOLET AND MICHEL WAUTELET
Université de l'Etat, Avenue Maistriau, 23   7000 Mons, Belgium.

ABSTRACT

We describe the oxidation of 1000 Å thick metal films on glass substrates when exposed to a scanning laser beam. For Cd and Cu films optical spectroscopy shows an energy gap of 2.45 eV and 2 eV respectively, in agreement with published data for CdO and Cu$_2$O. We measure the power threshold for complete oxidation in a single scan and deduce the maximum temperature, which is inconsistent with thermal oxidation data but corresponds to the m.p. of the metals. We point out the important contribution of the heat of formation to the temperature balance and demonstrate that in the case of Al this effect is sufficient to destroy any oxide formed.

INTRODUCTION

Though there remains some afterglow of a heated controversy it is now generally accepted that laser annealing of semiconductors is a thermal process. This does not, however, mean that the end-state obtained in a particular case will be the same as that resulting from a classical oven anneal. Where differences exist they can usually be reasonably attributed to time and distance scale effects, since heating and cooling rates, temperature gradients etc., can be many orders of magnitude greater, even for scanning CW beams, than is attainable by oven annealing which by comparison is essentially isothermal. In this respect we can also note that any energy liberated by exothermic reaction during the annealing step is in general not totally absorbed by the system in times comparable to the laser pulse duration or spot dwell times, and is therefore a further parameter influencing temperature.

Such effects are obviously most prominent for thin films on thermally insulating substrates, and are well exemplified by the so-called explosive crystallisation of α-Ge films using either pulsed [1] or scanning [2] laser beams, being in this case principally due to the liberation of the heat of crystallisation. Similarly, we have previously described [3] thin film fabrication of the semiconducting compounds CdTe, CdSe, AlSb and AlAs, by laser annealing of sandwich-like structures of the constituents, and have shown that the reaction, once initiated by the laser beam, is led to completion by the liberation of the heat of formation of these compounds. In fact -ΔH may be very large compared to the laser energy necessary to trigger the process, and the importance of the effect is such that the reaction can be completed up to 10^6 times more quickly than would otherwise be the case.

Some metal oxides also have large heats of formation, and we report here a study of the laser induced oxidation of thin films of Cd, Cu, and Al, by irradiation of these films in air.

EXPERIMENTAL RESULTS

Films of 1000 Å thickness of Cd, Cu and Al were vacuum evaporated onto sputter-cleaned glass substrates in a vacuum better than 10^{-6} torr. These films were then irradiated in air using a Kr$^+$laser operating on all red lines (647.1-676.4nm). Two optical arrangements were used, the first with cylindrical focussing to produce an approximately elliptically gaussian beam profile with $r_x \approx 5 \times 10^{-3}$cm, $r_y \approx 8 \times 10^{-2}$cm. The transmission efficiency η, i.e. the ratio of incident beam power after the optical system to indicated power output, was 0.61. In the second system, which became necessary to deliver the power density needed for the Cu and Al films, a spherical lens was used to produce a beam having $r_x = r_y \approx 1 \times 10^{-2}$cm, and $\eta=0.66$. The scanning speed v_x could be varied but in all the results to be reported was 0.5cm/s. The measurements made were the threshold hold beam power P_T for formation of the oxide, judged most simply by optical transparency, and the sub-threshold near-normal incidence reflectivity, R, of the films in the laser light.

Cd

Cd films of both 1000 Å and 2000 Å thickness were irradiated using the cylindrical lens system. At laser powers in excess of a 2.25W threshold, which was apparently independent of film thickness, a single scan produced a band some ~0.1 cm wide of material transparent to orange light. By partly overlapping successive traces we could produce large areas of uniformly transparent material whose optical absorbance characteristics are presented in fig. 1. The straight line fit to $(\alpha h\nu)^2$ vs $h\nu$ suggest a direct optical bandgap of 2.45 eV in good agreement with the published value of 2.5±0.1 eV [4] for CdO.

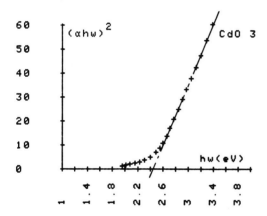

Fig. 1 Optical absorbance characteristic of a Cd film irradiated in air.

Irradiation in an inert gas atmosphere produced, rather predictably, either no change or, at higher laser powers, ablation of the Cd film. In a pure oxygen atmosphere there was no detectable change in the power threshold. These two mini-experiments confirm that the oxygen supply is indeed atmospheric, and is not rate limiting.

Repeated scanning in the same place at energies 10% below threshold produced a similar transformation after 5-10 traces, whilst at 15% below threshold there was no detectable oxidation effect.

The power threshold using the spherical lens system, for transformation in a single trace, was 0.45 W, with similar behaviour to that described above up to ~10% P_T. The measured reflectivity of our Cd films was 0.182.

Cu

Using the spherical lens system, irradiation of 1000 Å thick Cu films of reflectivity 0.915 showed a very sharp threshold at 2.0±0.1 W. The optical absorbance characteristics of a uniformly transformed region appear in Fig.2, indicating a direct gap at 2 eV, in excellent agreement with published data for Cu_2O [5]. Note that repeated scans some 2-5% below P_T did not result in oxide formation but only in a small change in surface reflectivity.

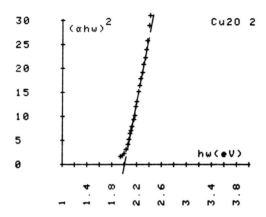

Fig. 2 Optical absorbance characteristic of a Cu film irradiated in air.

Al

Irradiation using the spherical lens system of 1000 Å thick Al films of R=0.86 (less than Cu in red light) showed a sharp threshold at P_T=4.5±0.1 W, with, like Cu, only a very faintly visible reflectivity change at sub-threshold power. However optical microscopy indicates ablation of the film rather than formation of the oxide and we were unable to detect oxide formation by optical spectroscopy or by X-ray analysis. We believe that the traces left after laser treatment show simply removal of the Al film from the substrate.

DISCUSSION

The growth of oxide layers on metals is a complex subject, with many parameters affecting the oxidation rate. Data for Cd is sparse, but oxide films of several hundred Å thickness appear to follow a parabolic law [6] where the layer thickness $z=K_p\sqrt{t}$. Remembering that the oxide layer will of course be somewhat thicker than the original metal layer the available published values of K_p [7] for Cd suggest that complete oxidation of a 1000 Å layer could be achieved in

~10 s at 400-550°C, but with no really good indication about what temperature would be necessary to oxidise the layer in times 10^3 or so less, i.e. comparable to the spot dwell time in our work. In theory a film twice as thick should take four times as long to oxidise at the same temperature, or, presumably, require a significantly higher temperature to oxidise in the same time.

Obviously the most interesting question concerns the maximum temperature, T_m, reached under the beam spot during the scan, although it is either necessary nor useful to attempt to obtain an exact solution to this non-trivial problem since so many parameters are imprecisely known. We can, though, make some estimates as follows.

As we shall show the thermal energy absorbed by the film itself is negligible compared to that dissipated in the substrate, so that the film acts simply as a photon/heat converter at the substrate surface, albeit with a somewhat larger effective spot size than the laser beam due to lateral heat conduction in the film. Since thermal diffusion in the substrate during the spot dwell time is limited to distances much less than the substrate thickness the problem reduces to that of surface temperature in a semi-∞ solid exposed to a scanning beam, and as such has been dealt with by a number of authors including Nissim et al. [8] . To minimize the error due to the lateral spreading effect we calculate the temperature rise ΔT for the cylindrically focussed beam on the Cd film. Taking the relevant values of r_x, r_y, P_T, R and η already given, and the thermal constants of the glass as C_p 0.25 cal/g, D=3.45x10^{-3}cm^2/s application of Nissim et al.'s formulae and graphs give ΔT=325 deg.C. Now the energy E_f absorbed by the film itself during the spot dwell time t_D=$2r_x/v_x$ is approximately that necessary to heat the volume of Cd $2r_y \times 2\sqrt{r_x^2+r_D^2} \times 1000$ Å by ΔT, where r_D=$\sqrt{4Dt_D}$. Taking the thermal constants of Cd from Table 1 we find E_f≈0.4mJ, which must be compared to the total energy E_a absorbed during the same time interval, i.e. $P_T\eta(1-R)t_D$≈23.6 mJ. Thus the film temperature is governed by the thermal behaviour of the substrate and, note, is virtually independent of film thickness in this range. We conclude that the peak temperature T_m induced by the laser is in the range 300-350°C, which seems hardly consistent with the oxidation data of [7] , but which coincides nicely with the m.p. of Cd at 321°C and with our model for the formation of compound semiconductor films. Here we showed that the reaction is triggered by partly melting the metal films, thus allowing rapid formation of a part of the compound, the liberation of whose heat of formation, $-\Delta H$, rapidly increases the temperature towards the m.p. of the compound, and so allows the reaction to be completed at this higher temperature. We postulate a similar situation here since $-\Delta H$ for CdO formation (corrected for formation from liquid Cd at 321°C)=63kcal/mole [7] , equivalent to ~12.5 mJ from the volume of film absorbing E_f, and as such directly comparable to E_f and E_a above. This extra energy will again be repartitioned in some way between the film and substrate but will evidently be sufficient to raise the temperature of the oxidising film well above the m.p. of Cd. Indeed we may remark that if a part of this liberated energy were not absorbed by the substrate then there probably would be no oxide, since a calculated 53 kcal/mole would suffise to heat, melt, vaporise and otherwise make disappear the film.

We conclude that the threshold power for oxide formation corresponds to heating the Cd film to its m.p. and so, using comparative data obtained with the spherical lens system, we can estimate T_m for the Cu and Al films. We note first, however, that the threshold for Cd is not very sharp since $-\Delta H$ is not very large, and in fact it may be that the partial transformation occuring up to 10% below P_T would be better associated with the onset of melting. (The agreement between the calculated T_m and the m.p. of Cd would also be better). In this case we should calibrate the spherical optics/substrate system by setting

$$\Delta T/P_T = 300 / 0.9 \times 0.45 \times 0.818 \times 0.66 \sim 1370 \text{ deg./W}$$

So for Al T_m=20 4.5 x0.14x0.66x1370~590°C which should be compared to the m.p. of Al at 660°C, but note that a reduction of only ~2% in R_{Al}, roughly corresponding to the changes seen at subthreshold power, would give a much better agreement here, and so we continue to associate the reaction threshold with melting of the metal film.

We refer now to Table 2 where, in addition to other parameters already defined, we tabulate the total energy E_a absorbed during the dwell time $2r_x/v_x$, the energy E_f absorbed by the film in the zone Πr_b^2, and the energy $E_{-\Delta H}$ that could be liberated by oxidation from the liquid metal of this same zone. We do not attach too much importance to the precise values of these figures which depend on the way the various parameters are defined but are interested in relative magnitudes. We see, for example, that E_f is no longer so negligible in comparison with E_a, owing to the smaller spot size, and that $E_{-\Delta H}$ assumes a relatively greater importance. These are but details. The important thing to notice is that whereas in this scheme $E_{-\Delta H} \simeq 5E_a$ for Cd, the ratio for Al is nearer 50, and the energy liberated, repartitioned as before between film and substrate, is easily sufficient to vaporise any oxide formed, which is why experimentally we observe only ablation tracks. The oxidation of Al is very exothermic, a point borne out by recent, more expensive, experiments in the South Atlantic where the aluminium superstructure of naval vessels led to uncontrollable conflagration.

We next consider the case of Cu, and see that owing to the very high reflectivity of these films T_m should not, according to our calculations, exceed ~175°C. The oxidation of Cu single crystals exposed to 760torr oxygen has been studied at 178°C by Young et.al. [9]. Depending on the crystal face the time required to oxidise a 1000 Å thick Cu layer varies from several hours to several months, at any rate rather longer than the dwell time of ~$2x10^{-2}$s. There is also evidence that the presence of water vapour markedly slows the oxidation rate [10]. Extrapolation of the data of [7] suggests formation at the rate we see cannot take place below the m.p. of Cu. We consider the possibility that if a very thin layer of oxide did form it could significantly change R, and hence the temperature and reaction rate, leading to a run-away process towards the m.p. of Cu and a reaction as described for Cd, with a similar $E_{-\Delta H}/E_a$ ratio. The value of R necessary to produce $T_m \simeq 1063$°C would be ~0.4, which is within the range of values of reflectivity we measure from Cu films very lightly oxidised on their front surface near a bunsen flame.

Note as well that such a process would presumably give a very sharp power threshold, which is precisely what we see despite the similarity of the $E_{-\Delta H}/E_a$ ratio to that of Cd. Thus such a proposal seems to be in agreement with, and is the most obvious explanation of, the observed behaviour, although it is evidently premature to rule out alternative mechanisms.

TABLE I
Specific heat, thermal diffusivity; heat of formation of the oxide and power threshold P_T for Cd, Al and Cu.

Metal	Oxide	C_p cal/gm/deg	D cm^2/s	$-\Delta H$ kcal/mole	P_T watt
Cd	CdO	0.055	0.462	63.1	0.45
Al	Al$_2$O$_3$	0.215	0.861	401	4.5
Cu	Cu$_2$O	0.092	1.14	40.5	2.0

TABLE II

Complement of reflectivity 1-R, calculated temperature rise ΔT, total energy absorbed Ea, energy absorbed by the film E_f and energy liberated by oxidation $E_{-\Delta H}$.

Surface	1-R	ΔT deg C	E_a mJ	E_f mJ	$E_{-\Delta H}$ mJ
Cd	0.818	300	8.22	1.31	44.5
Al	0.14	640[a]	15.6	6.35	686 !!!
Cu	0.085	154	–	–	–
Cu_2O	0.585[b]	1063	29	19.8	129

a) Assumed temperature rise after correction for surface reflectivity charge.
b) Value of 1-R necessary to give ΔT = 1063 deg.

CONCLUSIONS

We have described how thin metal films of Cd and Cu on glass substrates can be completely oxidised to CdO and Cu_2O by irradiation with a scanning laser beam, where the oxygen is supplied at a sufficiently high rate from the surrounding atmosphere, and demonstrated that large uniform areas may be obtained by scanning in a raster fashion. We show that the reaction cannot be explained by a simple thermal heating process which does not take proper account of the heat of formation of the oxide, but that the observations do appear to be reasonably consistent with a model previously proposed for the formation of compound semiconductors from metal films under similar conditions. We also explain, using the same model, why the laser induced oxidation reaction of thin Al films is self-destructive.

ACKNOWLEDGEMENTS

This work was supported by the R&D (Energy) Program of the Belgian Ministry for Science Policy.

REFERENCES

1. R. Andrew and M. Lovato, J. Appl. Phys. 50, 1142-1144 (1979).

2. G. Auvert, D. Bensahel, A. Perio, F. Morin, G.A. Rozgonyi and V.T. Nguyen in Laser and Electron Beam Interactions with Solids. B.R. Appleton and G.R. Celler eds. North Holland 1982 p. 535.

3. R. Andrew, L. Baufay, A. Pigeolet and L.D. Laude, J. Appl. Phys. 53, 4862-4865 (1982).

4. Handbook of Chemistry and Physics 59th Edition PE 103, R.C. Weast ed. CRC

Press Inc 1979.

5. V.F. Drobny and D.L. Pulfrey, p. 180 "13th IEEE Photovoltaic Specialists Conference" ed. by Institute of Electrical and Electronics Engineers, Inc. 1978.

6. Theory of Metal Oxidation Vol. 1., A.T. Fromhold Jr., p. 23, North Holland NY 1976.

7. The Oxide Handbook, G.V. Samsonov. ed. IFI Plenum NY 1973.

8. Y. Nissim, A. Lietoila, R.B. Gold and J.F. Gibbons, J. App. Phys. $\underline{51}$, 274-279 (1980)

9. F.W. Young, J.V. Cathcart and A.T. Gwathmey ... Acta Met $\underline{4}$ 145 (1956).

10. Oxidation of Metals, K. Hauffe, Plenum N.Y., 1965, p. 119.

Author Index

Abele, C.C., 185
Adler, D., 215
Allen, S.D., 207
Andrew, R., 283
Avouris, Ph., 257
Aylett, M.R., 177

Bauerle, D., 19
Baufay, L., 249, 283
Beneking, H., 193
Beri, A.C., 273
Bilenchi, R., 199
Boyer, P.K., 119
Brueck, S.R.J., 81, 161

Chen, C.J., 169
Chuang, T.J., 45
Collins, G.J., 119

Daneu, V., 57
Desai, H.D., 185
Deutsch, T.F., 129, 225
Donnelly, V.M., 151

Eden, J.G., 185
Ehrlich, D.J., 3, 235
Evans, H.L., 103

Gattuso, T.R., 215
George, T.F., 273
Gianinoni, I., 199
Gilgen, H.H., 29, 57, 109
Gorbatkin, S., 185
Greene, J.E., 185

Haggerty, J.S., 215
Haigh, J., 177
Herman, I.P., 9
Hwang, W., 103
Hyde, R.A., 9

Ibbs, K.G., 243

Jan, R.Y., 207
Johnson, A.W., 73
Johnston, W.D., 151

Karlicek, R.F., 151
Kirillov, D., 95
Kitai, A., 141
Krautle, H., 193
Krings, A., 193

Laude, L.D., 249
Lin, Jui-Teng, 273
Lloyd, M.L., 243
Longendorfer, D.H., 265
Lubben, D., 185

Marks, R.F., 257
McWilliams, B.M., 9
Merz, J.L., 95
Meunier, M., 215
Micheels, R.H., 265
Moore, C.A., 119
Mountain, R.W., 129
Muller, D.F., 135
Murphy, D.V., 81
Murphy, W.C., 273
Murri, R., 199
Musci, M., 199

Osgood, R.M., 57, 103, 169
Osmundsen, J.F., 185

Rao, G.B., 65
Pang, S., 161
Pigeolet, A., 249, 283
Podlesnik, D.V., 57
Pollak, R.A., 257
Poon, E., 103

Rauh, R.D., 265
Rhodes, C.K., 135
Ritchie, W.K., 119
Roche, G.A., 119
Rose, T.L., 265
Rothschild, M., 135
Roth, W., 193
Rytz-Froidevaux, Y., 29

Salathe, R.P., 29, 65, 109
Sanchez, A., 57
Silversmith, D.J., 129
Solanki, R., 119

Thacker, B.A., 35
Tisone, G.C., 73
Trigubo, A.B., 207
Tsao, J.Y., 3, 235

Wautelet, M., 283
Weisberg, A.H., 9
White, J.C., 35
Wolga, G.J., 141
Wood, L.L., 9
Wood, T.H., 35

Yang, E.S., 103

Subject Index

A

Adlayers, 233
Adsorption process, 273
Adspecies, 277, 280
Aluminum oxide, 119
Al, 119, 155, 283
AlAs, 283
Al_2O_3, 119
$Al(CH_3)_3$, 136
$Al_x Ga_{1-x}$, 109
AlSb, 283
Amorphous semiconductors, 215
Aqueous electrolyte, 268
Ar+ and Kr+ lasers, 21 (See also Laser entries)
ArF radiation, 226
Argon-ion laser, 18, 38, 73
As_2, 154
As_4, 154
AsH_3, 154

B

Band-to-acceptor level recombination, 111
Band to band recombination, 111
Barrier height, 103

C

Cadmium spheres, 175
Cd, 283
CdO, 284
CdS, 57
CdSe, 283
CdTe, 252, 283
Cu, 283
Cu_2O, 285
CF_2 radical(s), 161, 162
CF_4, 50, 54, 161
Chemical
  reaction rates, 3
  vapor deposition (CVD), 151, 215
Chemisorbed, 172
Cl_2, 46, 50, 155
CO_2 lasers, 207
CO_2 laser-induced pyrolysis of silane, 215
Conductivity, 220
Cr, 119
Cross section, 275
Crystallite size, 82
C, Si and Ni, 24
cw CO_2 lasers, 21

CW laser heating, 101

D

Deposition rate, 218
Desorption process, 273
Dielectric properties, 133
Dimethyl cadmium, 35, 169
Dimethyl mercury, 171
Dimethyl zinc, 171
Direct
  chemical etching, 57
  gap semiconductors, 109
  writing method, 21, 35
Dissociation, 243
Dry etching, 161

E

Electroless imaging, 265
Electron
  -phonon coupling, 279
  spin resonance (ESR), 219
Enhanced impurity diffusion, 235
Etching (See entries under specific types of etching)
Excimer laser(s), 119, 135, 185

F

Fano-type interference, 96
Fe, 210
Finite dimensions, 82
First-principles theory of pyrolytic deposition, 19
Fluorocarbon plasmas, 155

G

GaAs, 57, 65, 73, 109, 154
  Cr-doped, 74
  epitaxial, laser stimulated growth of, 193
GaCl, 154
Gallium, 177
  trimethyl, 180
Ge, 185
Grain boundaries, 103
  sizes, 185

H

HNO_3, 73
Hydrogenated amorphous silicon (a-Si:H), 200

I

Implantation, 243
InCl, 154
InMe$_3$, 179
Inf, 152, 225
Indium, 177
  cyclopentadienyl (InCp), 180
  phosphide, 177
  trimethyl, 180
In-situ measurement, 60
Interface charge density, 103

K

KOH, 73
Kr+ laser, 284
Kr-ion laser, 65, 207
  radiation, 70

L

Laser, 243, 283
  chemical processing, 3
  CVD, 121
  doping, 225, 235
  -driven pyrolysis, 12
  enhanced chemical etching, 45
  heating, 95
  induced chemical vapor deposition (LCVD), 21, 141, 185, 207
  induced etching, 48
  induced fluorescence (LIF), 151, 152, 161, 162
  induced transitions, 275
  nitride, 132
  photochemistry, 259
  pyrolysis, 21
  spectroscopic techniques, 151
Lattice temperature, 98, 111
Light-induced etching, 65
Light-stimulated breakdown, 177
Light-stimulated decomposition, 177
LPCVD, 132 (See also Laser entries)
Local field enhancement, 174

M

Manganese carbonyl, (Mn$_2$(CO)$_{10}$), 141
Maskless etching, 45, 48
Me$_3$InPMe$_3$, 180
Metal
  -alkyl, 169

Metal (continued)
  deposition, 12
  micropatterning, 12
  oxides, 283
Metallic dots, 252
  films, 119, 212, 249
Metallo-organic, 177
Microfabrication, 3
Micron-scale widths, 12
Microstructures, 21
Minimum scan rate Vmin, 17
Mo, 119
MOCVD, 177
MOS (metal-oxide semiconductor), 11
Multiple photon absorption, 46, 49
Multi-photon collisionless processes, 216

N

N$_2$O, 185
Nd-YAG laser, 250
NH$_3$, 185
Ni, 208
Nickel, 13
  carbonyl, 12
Ni(CO)$_4$ in He, 22
Ni rod, 26
Niobium, 257
  oxide, 257, 260

O

Optical
  absorption, 215
  coefficients, 215
  diagnostics, 81
  fiber, 250
  gap E, 220
  microanalysis, 81
  spectroscopy, 151
Optically
  print, 249
  write, 249
Organometallic, 35, 135
  molecules on surfaces, 169, 243
Oxidation, 257
Oxygen impurity, 103

P

P$_2$, 154
PH$_3$, 154
Phonon line, 95
Phosphorous trimethyl complex, 180

Photo
 conductivity, 103
 electrochemical deposition, 265
 dissociation, 29, 33, 187
 -induced surface reactions, 273
 luminescence, 109
Photolysis, 177, 243
Photolytic mechanisms, 233
Photoreactions, 169
Photoresist, 135
Photox SiO_2, 122
Physical ablation, 48
Physisorbed layers, 169
Plasma chemistry, 257
 deposition (PD), 151
 etching (PE), 45, 48, 161
 oxidation, 258
PM junction, 243
Polycrystalline, 87
 silicon, 103, 226
Polyester film (Mylar), 54
Polyethylene terephthalate (PET), 54
Polymetallic multilayered films, 249
Polymethyl methacrylate (PMMA), 54
Prenucleation, 18, 35
Pressure broadening, 216
Pyrolysis, 177, 243
Pulsed CO_2 laser, 257
Pulsed Nd-YAG laser, 193
Pyrolytic LCVD, 21, 23
 mechanisms, 233

Q

Quartz substrates, 29

R

Radiative transitions, 109
Raman
 enhanced, 81
 scattering, laser, 151, 153
 techniques of, 26, 95
 spectroscopy, 81
Reactive ion etching (RIE), 151
Resonant absorption, 199

S

Semiconductor processing, 151
Semiconductoring, 81, 151, 152
SF_6, 46, 47, 49, 50
Si, 46, 50, 95, 155, 185, 211, 225, 265
SiF_4, 46, 47

SiH_4, 185
Si films, 81
Si GaAs, 58 (See also GaAs entries)
SiH_4, 24, 199
SiO_2, 46, 50, 119, 129, 185
Si-on-insulator, 81
Si-on-sapphire, 81
$SiSF_6$, 46
SiN_4, 119, 129, 185
 laser-deposited, 133
Si ribbons, 233
Si-XeF_2, 47
Silane pyrolysis, 216
Silanol, 135
Silicon, 135 (See Si entries)
 dioxide, 119
 nitride, 119
Spectrophotometric measurements, 203
SOI, 83
Solar cells, 225
Solid surfaces, 273
SOQ, 82
SOS, 82
Spectroscopy, 169, 177
Stimulated growth, 193
Stress, 81
Structure Resonances, 91
Submicrometer
 gratings, 57
 -linewidth surface relief, 235
Surface band, 274
 charge, 277
 electron density distribution at, 280
 interaction potential, 278, 280
 processes, 273
 states, 274
 excited, 277

T

Temperature, 109
 probe, 95, 101
Theoretical, 273
Thermal capture cross-section, 103
Theory of laser-induced pyrolytic deposition processes, 13
Thin film electroluminescent (TFEL), 141, 283
Three dimensional structures, 21
III-V compound(s), 65, 177
 semiconductor, 151
$TiCl_4$, 136, 138
Transition rate, 275

T (continued)

Trap energy, 103
Triethyl Boron (TEB), 243
Trimethyllaluminum (TMA), 124
Trimethylgallium, 29, 30
Tunable dye laser, 154

U

ULSI (ultra-large scale integrated) patterns, 11
UV
 excimer lasers, 225
 laser, 129, 243
 light, 31

W

W, 119, 208, 211

X

XeF laser, 227
XeF$_2$, 50
X-ray diffraction, 203

Z

Zinc, 65
 oxide, 119
Zn, Al and Ni from Zn, 18
ZnO, 119
ZnSiMn, 141

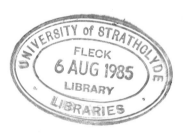